The Psychic Immune System

The Psychic Immune System

A Hidden Epiphenomenon of the Body's Own Defenses

Jerry Kroth

LEXINGTON BOOKS
Lanham • Boulder • New York • London

Published by Lexington Books
An imprint of The Rowman & Littlefield Publishing Group, Inc.
4501 Forbes Boulevard, Suite 200, Lanham, Maryland 20706
www.rowman.com

Unit A, Whitacre Mews, 26-34 Stannary Street, London SE11 4AB

British Library Cataloguing in Publication Information Available

Library of Congress Cataloging-in-Publication Data Available

ISBN: 978-1-4985-2891-7 (cloth: alk. paper)
ISBN: 978-1-4985-2892-4 (electronic)

∞™ The paper used in this publication meets the minimum requirements of American National Standard for Information Sciences Permanence of Paper for Printed Library Materials, ANSI/NISO Z39.48-1992.

Printed in the United States of America

Dedicated to the late Norman O. Brown, author of *Love's Body*

Contents

List of Figures and Tables ix
Acknowledgments xi
Introduction: Invisibility 1

Part I: Dark Matters **3**

1 Two Strains of Plague 5
2 On the Shore with Thucydides 31
3 Nuclear Winter 47

Part II: Epiphenomenon **77**

4 An Overview of the Physical Immune System 79
5 The *Innate* Psychic Immune System: Fight-Flight, Competition, and Territoriality 85
6 The *Innate* Psychic Immune System: Cooperation, Nonviolence, and Reciprocal Altruism 111
7 The *Adaptive* Psychic Immune System 131
8 The *Artificial* Psychic Immune System 163
9 The *Invisible* Psychic Immune System 183

Part III: An Experimental Test of the Theory **205**

10 Hypothesis Testing: Where the Rubber Meets the Road 207
11 How Global Warming Might Test the Theory of the Psychic Immune System 227

Bibliography 257
Index 279
About the Author 283

List of Figures and Tables

Figure 0.1	1
Figure 2.1 Mathematical Models of Epidemics	36
Figure 2.2 Psychic Epidemic Mortality Curves	39
Figure 2.3 Comparing Physical and Psychic Epidemics	40
Figure 2.4 Physical and Psychic Epidemic Curves	42
Figure 5.1 Overview of Physical Immune System and Psychic Immune System as an Epiphenomenon	85
Figure 9.1 Remission Curve for Psychic Epidemics	190
Figure 9.2 Remission Curves for Psychic Epidemics (Iraq) and Physical Epidemics (Spanish Flu)	194
Figure 9.3 Contemporary Psychic Epidemic Mortality Curves	198
Table 1.1 Humanity's Greatest Plagues	6
Table 1.2 Psychic Plagues	11
Table 1.3 Physical and Psychic Epidemics Compared	20
Table 3.1 Major Nuclear Incidents	60

Acknowledgments

The author wishes to thank journalist John Leighty for his care and attention in proofreading the manuscript, and to Ann Janowsky, Dept. of Immunology, University of Iowa, for fact-checking the medical aspects of this text.

Introduction

Invisibility

This text is about something right in front of us, except that it isn't easily seen. If one takes a step back to look at things from a more distant perspective, using a fresh mindset that transcends more traditional and comfortable inclinations, a glimpse of an unknown and even magical reality slowly appears.

If you look carefully at this picture, at first glance it appears to be just a series of vertical black and white lines. But when you step back about four feet and look at it from a distance, what is hidden becomes visible.

Figure 0.1 Optical illusion courtesy of Niels Schumm, Blommers/Schumm ©blommers/schumm

It is undetectable until we see it with new eyes.

The adventure upon which we embark is controversial, unconventional, mercurial, and always precariously balanced on a gossamer tightrope of intangibility. We will cover familiar stories, in many cases topics we thought we understood—even well—like the Cuban Missile Crisis, but when looked at from a more distant perch, a wholly new reality comes into focus.

Science may provide a better metaphor. Physicists have been explaining the universe with concepts that are often immeasurable and invisible too, and, because of their incorporeality, those ideas ran headlong into weighty criticism or outright condemnation. Concepts like dark matter, dark energy, WIMPS, neutrinos or that quintessentially insubstantial Higgs boson were all brought into the world amidst howls of ridicule.

Wolfgang Pauli proposed the existence of the neutrino, but his quantum speculation was not only invisible, it was also immeasurable. The attacks were almost too much to bear. His theories, his critics said, were so unclear, untestable, and unable to be evaluated, they did not properly belong *even within the realm of science*. "They were worse than wrong, because they could not be proven wrong . . . it is not even wrong!" one critic bellowed.[1] Pauli suffered from the disparagement, went through a divorce, entered therapy, but to everyone's surprise, the invisible, indiscernible neutrino, postulated in the 1930s, was observed in 1951.

Ridicule turned to praise. Einstein nominated him for the Nobel Prize. It was awarded. He accepted. The invisible became visible.

We are embarking on a similar journey, but in psychology, not physics. We are in search of another hidden variable. When we alter our perspective and crane our necks to try to find a more panoptic frame of reference, something glimmering out of the shadows appears, lying behind our reality, shaping and influencing it in a way beyond anything we ever imagined.

NOTE

1. R. Peirls, "Wolfgang Ernst Pauli, 1900–1958," *Biographical Memoirs of Fellows of the Royal Society*, 1960.

Part I

Dark Matters

ONE

Two Strains of Plague

Humanity has endured four major plagues that threatened its survival.[1] The first was the plague of Justinian in the Roman Empire around 541 AD which killed twenty-five million people. The second was the Black Death—bubonic plague—which ravaged Europe between 1338 and 1351 killing close to one hundred million people. The Black Death was zoonotic, meaning that it jumped from animals, in this case fleas, rodents, or gerbils, to humans. It killed two-thirds of those infected within a few days. Italian merchants traveling from the Black Sea imported it to Western Europe.[2]

The third plague comes wrapped in denial and a slightly airbrushed view of history. Americans know less about it than they should since most were educated with a Eurocentric bias. This is the story of white men "conquering" barbarian lands, establishing colonies in the "New World" and bringing "civilization" to backward—read "savage"—peoples. That set of skewed perceptions spared most Americans from two major insights: First, there were more human beings in North and South America when Columbus discovered it than were living in Europe,[3] a fact that surprises most people.

Second, in the four hundred years since Columbus imported his civilizing influences, more than 90 percent of the native population in North and South America succumbed to diseases to which they had no immunity, namely small pox, measles, and typhoid. David Stannard in *American Holocaust* calls this the most massive act of genocide in the history of the world and alleges one hundred million native people perished.[4] Others say Stannard exaggerates. A more reasonable guesstimate is thirty million people lived in the Americas at the time of Columbus, and 80 percent fell victim to European diseases.[5]

Most of these Native American epidemics occurred from 1590 to 1750, although a second wave hit between 1837 and 1870.[6] The epidemics repeatedly attacked Plains tribes, and the most prevalent diseases were measles, scarlet fever, typhoid, typhus, pertussis, tuberculosis, cholera, diphtheria, and chicken pox.[7]

In addition to these three major plagues impacting the human race, there were minor plagues in Russia, Italy, and Yugoslavia, but humanity's next mega plague originated in the United States in 1918. It took seventy-five million lives. About a third of the world's population—more than five hundred million people—were infected.[8]

From the perspective of the existential threat to the human race, the Black Death was the worst, killing 28 percent of all people on earth, and 60 percent of the population of Europe.[9]

Following is table 1.1 summarizing humanity's great plagues.

Plague	Lives lost	Percent of humanity lost	Human population at the time
Justinian 550-750 AD	25 million	14 percent	190 million
Bubonic plague 1348-1350 AD	100 million	28 percent	360 million
Native Americans 1590-1750 and 1837-1870	24 million (est.)*	6 percent	425 million
Spanish flu 1918-1919	75 million	4 percent	2 billion

Table 1.1 Humanity's Greatest Plagues
Source for world population estimates: http://www.worldhistorysite.com/population.html.
***Others believe the population estimates cited by Stannard to be overstated, so we are using these more conservative estimates. Note that lesser plagues occurred which are not listed here, most notable among them is the "Modern Plague" which impacted China from 1850 to 1894 and killed some 12 million people. The disease was a variant of the bubonic plague. Source: Pryor, E. G. (1975). "The Great Plague of Hong Kong." Journal of the Hong Kong Branch of the Royal Asiatic Society (Hong Kong: Royal Asiatic Society of Great Britain and Ireland-Hong Kong Branch.) 1975: 69.**

THE SPANISH FLU

Dr. Victor Vaughn, the president of the American Medical Association in 1918 was so shocked about the spreading influenza. He said "If the epidemic continues its mathematical rate of acceleration, civilization could easily disappear from the face of the earth."[10] Although not as threatening as the Black Death, the Spanish flu is worth a moment, because it has been studied extensively.

The flu occurred in the United States, not in Spain, and has much to teach about diagnosis, fear, panic, resistance, and the human immune system. It started when Canadian geese, migrating south, dropped excrement on pig farms in Kansas.[11] Once ingested, the pigs incubated the virus. Farmers routinely burned pig dung, unwittingly creating an airborne virus that was inhaled by members of a nearby U.S. military base. A number of soldiers died from the flu, which then seemed to disappear rapidly.

A few months later, however, as soldiers were boarding ships to fight in World War I, a stronger, mutated strain appeared. When the convoy arrived in France, 10 percent of the soldiers on the troop ships were dead and others were sick when they disembarked. American ships took supplies to Murmansk, Russia, and the flu spread throughout that nation, ultimately killing more than half a million Russians.

The global pandemic killed twenty-five million people in the first twenty-four weeks, more than the number of people who died from AIDS in twenty-four years. India had the highest casualty toll, seventeen million. In Japan 390,000 died. In isolated areas, particularly in Alaska where immunities to this influenza were nonexistent, entire villages were wiped out. The overall mortality rate was between 10 to 20 percent of those infected.[12]

In Philadelphia, death rates seemed to double every week. On October 16, 1919, 4,597 people were put in caskets and buried. In San Francisco, a law was passed requiring people to wear masks in public. Every gathering, whether a parade or a baseball game, became a transmitter of the virus. Altogether, 650,000 Americans died from the disease in the span of nine months,[13] more than five times the number of American soldiers who died in World War I. At the time, viruses were unknown so the methods of handling the pandemic were mysterious, often based on little more than superstition. When sick people were taken to the hospital, they infected doctors, nurses, and other patients. The closer the proximity, the deadlier the result.

In Western Samoa, people had little resistance to the disease that infected 90 percent of the islanders, killing 30 percent of adult men, 22 percent of women, and 10 percent of the children. Adjacent Eastern American Samoa, however, escaped the flu. There, the governor quarantined the island and blockaded all incoming ships. The atoll was one of the few places on earth, along with some isolated villages in the Amazon rainforest, which were spared.[14]

Just as suddenly as it had appeared the pandemic vanished. The flu crested between October and November of 1918, and seemed to be entirely gone by June of 1919.[15] Curiously, the most vulnerable people were in the prime of their life—strong young men and women in their twenties and thirties. Many older people seemed to have immunity, perhaps from exposure to an earlier strain.

Since viruses were unknown, there was no genuine science to quell the pandemic. In the 1990s, fluid was carefully extracted from the frozen bodies of Inuit preserved in the tundra who had died from Spanish flu. These lung samples revealed the flu was avian in origin and ultimately morphed into a virulent strain of swine flu.

A 2014 study showed the immune system played a dramatic role in who became infected. Investigators believe a proto-virus circulated after 1900. "People under the age of twenty-five were protected from the new virus because they had already been exposed to its weaker version."[16] and thus had a significant immunity to the pandemic while others did not.

THE SELF-PRESERVATIVE INSTINCT AND THE IMMUNE SYSTEM

The human immune system has a memory function that allows for such traumatic and species-threatening events to be encoded, stored, and used again when a new or similar threat appears:

> After defeating an infection, the immune system creates a memory of the vanquished attacker to make it easier to identify and eliminate in the future. . . . Cells that store these memories, termed memory T cells, enhance their own survival by packing themselves full of energy generators known as mitochondria. The extra mitochondria help the cells live a long time, which in turn extends their ability to help recognize a returning invader.[17]

The magic of the body's defense system is that today about 10 percent of the European population *has an immunity* to HIV infection.[18] This has puzzled scientists.

Why is HIV immunity higher in Europe than elsewhere? One theory is that the bubonic plague that ravaged Europe *strengthened* the immune system of survivors so that a variant or immunological *memory* of the plague may be providing extra resistance against modern day HIV exposure.[19]

A competing interpretation is that a mutation in the CCR5 receptor gene provided immunity against the plague and that same mutation persists today leading to decreased susceptibility to HIV infection in people of European descent. Dr. Steven O'Brien notes: "This mutation, dating back 700 years, may have been a selective advantage during the bubonic plague, as it is today, with the onslaught of HIV."[20]

Others argue that smallpox outbreaks in the Middle Ages, not the bubonic plague, were responsible for HIV immunities in Europe today.[21] Regardless of the theory, one scientist opines "Nature's past successes often remain part of our genetic toolbox."[22]

Decades later, those who survived the Spanish flu were tested in two independent studies and their immune systems still contained virus-specific antibodies.[23]

> Nearly 90 years after the outbreak of the 1918 Spanish flu, survivors of the pandemic still carry functional antibodies against the virus in their blood, demonstrating the longevity of immunological memory in humans. What's more, these antibodies are able to protect mice from lethal infection with the reconstructed 1918 virus.[24]

Psychic Memories?

Psychiatrist Carl Jung argued the human psyche has a similar memory function for protection: "Just as the body bears the traces of its phylogenetic development, so does the human mind."[25] Jung conjectured that the psyche retains memories or has some kind of *template* of ancestral events. The belief that not just the physical immune system, but the human psyche itself—the unconscious, or the collective unconscious—possesses ancestral footprints influenced psychoanalysts far beyond Jung. Karl Abraham elucidated it further:

> And just as certain psychic products of the healthy and sick individual are reminiscent of that early stage of his childhood, so in its legends and fairy tales does the race as a whole preserve the traces of its remotest past.[26]

Abraham says that folktales and myths *encode* human experiences and preserve them from ancient times. For example, "Ring around the rosy, pocket full of posy," traces back to the bubonic plague.[27] Children sing these verses and, in turn, pass on a memory trace to the next generation entirely unconscious of the roots or origins of this human trauma. They simply sing the song and perpetuate the remembrance, while their parents remain quite unaware the verses are rooted in a plague that ravaged humanity six hundred years earlier.

If one asks why this process occurs, the best answer seems to be that oral cultural transmission through myth, fable, fairy tale, and metaphor has adaptive significance, as if the recitation triggers a genetic or unconscious impression of an event, disease, or condition that threatened our species.

When 25 percent of the European population died from the Black Death, a symbolic ring-around-the-rosy memory trace seems propitious from the standpoint of evolutionary psychology. These rhymes may also contain more information than one might think. During the devastating Spanish flu of 1918, another rhyme appeared:

> I had a little bird
> And its name was Enza
> I opened the window

And influEnza.

President Wilson, who almost died from it, murmured this verse in the Oval Office as did so many others across the nation. With more than a half million Americans dying in the epidemic's ravaging nine months, the rhyme not only memorializes the event, but its most elegant component is *it actually hints the disease was bird-borne.*

The bird-borne virus incubated in a pig's gut, mutated, and then spread to human beings. The rhyme about the bird, *Enza,* not only recalls the trauma, but provides a diagnostic clue—completely unknown in 1918—that the pandemic was of avian origin, a fact not discovered until the 1990s.

A SECOND STRAIN OF PLAGUE

Carl Jung called war a "psychic epidemic," and noted human beings have been torturing each other in violent conflicts for all of recorded history. Thus, another category of epidemics and plagues to consider that were not physical but psychic in origin.

Outbreaks of these human-borne plagues populate history books. Let us examine the worst human-caused psychic plagues with the same lenses used to analyze disease outbreaks. The following table 1.2 lists the most to least lethal epidemics that have occurred to the end of the twentieth century.

Human plague	Total deaths	Percent of inhabitants exterminated	Percent of human race exterminated
World War II	60 million	6.4 percent of Europe	2.5
Maoist China	38.6 million	4 percent of China	0.5
Timur dynasty	17 million**	NA	4.6*
World War I	16 million	3.9 percent of Europe	0.08
Genghis Khan/ Mongols	15 million**	NA	4*
An Lushan rebellion	13 million	16 percent	5
Congolese genocide	10 million	8 percent of Africa	0.04
Atlantic slave trade	8 million	8 percent of Africa	0.1
Stalinism	6 million unrelated to WWII	3 percent of Russia	0.02
Ottoman empire genocides	2.3 million	16 percent	0.001
Cambodian genocide	1.7 million	24 percent of Cambodia	0.0004
Total/Average	187.6	8.1	1.53

Table 1.2 Psychic Plagues
Estimate based on a hypothetical world population of 375 million; source http://www.timelines.info/history/ages_and_periods/population_through_the_ages/. Genghis Khan atrocity total is said to be 15 million, while Timur's is estimated at 17 million. "Selected death tolls: Timur Lenk (1369–1405)." Necrometrics.com; Jones, Adam (2010). Genocide: A Comprehensive Introduction. New York: Taylor & Francis, 2010) 194. http://necrometrics.com/20c5m.htm See J.J. Saunders. The history of the Mongol conquests, New York, Routledge & Kegan, 1971; also: M. S. Asimov and C. E. Bosworth, History of Civilizations of Central Asia,UNESCO Regional Office, 1998. Note some authors are critical of such lists of atrocities arguing that precise historical data, especially on pre-twentieth century atrocities is often misleading or inaccurate. An interesting article on this is given at http://bedejournal.blogspot.com/2011/11/steven-pinker-and-an-lushan-revolt.html. See also Matthew White, The 100 deadliest episodes in human history. (New York: Norton, 2011).

These events are generally agreed to be the most homicidal moments in human history since the time of Christ. In discussing these convulsions of destructiveness, one caveat to observe is that in this chapter the problem of human violence, the origin of war, or the causes of genocide will not be solved. Not only would that be presumptuous, but it is not the intent of the discussion. Instead we are looking for something else that bears upon the thesis of this book, but before embarking on that mission, it is necessary to review a short history of these psychic epidemics.

The An Lushun Rebellion

Harvard psychologist Steven Pinker says the An Lushun rebellion (755–763 AD) killed about a sixth of the world's population, and may have been the largest atrocity ever committed by mankind. Others dispute his numbers and a more conservative estimate puts the death toll at about thirteen million.[28] It is not known why so many people died in this turbulent eight-year period of the Tang dynasty in China, but many deaths may have resulted from famine, not merely a homicidal impulse.[29]

An Lushan was Turkish, or perhaps Mongol, and deployed an army of between one hundred and sixty thousand and two hundred thousand troops. As part of his conquests, he virtually massacred the entire city of Kaifeng. After early successes, he declared himself emperor of what he called the Great Yan.[30] His reign, however, did not last long.

In 757, An Lushan was killed by his son An Qingxu. The late general's paranoia was taking a toll to the entourage and due to this his son took over the rebellion. "An Qingxu was then assassinated by general Shi Siming who was the follower and childhood friend of Lushan . . . Shi Siming . . . also was killed by his own son in 761. The son, Shi Chaoyi, proclaimed himself the new emperor . . . but he was unpopular. On February 17, 763, Tang troops cut off the self-proclaimed Yan emperor Shi Chaoyi. Rather than facing capture, Shi committed suicide, bringing the An Lushan Rebellion to a close."[31] At least thirteen million human beings died at the hands of An Lushan and his descendants.

Genghis Khan and Timur-the-Lame

The Mongol empire, the largest in the history of the human race—over twelve million square miles—began about 1204 AD and lasted until 1370. It brought remarkable changes to human society: economic development, modernization of trade, encouragement of arts and literature, advances in medicine and astronomy, development of trade routes, unification of China, a freedom of religion policy, and advances in architecture, poetry, and painting.[32]

As one writer opines, however,

> This all started with Genghis Khan, the founder of the Mongol Empire. Genghis realized that there was a way to steal from civilized people without all the work of seasonal raiding. You raid them just once, quickly and brutally: you massacre their people and burn their cities to the ground. . . . Then you tell them to pay you, or you'll do it again. And as long as they keep paying you, they're under your protection, in much the same way as someone pays the Mafia for protection. Under the leadership of Genghis Khan and his successors, the Mongols expanded this extortion racket, demanding tribute from cities across Asia and Eastern Europe.[33]

Khan said, "I am the punishment of God. . . . If you had not committed great sins, God would not have sent a punishment like me upon you."[34] Indeed, the barbarity of Genghis Khan represents a milestone in human cruelty. Writer Diana Lary argues that the Mongols brought terror and panic to Europe on a scale not seen again until the twentieth century. "Terror and mass extermination of anyone opposing them was a well-tested Mongol tactic."[35]

The table that appeared earlier only cited lower level estimates of the amount of human carnage attributed to the Mongols. There is a great variance in statistics among scholars. Allen Godby in *The Lost Tribes* contends Genghis Khan killed twenty million people. Jeremiah Crin in *The Mongols: A History*, gives a number of eighteen million. Some estimates go much higher. A short review of these atrocities follows: [36]

- Two million Hungarians perished under the Mongols.
- More than half a million Russians died due to Mongol conquests from 1223 to 1240 AD The "Golden Horde,"as it was called, ruled Russia for 250 years.
- Khan massacred more than four million people in his conquests of Maru, Herat, and Neisabour, and built a pyramid in Baghdad out of 90,000 skulls.
- Mongol invaders slaughtered at least 700,000 people in Persia and killed 800,000 others in Baghdad alone. Some say two million Persians may have died overall at the hands of the Mongols.

The Mongol empire extended from modern day Korea to Poland, and today it would include thirty-two countries.[37] After Khan's death in 1227 AD, the Mongols continued to expand, but gradually fragmented as his progeny squabbled. The Russians overthrew the Golden Horde in 1380, although parts of Russia remained under their control until 1480. Historians generally define the end of the Mongol empire as 1370. The causes for the end of the Mongol empire are many. One, certainly, is the beginning of the Black Death in Europe.[38] Another is the fractious fighting of Khan's descendants.

TIMUR THE LAME

Timur and the Timurid dynasty is not synonymous with Genghis Khan. Khan's empire stretched much farther. Timur attempted to reconquer lost areas, but never fully succeeded. His barbarity, however, exceeded even the great Khan. Often he tried to consider himself a descendant of Genghis Kahn, but that connection was at best dubious. Nonetheless,

> he sought to conquer the Golden Horde but only managed to attack his Mongol brothers from the east while the Russians began attacking them from the west. . . . Timur the Lame set out to ensure that his lineage would contain the blood of Genghis Khan by having his family intermarry with some of Genghis Khan's true descendants. He did not follow Genghis Khan's ways, however. Timur slaughtered people without reason and found perverse pleasure in torturing and humiliating his prisoners. When he conquered Turkey and seized the Seljuk sultan, he forced the sultan's wives and daughters to serve him dinner naked while the defeated ruler watched. He also forced the sultan to watch his sexual assaults on these women and to pull Timur's royal chariot harnessed like a draft animal. Timur displayed the sultan in a cage.[39]

Timur slaughtered 100,000 people in Delhi in 1398, piled five thousand human heads into minarets at Zirih, massacred seventy thousand people in Isfahan, similarly stacking their skulls into minarets, and buried four thousand Christian soldiers alive.[40] His victories gave him large swaths of Central Asia, Uzbekistan, Turkmenistan, Kazakhstan, Persia, and Syria, but his dynasty never reached the magnitude of the Mongol empire.

Regarding Timur's atrocities, numerous writers like Peter Ford, Stephen Kinzer, David Carpenter, Jonathan Fenby, H. D. S. Greenway, Allen Godbey, Israel Smith Clare, and Ian McWilliam make independent estimates for the carnage ranging from seven million to twenty million people. The consensus is seventeen million deaths.[41]

On an expedition to conquer China, Timur died and his empire quickly disintegrated as Shah Rukh (Shahrukh Mirza) consolidated rule and a relative period of peace followed from 1409 to 1447. As the dynasty crumbled, a strange tranquility followed with a cessation of wars of conquest and a gradual prospering of arts and science.[42]

The most horrific barbarities are dated to the period of 1206–1327 for Khan[43] and from 1370 to 1405 for Timur, even though both lasted much longer, Timur's extending until 1506.[44] These two bloodthirsty periods covered 121 years and thirty-five years, respectively.

The Atlantic Slave Trade (1700–1850)

While slavery existed in the Islamic world and dates back to the Roman Empire, the largest forced movement of people out of Africa to the

West happened between 1700 and 1870, although some came as early as 1600. The demographics of American slavery are also instructive.[45]

- About half of all slave babies died in infancy, twice the rate for whites.
- By the age of seven, more than 40 percent of boys and half the girls were assigned to adult field jobs.
- Slaves frequently suffered from blindness, bowed legs, skin lesions, tetanus, rickets, convulsions, and other maladies caused by deficiencies of thiamine, essential nutrients, and protein deficiency.

Varying estimates have been given for how many people perished as a direct result of enslavement. Some authors estimate four million died. Jan Rogozinski in *A Brief History of the Caribbean,* argues the figure is closer to eight million. Slaves who died, or who were merely sick on the voyage, were often thrown overboard:

> Of the, say 50 or so people that board the ship, generally 25–35% die in the miserable conditions of the "middle passage" from disease, murder (mutiny was common) or suicide along the way. It was not uncommon for Africans to jump overboard or refuse to eat and die to avoid life as a slave. It is said that sharks often followed slave ships because so many bodies were thrown overboard. There are also numerous examples of slavers throwing their cargo overboard to collect the insurance.[46]

Eight months after the civil war, the 13th Amendment to the Constitution formally put an end to the practice of slavery, certainly one of the darkest periods in American history.

The Congolese Genocide (1885–1908)

King Leopold II is not well known. His atrocity began as Belgium colonized the Congo. The "Belgian Congo," as it was known, became an area rich in natural resources, especially rubber. In 1891, Leopold signed legislation reducing the native population to serfs. Male rubber tappers were maliciously treated. Leopold's men held women and children of his laborers hostage until they met their quotas.

> Those who refused or failed to supply enough rubber often had their villages burned down, children murdered, and their hands cut off. Yielding to international pressure, the Belgian parliament in 1908 annexed the CFS as the Belgian Congo, effectively removing Leopold from power. Just prior to releasing sovereignty, Leopold destroyed all evidence of his activities, including the archives of its Departments of Finance and the Interior. The Belgian parliament refused to hold any formal commission of inquiry into the human rights abuses that had occurred.[47]

From 1885 to 1908, the Congolese native population decreased by about ten million people. The population of the continent of Africa was correspondingly reduced by 8 percent and the human race by roughly four-tenths of 1 percent. Leopold disappeared from the scene in 1908, but as one writer claims, "the slashing of the territory's population through a combination of disease, famine, slave labor, suppression of rebellions, and diminished birth rate indisputably occurred on a genocidal scale."[48]

Ottoman Genocides: Armenia, Greek (1914–1922)

The Ottoman Empire lasted almost six hundred years and covered a huge expanse of territory. As the empire began to collapse, however, three Ottoman-inspired genocides occurred very close in time. First was the massacre of 1.5 million Armenians beginning in 1914 that involved killing the able-bodied male population and the deportation of women, children, and the elderly.[49] The Greek genocide followed with ethnic cleansing, death marches, executions, and deportations between 1914 and 1922 when 348,000 Greeks perished. During this same period, close to three hundred thousand Assyrians were also the victims of genocidal campaigns mostly aimed at Christian minorities.

All three murderous events happened in a seven-year period as the Ottoman Empire came to its close. The atrocities were directed by the "three Pashas," Mehmed Tallat, Ismail Enver, and Ahmed Djemal.[50] As one of their officials, Rafet Bey, said, "We must finish off the Greeks as we did with the Armenians . . . today I sent squads to the interior to kill every Greek on sight."[51]

The Ottoman Empire ended in 1922 when Mustafa Ataturk founded the first secular Turkish state. Ataturk called these genocides "shameful acts" and he became known as a "truly great personality in the Islamic world . . . and a great statesman."[52]

World War I (1914–1918)

The next major psychic plague begins with the assassination of Archduke Ferdinand of Austria by a Yugoslav nationalist in June of 1914. Because of a huge network of interweaving alliances, most of the countries of Europe became embroiled in what was called The Great War. It pitted the Allies (Britain, France, and Russia) against the Central Powers (Germany, Austria-Hungary, and Italy).

The United States joined the Allies and declared war on Germany in 1917. An armistice was signed on November 17, 1918. There were sixteen million deaths and twenty million wounded. The population of Europe was about 410 million people, so the death toll consumed 3.9 percent of the continent's inhabitants.[53] On a global scale, the Great War reduced the human population of roughly 1.8 billion by slightly less than 1 percent.

World War II

World War II is usually dated from 1939 until 1945, although the Japanese invasion of China occurred in 1937. It is known as the most widespread conflict in history with one hundred million military personnel participating in two major venues, the Asia-Pacific region and Europe. Total military and civilian casualties are estimated at sixty million dead and more than one hundred million wounded.[54] This included six million Jews, virtually 75 percent of all European Jewry.

More than one million Jewish children were murdered along with two million Jewish women. In addition, Polish Christians, the disabled, prisoners of war, and gypsies were exterminated to bring the holocaust—or victims of premeditated murder—to eleven million people.[55] All told, the European population was reduced by more than 6 percent, and humanity itself winnowed down by 2.5 percent over this six-year eruption of what many regard as our greatest episode of collective insanity.[56]

Stalinism

Stalinism produced a high number of human casualties in Russia in addition to those killed in World War II.[57] A recent scholarly look comparing the deaths occurring under Stalin and Hitler by Timothy Snyder is of interest. Synder was able to have unprecedented access to Soviet records after the fall of the USSR, and some of his findings are surprising:

> It turns out that, with the exception of the war years, a very large majority of people who entered the Gulag left alive. Judging from the Soviet records we now have, the number of people who died in the Gulag between 1933 and 1945, while both Stalin and Hitler were in power, was on the order of a million, perhaps a bit more. The total figure for the entire Stalinist period is likely between two million and three million. The Great Terror and other shooting actions killed no more than a million people, probably a bit fewer. The largest human catastrophe of Stalinism was the famine of 1930–1933, in which more than five million people died. . . . In early 1930, Stalin had announced his intention to "liquidate" prosperous peasants ("kulaks") as a class so that the state could control agriculture and use capital extracted from the countryside to build industry.[58]
>
> Thousands were shot by the police and many tens of thousands deported. In 1937 what is known as the Great Terror was announced.
>
> Because we now have the killing orders and the death quotas, inaccessible so long as the Soviet Union existed, we now know that the number of victims. . . The total figure of civilians deliberately killed under Stalinism, around six million, is of course horribly high. But it is

far lower than the estimates of twenty million or more made before we had access to Soviet sources.[59]

Stalin, quite independent of the severe losses incurred by Russia in World War II, liquidated through terror or famine some six million people, 3 percent of the nation's citizens. The deaths reduced the earth's population by two-tenths of 1 percent.

Maoist China

Maoism also produced impressive casualty figures. Scholars estimate 1.5 million perished during the Cultural Revolution and another million due to land reform and the "suppression of counter revolutionaries." The greatest death toll, however, was caused by the Great Famine,[60] largely induced by forced agricultural reforms similar to Stalin's experiment in the Ukraine.

Some thirty-six million Chinese people died of starvation in a few short years (1958–1961). This may have been the greatest famine in the history of the world, as well as one of the most censored and suppressed.[61] [62] Mao exterminated roughly 4 percent of the Chinese population or, with the global population at the time estimated at about three billion, about 1 percent of the human race.

Pol Pot's "Kampuchea"

Saloth Sar changed his name to Pol Pot and walked onto the stage of human barbarism for three short years, 1975–1978. Pol Pot was a paranoid, delusional village boy who tried to create a communist utopia by force and murder. He had a desultory view of Maoism and sought to "step-leap" from feudalism to utopian communism by force of arms—skipping all the intervening steps described in Marxist theory.

His attempt to imitate the Chinese Communist's Cultural Revolution resulted in the Cambodian genocide. Pol Pot's Khmer Rouge killed between 1.7–2.3 million people, burying them in mass graves—and all in the space of thirty-six months.[63] His killing fields and extermination camps transformed the country into a gigantic gulag and reduced the population of the country by close to 24 percent. On a per capita basis, the Cambodian genocide represents one of the greatest human atrocities of all time.

THE QUESTION WE ARE ASKING

One can, of course, opine about the causes of war and genocide. One can look at individual psychopathologies (Hitler, Pol Pot, Timur, Mao) and attempt to conjure up psychiatric explanations for these holocausts. One can resort to sociological, historical, or political explanations about the causes of war, but that is not within the scope of this short chapter. Our interest is far more obscure and nuanced.

Physical vs. Psychological Plagues

When looking at the major *physical* plagues that infected humanity, what is observed is an increase in resistance. Immunities appear to be developing against these plagues. And human "strategies" develop to enhance immunity and protection (quarantines of populations and increased sanitation, for example, with the Spanish flu).

To introduce this conundrum in slightly more technical terms, there is a phylogenetic self-preservative system, particularly the physical immune system that protects the human race from epidemics, disease, and eventual extinction. This self-preservative system not only operates at the unconscious or autonomic level (through the immune system and its resistances), but also operates at the conscious level. Populations quarantine afflicted groups, wear masks, try to disinfect, increase prophylactic measures, and engage in hygienic behaviors even though they may not know the cause of the disease ravaging their community.

But that is about physical disease and physical pandemics. What about psychic epidemics, wars, and barbarities that have also been a scourge of the human race? Are any such self-preservative mechanisms operating at a *psychological* level?

Just as a disease or antigen running through our bloodstream is attacked by our physical immune system, is there a psychological immune system which similarly mounts a defense or resistance against psychic epidemics: genocides, barbarity, atrocities, exterminations, and evil?

That is the central question pursued in this text. As we begin to work toward an answer, consider a comparison chart (table 1.3) of the physical and psychological epidemics already discussed:

Physical epidemic	Duration	Psychic epidemic	Duration
Plague of Justinian	200 years	World War II	6 years
Black Death	2 years	World War I	4 years
Native American plagues	193 years	Stalinism	18 years*
Spanish flu	9 months	Maoist China	27 years
Average	99 years	Congolese genocide	23 years
		Cambodian genocide	3 years
		Mongols	121 years**
		Timur-the-lame	35 years **
		Atlantic slave trade	150
		Ottoman genocides	8
		An Lushan rebellion	8
		Average	37 years **

Table 1.3 Physical and Psychic Epidemics Compared
***Stalin's purges began in the mid 1930s and until his death covered a period of 18 years.**
****These estimates for duration are not synonymous with the length of each empire, but with the period where incidence of extermination occurred and excluding the more peaceful periods of each dynasty.**

What can be seen from the chart is that the physical plagues hurling themselves at humanity lasted considerably longer than psychic epidemics, ninety-nine years versus thirty-seven years. One can also see that physical epidemics end as resistance to the disease develops or as prophylactic measures enhance immunities. But how do psychic epidemics end, and why do they end?

Genghis Khan's descendants continued to rape and pillage, but the fractious disputes depressed the empire, and gradually, "the Mongols became *less warlike.*" Under Kubla Khan, grandson of Genghis Khan,

> The Mongol rule brought prosperity and stability to the large empire as Marco Polo described in his famous book. Kublai's Empire stretched from the far north of Mongolia to far into Central Asia and at times it stretched south into parts of Vietnam . . . Marco Polo's account of his travels is well-known in the West. . . . He invited the Pope to send 100 priests in 1270 or 1271. Marco Polo described some cities he visited as being bigger and richer than any city in Europe or the world.[64]

Kubla Khan died in 1294 and was succeeded by grandsons and nephews (Khaishan, Ayrubarwada, Shidebala, and Hulagu Khan); some like Hulagu were particularly vicious,[65] some self-indulgent, while others supported education and painting. In general, though, most of the prior barbarities ended.

Just as the Mongol dynasty retreated from barbarity, Timur's genocidal practices diminished upon his death as well. His sons and grandsons bickered, just like Khan's, and similarly shepherded in the decline and fall of the Timurid dynasty.

One of Timur's sons, Shah Rukh, brought peace and even culture to what remained of this brutal empire. He expanded and cultivated Persian poetry, the "golden age" of Persian painting, and architecture while his wife built mosques, theological colleges, and commissioned important works in history and geography.[66]

What an incredible turn of events! The atrocities and barbarities ended, and a period of peace, tranquility, and even art came front and center.

Leopold's orgy of violence in the Congo sounded its death-knell as well by sheer embarrassment and an international outcry against his human rights abuses, led in part by Mark Twain:

> In articles in church magazines and in speeches throughout the United States and Europe on visits home, they described what they saw: Africans whipped to death, rivers full of corpses, and piles of severed hands . . . detail that quickly seared itself on the world's imagination. Army officers often demanded of their men a severed hand from each rebel killed in battle. . . . Alice Harris, a British Baptist, took photographs of the atrocities she witnessed. William Morrison, a white man, and William Sheppard, the first black missionary in the Congo, were Presbyterians from Virginia.[67]

Ditto for a young official named Edmund Morel who noticed that ships carrying rubber sailed off to Belgium, but nothing was sent back to pay Congo people for the commodity:

> instead, the ships carried soldiers, and large quantities of firearms and ammunition. Standing on the dock, Morel realized that he had uncovered irrefutable proof that a forced labor system was in operation 4,000 miles away. Morel soon quit his job and in short order turned himself into the greatest British investigative journalist of his time . . . he devoted his formidable energy and skill to putting the story of forced labor in King Leopold's Congo on the world's front pages.[68]

Through the power of the pen, Leopold's genocide ended. Abuses continued in the Congo for years after, but nothing as horrific as during Leopold's reign. The Congolese genocide officially halted with Leopold's departure. Again, a strange and happy ending to an era of savagery and barbarity.

In Cambodia, in the midst of Pol Pot's auto-genocide, he made the decision to attack Vietnam. This was an act of suicidal idiocy, because Vietnam was ten times more populous. Vietnam routed the invaders and put in place its own government in Cambodia, driving the Khmer Rouge into the jungles where they stayed until Pol Pot's death. Once again, the atrocities and killing fields came to an abrupt end.[69] The whole convulsion of Pol Pot's cruelty lasted only about three years. Another happy outcome.

Hitler's bunker was assaulted by the Russians; Hitler committed suicide; the concentration camps were liberated, and Auschwitz closed. From beginning (1939) until the end (1945) only six years passed. Once again we see a swift end to one of the darkest moments of human butchery and premeditated murder. The killings ceased, and another psychic epidemic comes to a happy conclusion.

After Stalin's death, the Russian gulags were emptied. Under Khrushchev, the gulag population declined by two-thirds in what was called the *thaw,* a vast program of de-Stalinization.[70] Stalin's reign of terror lasted twenty-eight years.

As we review this history—and crane our necks toward a more global perspective—something previously unnoticed appears, happy endings, and they are even becoming predictable.

Mao died and was replaced by a succession of bureaucratic leaders far more interested in economic development than prison camps, executions, and famine. Subsequent leaders—Deng Xiaoping, Jiang Zemin, Wen Jiabao, Hu Jintao, Xi Jinping—had no particular thirst for barbarity. Under new leadership, China's gross domestic product (GDP) multiplied twenty-three times from what it was when Mao died three decades ago.

Although China executed an estimated five thousand prisoners in 2009, that is a far cry from the atrocities that took place under Mao,[71] whose reign of terror lasted only about as long as Stalin's.

What If?

Eventually, these human-borne psychic pandemics all came to an end. The question to might pose is this: How do we know these outcroppings of human barbarity will end rather than continue to grow and multiply similar to how a cancer metastasizes, overtakes its host, and ultimately consumes it?

Numerous books explore what might have happened if righteousness and reason did not triumph over humanity's dark side. Here are a few: *Third Reich Victorious: Alternate Decisions of World War II,* by Peter Tsouras; *Disaster at D-Day: The Germans Defeat the Allies,* by Peter Tsouras; *If Britain Had Fallen: The Real Nazi Occupation Plans,* by Norman Longmate; and *What If?: The World's Foremost Military Historians Imagine What Might Have Been,* by Robert Cowley.These books explore the doomsday hypothesis of what could have happened if sanity and nonviolence did not triumph over cruelty and butchery.

For example, scholars assembled in the text *What if* speculated on what might have happened if Hitler won World War II. The consensus is he would have likely extended his exterminations to include the whole of

Eurasian Jewry, and might have taken his cause to Palestine to finish the job. Recall one of Hitler's statements:

> If I am ever really in power, the destruction of the Jews will be my first and most important job. As soon as I have power, I shall have gallows after gallows erected, for example, in Munich on the Marienplatz as many of them as traffic allows. Then the Jews will be hanged one after another, and they will stay hanging until they stink. They will stay hanging as long as hygienically possible. As soon as they are untied, then the next group will follow and that will continue until the last Jew in Munich is exterminated. Exactly the same procedure will be followed in other cities until Germany is cleansed of the last Jew![72]

If Hitler triumphed in World War II, one can imagine him taking his psychotic mission well beyond the borders of Germany to the farthest reaches of his delusions. We can envisage ethnic cleansing of the whole of Eurasia and large parts of the Middle East and North Africa of Jews, the retarded, the disabled, gypsies, and probably blacks in an orgy of multiple racist extinction crusades across an ever-enlarging Reich. But as luck would have it, those eruptions of evil, murderousness, and genocide *came to an end.*

Was It Just Luck?

We know physical plagues and pandemics finally dissipate when the human immune system kicks in or resistances develop, but what brings psychic traumas to an end?

Is It Luck?

Why didn't Stalin's era of persecution and the Great Terror continue after his death? Why didn't some equally noxious, iron-fisted totalitarian regime follow and enlarge the gulags, intensify the persecutions, further tighten censorship, and increase the suppression of the population, not just in the USSR, but throughout the Soviet empire?

Why is it Stalinism did not enlarge, magnify, and enforce the collectivization of agriculture throughout the whole of Eastern Europe? Instead of having a mere six million perish at Stalin's hand, why didn't three times that many succumb to even more perverted forms of "neo-Stalinism" to be carried on by another Stalinist doppleganger?

It didn't happen that way. After Stalin's passing, life changed for a generation of Russians.

Why didn't Maoism, the Red Guards, and the Cultural Revolution proliferate after Mao's death rather than wither and disappear? Why didn't Mao become a role model for all Chinese communists so that brigade after brigade of Red Guards would continue his mission and destroy all vestiges of capitalism, all monuments to the past, and all private farm plots? Why didn't ever-increasing numbers of the next generation wave their red books as the whole of China further descended into the grips of ideological insanity, cruelty, and famine?

It certainly could have happened that way, but it didn't. The gang of four, which included Mao's wife, was repudiated and China followed a completely different trajectory.

Again, why didn't Leopold's colonial enslavement and persecution of the Congolese gain an even larger foothold after his death? The African continent could have been savagely raped and exploited by multiple greedy Leopolds. Why didn't this occur?

While there was an era of racist colonial masters that followed Leopold, none came close to his ferocity. What if one observed a snowballing rather than a decline of human malevolence, racism, and barbarism in the Congo?

Instead of ten million people slaughtered in Africa at the hands of white devils like Leopold, why wasn't there a period of "neo-Leopoldism" populated by dozens of wannabe white slave-masters *furthering* the savagery and greed? Millions more could have perished under the yoke of a genocidal movement inspired by Leopold's atrocities. History could have unraveled in this way, but it didn't.

Pol Pot's ambition was to cleanse Cambodia of all vestiges of capitalist residue. He wanted to step-leap and accelerate a Kampuchea's Marxist evolution. In pursuit of that aim, all libraries were closed, money and currency were eliminated, and all signs of capitalist decadence were destroyed. Anyone who spoke French, a leftover from colonial exploitation, would be killed; ditto for people who wore glasses, men who sported beards, and anyone who ever owned a small business or employed a maid.

Mirrors were forbidden because "vanity" was a sign of capitalist degeneracy. Off to the killing fields they went.[73] All members of society were required to wear black. All had their names changed to monosyllabic appellations. All references to "father," "mother," "grandfather," or any signs of respect for elders (and the past) were capital offenses.

Most women in Cambodia stopped menstruating as the entire population suffered from varying degrees of starvation. To create a new generation of "pure Khmer," Pot Pol matched boys and girls to marry and fed his "breeders" extra rice and protein so they could repopulate the country and carry forward his utopian delusions.

Pol Pot's Kampuchea was *Brave New World, Big Brother, Animal Farm, and Auschwitz* rolled into one paroxysm of collective psychosis. Had he not invaded Vietnam and been overthrown, Pol Pot's experiments in racial cleansing would have persisted. What if he had prevailed?

Had the Khmer Rouge remained in power, most of the population of Cambodia over the age of fifteen would likely have been liquidated so Pol Pot's "pure Khmer" could rise like a phoenix from its ashes.[74] Another two to four million people might easily have perished in his psychotic crusade. However, history did not turn out that way. Like our other eruptions of barbarity, this psychic pandemic came to an end as well.

After Genghis Khan, why didn't the savagery of his regime not continue and expand? His death, one historian explains "meant the end of the Mongol Empire," despite the fact that numerous, clashing Khanates continued to survive.[75] Why did the tilt of history not favor further genocide, even larger savage hordes, more and more skulls piled into minarets? Why did history so predictably tilt toward peace?

The three Pashas at the conclusion of the Ottoman Empire ravaged the Armenians, the Assyrians, and the Greeks, and were the bloodthirsty overseers who crucified and raped Christian women and "cleansed" the empire of heretics. What might have happened if they continued? How many more Christians, Jews, and other groups would have been exterminated among the twenty-four million inhabitants of the Ottoman Empire that stretched from North Africa to Baku?

The three pashas did not increase their power, but their villainy withered, died out, and was replaced by sanity, rationality, and peace in the creation of the first secular state of Ataturk's Turkey.

Why did these frenzies of murder, beheadings, crucifixions, and genocides come to an end instead of intensify and proliferate? Was it luck? Was it a miracle? Was it chance? Why?

We rarely ask such questions, but when we do, we start to wonder whether a force exists in human psychology that prevents such collective human cancers from metastasizing further.

Why is the average life expectancy of these human-designed psychic epidemics only about thirty-seven years instead of centuries? Is there an invisible psychic force that resists and fights outbreaks of inhumanity in a manner similar to how our body's immune system activates to ward off disease, physical threats, and pandemics? To put it differently: Is there a human *psychological* immune system that develops antibodies, immunities, or resistance to outbreaks of mass psychosis, lunacy, murderousness, barbarity, and war?

This is the key question pursued in this text, and it closely follows an observation made by Mahatma Ghandi:

> When I despair, I remember that all through history, the way of truth and love have always won. There have been tyrants and murderers, and for a time, they can seem invincible, but in the end, they always fail. Think of it . . . always![76]

THE SEARCH FOR THE HIDDEN VARIABLE

In a way, we are like nuclear physicists pouring over tracings from collisions in an accelerator. We theorize about how to explain the mysterious results we see, but, like Wolfgang Pauli, our explanations take us to hidden variables we can't measure or visualize.

In this case, however, the collisions and tracings observed are psychological. How come Hitler didn't develop the atomic bomb first and win World War II, or Leopold's heirs create even more genocidal Beelzebub's? Why wasn't Stalin succeeded by darker, gloomier, and more draconian overlords? Why didn't the progeny of Maoism become even more treacherous despots? Why didn't Pol Pot's Orwellianism thrive and expand?

Genghis Khan, upon his death, said to his sons, "With heaven's aid I have conquered for you a huge empire. But my life was too short to achieve the conquest of the world. That task is left to you."[77] Why wasn't his task completed? What brought an end to his lethal ambitions?

In probing these psychic tracings and human collisions, we are gradually coming upon a theory, or a hypothesis or, perhaps, just a question: Is some force operating in human collective psychology—a positive *press* lurking in the background of the human landscape—some kind of counterforce that acts as a shield against outbreaks of violence, insanity, villainy, destructiveness, darkness, and evil?

If there is such a psychic defense, and if our hypothesis, theory, or question has any meaning, all we know about this force is that it is unknown, unnamed, unmeasured, and, as far as we can tell, so far invisible.

In the next chapter, we will attempt a closer look into this epiphenomenal ether.

NOTES

1. George Kohn, *Encyclopedia of Plague and Pestilence* (New York: Infobase Publishing, 2007).
2. B. Schmid, E. Buntgen, et al., "Climate-driven Introduction of the Black Death and Successive Plague Reintroductions into Europe," (2010), PNAS, doi: 10.1073/pnas.1412887112, http://www.pnas.org/content/112/10/3020.abstract
3. National Geographic, "America before Columbus," (2010), http://topdocumentaryfilms.com/america-before-columbus/.
4. David Stannard, *American Holocaust* (New York: Oxford University Press, 1992), http://www.amazon.com/American-Holocaust-Conquest-New-World/dp/0195085574
5. La catastrophe démographique" (The Demographical Catastrophe"), July–August, 2007, https://odzworld.wordpress.com/casualties-of-important-events/native-american-deaths/.
6. M. Halverson, "Native American Beliefs and Medical Treatments During the Smallpox Epidemics: An Evolution." Archiving Early America, 1995, http://www.earlyamerica.com/review/2007_summer_fall/native-americans-smallpox.html
7. John M. Francis, *Iberia and the Americas Culture, Politics, and History: A Multidisciplinary Encyclopedia* (Santa Barbara, CA: ABC-CLIO, 2005).

8. J. Taubengerger and D. Morens, "1918 Influenza: the Mother of All Pandemics"Centers for Disease Control and Prevention, (2006).

9. Suzanne Austin Alchon, *A Pest in the Land: New World Epidemics in a Global Perspective* (Albuquerque: University of New Mexico Press, 2003), 21.

10. U.S. Medicine, the voice of Federal Medicine, (2014), http://www.usmedicine.com/editor-in-chief/if-the-epidemic-continues-its-mathematical-rate-of-acceleration-civilization-could-easily-disappear-from-the-face-of-the-earth-within-a-few-weeks/.

11. G. Vanga and V. G. Westover "Origin of the 1918 Spanish Influenza Virus: A Comparative Genomic Analysis." *Molecular Phylogenetics and Evolution* 47, no. 3 (2008): 1100–10.

12. Gina Kolata. *The Flu: The Story of the Great Influenza Pandemic* (New York: Touchstone, 1999).

13. Flu.gov (2015), http://www.flu.gov/pandemic/history/index.html

14. Cited in Kroth, J., *Psychology Underground* (Akron, OH: Academic Press, 2001).

15. H. Nicholls, "Pandemic Influenza: The Inside Story." *Biology*, vol. 4 (2006).

16. Carl Zimmer, "In 1918 Flu Pandemic, Timing was a Killer," *New York Times*, April 30, 2014.

17. Michael Purdy, "Immune System Memory Cells Have Trick for Self Preservation," (2012), http://news.wustl.edu/news/pages/23214.aspx.

18. Randy Dotings, "Genetic HIV Resistance Deciphered," (2005) http://www.wired.com/medtech/health/news/2005/01/66198?currentPage=all .

19. Michael Hopkin, "Did Black Death Boost HIV Immunity in Europe," *Nature*, March 11, 2005, doi:10.1038/news050307-15

20. WGBH Educational, "Double Immunity," (2001), http://www.pbs.org/wgbh/evolution/library/10/4/l_104_05.html.

21. Michael Hopkin, "Did Black Death Boost HIV Immunity in Europe."

22. WGBH Educational, "Double Immunity."

23. Tina Hesman Saey, "Glu Immunity Prompted, YearsLater." *Science News* September 21, 2013.

24. X. Yu et al., "Neutralizing Antibodies Derived from the B cells of 1918 Influenza Pandemic Survivors," Nature, 455:532–36, 2008.

25. C. J. Jung, *Psychological Reflections* (Princeton, NJ, Princeton University Press, 1973), 93

26. Karl Abraham, *On Character and Libido Development* (New York: W. W. Norton, 1966), 66

27. Karl Abraham, *On Character and Libido Development*, 66.

28. "Selected Death Tolls for Wars for Wars and Atrocities before 20th Century," (2015) http://necrometrics.com/pre1700a.htm#AnLushan.

29. New World Encyclopedia (2015), http://www.newworldencyclopedia.org/entry/An_Lushan.

30. Jiu-Hwa Lo Upshur, "An Lushan's Rebellion," in Marsha E. Ackermann, Michael Schroeder, Janice J. Terry, Jiu-Hwa Lo Upshur, and Mark F. Whitters, eds., *Encyclopedia of World History: The Expanding World, 600 CE to 1450*, vol. 2. (New York: Facts On File, Inc., 2008); *Ancient and Medieval History Online* (New York: Facts On File, Inc, 2008), http://www.fofweb.com/activelink2.asp?ItemID=WE49&iPin=WHII014&SingleRecord=True (accessed July 22, 2015).

31. Kallie Szczepanski, "What Was the An Lushan Rebellion?" (2015), http://asianhistory.about.com/od/ancientchina/f/What-Was-The-An-Lushan-Rebellion.htm See also: http://ozebook.com/wordpress/archives/26016.

32. Harold Lamb, *Genghis Khan Emperor of all Men*, http://www.goodreads.com/book/show/224038.Genghis_Khan.

33. Max Pfingstein "Mongolians and their Contributions to Western Civilization," study.com, accessed 2015, http://education-portal.com/academy/lesson/mongolians-and-their-contributions-to-western-civilization.html#lesson.

34. http://www.goodreads.com/quotes/463440-i-am-the-punishment-of-god-if-you-had-not-committed.

35. David Nicolle, *The Mongol Warlords: Genghis Khan, Kublai Khan, Hulegu, Tamerlane* (New York: Firebird, 1990,) 2, http://www.biblio.com/book/mongol-warlords-genghis-khan-kublai-khan/d/707025332.
36. Sources for this list are http://www.parallelsixty.com/history-russia.shtml. Also: http://home.arcor.de/mustangace/sca_class_mongols.htm; Edward Gibbon, *Decline and Fall of the Roman Empire* (London, Stahan and Cadell, 3 & 6, 1776); Battuta's Travels, *Part Three, Persia and Iraq*; see also "The History of Russia" http://www.parallelsixty.com/history-russia.shtml; Jeffrey Hays, "Tartars and Mongols," (2012), http://factsanddetails.com/asian/cat65/sub423/item2692.html.
37. David Morgan. *The Mongols and global history.* (New York: Blackwell Publishing, 2007).
38. Ole Jørgen Benedictow, *The Black Death, 1346-1353: The Complete History* (2008), London, Boydel & Brewer, p. 382
39. Morris Rossabi, "The Mongols in World History," http://www.google.com/search?client=safari&rls=en&q=collapse+of+mongols&ie=UTF-8&oe=UTF-8
40. *First Encyclopaedia of Islam: 1913–1946* (New York: Brill, 1993) http://books.google.com/books?id=ro--tXw_hxMC&dq=timur+buried+4000+christians+alive&source=gbs_navlinks_s.
41. Stephen Kinzer, "A Kinder, Gentler Tamerlane Inspires Uzbekistan," *New York Times*, November 10, 1997
42. Rajkai Timor "The Timurid empire and the Ming Ching China," doctoral dissertation, accessed 2015 http://doktori.btk.elte.hu/hist/rajkai/diss.pdf
43. Sinor, Denis. "Inner Asia: History, Civilization, Languages; A Syllabus." Bloomington: Indiana University, (1969).
44. Luke Pring, "Empire History" (2015), http://empirehistory.weebly.com/timurid-empire.html.
45. Gilder Lehrman, Institute of American History, accessed 2015, http://www.gilderlehrman.org/history-by-era/slavery-and-anti-slavery/resources/facts-about-slave-trade-and-slavery.
46. Jack Crawford, "The Missing 100 Million," (2015) http://www.mobilization2-21.com/missing.htm.
47. Yale University, Genocide Studies Program, (2015), http://www.yale.edu/gsp/colonial/belgian_congo/index.html.
48. Mark Dummett, "King Leopold's legacy of DR Congo violence," 2004, http://news.bbc.co.uk/2/hi/africa/3516965.stm.
49. Vicount James Bryce and Arnold Toynbee, *The Treatment of Armenians in the Ottoman Empire, 1915–1916: Documents Presented to Viscount Grey of Falloden, Uncensored Edition,* Ara Sarafian, ed., (Princeton, NJ: Gomidas Institute, 2000).
50. Emin Ahmed, *Turkey in the World War* (New Haven, CT: Yale University Press, 1930).
51. Manus I. Midlarsky, *The Killing Trap: Genocide in the Twentieth Century* (UK: Cambridge University Press. 2005), 342–43.
52. Sukru Hanioglu, *Ataturk: An Intellectual Biography,* (Princeton, NJ: Princeton University Press, 2011), 129.
53. United States Census Bureau, http://www.census.gov/population/international/data/idb/sysmessage.php.
54. Dan Alex, "Second World War History," accessed 2015, http://www.secondworldwarhistory.com/world-war-2-statistics.asp
55. Teresa Pensac Schwartz, *Holocaust Forgotten,* (2012), http://www.holocaustforgotten.com/non-jewishvictims.htm.
56. Michael Clodfelter, *Warfare and Armed Conflicts—A Statistical Reference to Casualty and Other Figures, 1500–2000.* 2nd ed. (New York: McFarland & Co., 1998).
57. Josef Zisels and Halyna Kharaz, "Will Holodomor Receive the Same Status as the Holocaust?" "Maidan" Alliance (2012), http://eng.maidanua.org/.

58. Timothy Snyder, "Hitler vs. Stalin: Who Killed More," *New York Review of Books,* July 2011, http://www.nybooks.com/articles/archives/2011/mar/10/hitler-vs-stalin-who-killed-more/?pagination=false.

59. Snyder, "Hitler vs. Stalin: Who Killed More."

60. Jonathan Fenby, "Mao's Great Famine by Frank Dikötter" *The Guardian,* September 2010.

61. Demographic Consequences of the Great Leap Forward in China's Provinces," *Population and Development Review* 13, no. 4 (1987): 639–70.

62. Yang Jisheng, "China's Great Shame," *New York Times,* November 13, 2012.

63. Yale Genocide Studies Program, 1994–2008, http://www.yale.edu/cgp/.

64. Timothy May *The Mongol Conquests in World History* (London: Reaktion Books, 2012).

65. J. A. Boyle, ed., *The Cambridge History of Iran: Volume 5, The Saljuq and Mongol Periods* (Cambridge, UK: Cambridge University Press, 1968).

66. "Timurids," *The Columbia Encyclopedia, 6th ed.,* (New York: Columbia University, 2006).

67. "Leopold II and the Congo Free State," accessed 2015," http://leopoldandcongo.wiki.elanco.net/Missionaries.

68. "Leopold II and the Congo Free State."

69. Ben Kiernan, "The Original Cambodian" *New Internationalist,* 1993, 242.

70. William Tompson, *J. Khrushchev: A Political Life* (New York: St. Martin's Press, 1995).

71. Maureen Fan and Ariana Cha, "China's Capital Cases Still Secret, Arbitrary," *Washington Post,* 2008.

72. http://ess.uwe.ac.uk/genocide/statements.htm.

73. J. Kroth "Saloth Sar," *Omens and Oracles: Collective Psychology in the Nuclear Age* (New Haven, CT: Praeger, 1991).

74. Kroth "Saloth Sar."

75. All Empires, online history community, (2010), http://allempires.com/article/index.php?q=The_Mongol_Empire.

76. Mahatma Ghandi, *An Autobiography: The Story of My Experiments with Truth* (Boston: Beacon Press, 1990), http://www.un.org/events/nonviolence/2008/.

77. Michael Prawdin, *The Mongol Empire,* (New Brunswick, NJ: Transaction Publishers, 2009), 224

TWO

On the Shore with Thucydides

In 430 BC, Thucydides in Athens noticed that if people contracted a disease and survived, they could then nurse people who had the ailment without getting sick again. That was humanity's incipient awareness of the immune system. Unfortunately, the idea was not picked up again for 2,300 years.

Instead, the "miasma" theory held sway. It said that putrid air and decomposing matter caused diseases, especially epidemics. Contagions came from the air. As Vitruvius in Rome described it:

> For when the morning breezes low toward the town at sunrise, if they bring with them mist from mashes and, mingled with the mist, the poisonous breath of creatures of the marshes to be wafted into the bodies of the inhabitants, they will make the site unhealthy.[1]

Germs, microorganisms, and vaccines were unknown. So was the immune system.

In China, despite its three-thousand-year history of medicine, the situation was similar. Miasma had its heyday here too as early Chinese chronicles considered cold, influenza, malaria, and dysentery to originate from the air, fog, putrefied dust and gases in the atmosphere.[2]

Smallpox

In 1796, Edward Jenner experimented with cowpox by infecting an eight-year-old child with it in hopes it would provide protection against smallpox. It worked. Vaccination is a way to stimulate the immune system in order to provide protection against subsequent infection. While a smallpox vaccine was underway, the notion of some kind of immune system "that was stimulated" to fight disease wasn't yet grasped by human consciousness. Nonetheless, an awareness was emerging that the body carries ancestral information from past events that can be deployed to defend against new infections.

Alexins

In 1890, Hans Buchner's humoral theory held there were "protective substances" existing in bodily fluids capable of killing microorganisms. This was the first statement officially declaring the existence of a positive force in human biology, which has come to be known as the immune system. Others working at the same time as Buchner are credited with similar insights—Louis Pasteur, Paul Ehrlich, Elie Metchnikov, and Joseph Lister.[3]

From Alexins, the knowledge base exponentially grew to include cell types such as dendritic cells, macrophages, regulatory T cells, B cells, cytotoxic T cells, natural killer cells and helper T cells. Today, the human immune system is widely accepted. It is subdivided into parts, an innate immune system, which protects through evolution and natural selection, and an adaptive one that protects by its gradual build-up of antibodies to diseases that have been encountered.

Today, scientists have genetically engineered mice with human immune system characteristics so they can study how various drugs interact with diseases and to enhance their therapeutic effect. Humanity has come a long way since Alexins, but it is worth noting that our knowledge of this positive force in human physiology—a force that shields and protects humanity from threats and disease—is little more than a century old.

In our present understanding of psychology, we are standing on the same shore as Thucydides two millennia ago and looking out across a mysterious horizon. We only see tracings and hints that some kind of positive force exists in the background of human psychology. Nothing definite. Nothing we can put our fingers on.

Something appears to operate in a protective way. Something seems to mitigate or attenuate horrific eruptions that periodically appear on the human landscape. Whatever it is, this entity moves humanity in a positive direction and out of its episodic negative fugue states, which we call war, genocide, tyranny, or just garden variety barbarism. This something defuses or minimizes the worst that our species produces, and this deflected chaos is the first important observation made during our prior review of mankind's atrocities.

However, from our vantage point on the shore, standing next to Thucydides, looking out, all we see are faint outlines. It is just as easy to think this psychic immune factor is a mirage, and the human race merely "lucked out." Beyond opaque silhouettes, little is known about this psychic force, or even if it is a force, or a system, an entity, a mechanism, a process, or some kind of "field."

We have no idea how it works, know nothing of its internal dynamics, and, frankly, don't even have words to name it. We are at the stage of alexins, with nothing more than a theory that inside the serum of human collective psychology is some protective substance, field, force, or system that happily has humanity's back.

It seems prudent, therefore, to backtrack and learn more about the self-preservative network, the physical immune system, and how it works, before speculating too expansively on any *psychic* immune system and its elusive mechanisms.

Self-Preservation and the Physical Immune System

Eman Farouk opines,

> Break a bone . . . and as the broken part heals it becomes the strongest part in it . . . get hit by a virus, survive that, and it can never get you again . . . observe how your skin that gets rubbed on a surface often becomes thicker and more rough with time . . . you can't be stronger if life doesn't try you every now and then, and after each trial, it promises a stronger more immune version of you.[4]

Humans are blessed with a whole sequence of self-preservative instincts. We immediately and reflexively retreat from a very cold or very hot object. From blinking to sweating, fight to flight, we are programmed to react to danger and injury.

A baby when touched on the cheek immediately turns toward the object and begins to suck (the rooting reflex). When hungry, the baby cries, and the mother is quite literally neurologically programmed to hear that cry and respond to it, as if both mother and child were "wired" for the survival and well-being of the child. When males and females are exposed to a child's cry against a background of white noise, females hear the noise far more readily than males do, and a woman's brain regions respond differently than that of a man.[5] This phenomenon occurs whether or not the woman is a mother.

Our tongue's response to bitter taste evolved to protect us from ingesting plants that could be poisonous. We have a knee-jerk reflex that prevents injuries to our joints.

> If we stand on a nail, pain sensors in our foot are activated, causing contraction of the hamstrings and calf muscles which lift our foot off the nail. Without such a reflex, we might carry on walking normally and do much more damage. The sensors in our feet respond not just to pain, but also to pressure and light touch. Notice the way we flinch when tickled, and find it difficult to walk with a pebble or other small object in our shoe.[6]

Not only are we wired for survival, but as first noticed by Thucydides, the crown jewel of our self-preservative network is the body's immune system. Here are some of its constituents: the tonsils are immune organs where the adaptive response to pathogens in the throat are generated. The thymus is the site of T cell development. Once developed the T cells leave the thymus where they can be activated in response to stimuli. The spleen is a reservoir of white blood cells that migrate to remove dead cells and heal wounds. Lymph nodes contain lymphocytes to make antibodies that target pathogens for destruction. The immune system works tirelessly to prevent and clear infections as it fights off invasive bacteria, parasites, viruses, toxins, pollution, and fungi.

Aiding and Abetting the Immune System

The nervous system is partitioned into autonomic (involuntary) and voluntary systems. The latter controls movements like walking and talking, while the involuntary nervous system, acting outside of conscious control, regulates salivation, heartbeat, digestion and other visceral functions. The immune system generally operates autonomically.

By the way, since this text is ultimately a psychological enterprise, let us use a psychological term here—unconsciously. Indeed, the autonomic nervous system and the immune system operate autonomically and unconsciously.

One can certainly lessen the burden on the immune system with voluntary, intelligent, and conscious behavior—by taking care of ourselves, washing and bandaging wounds, exercising regularly, eating a diet high in fruits and vegetables, avoiding infections, inventing and using appropriate vaccines, developing antibiotics,[7] and, of course, not smoking. So both voluntary and involuntary processes—conscious and unconscious—are involved in physical preservation, survival, and immunity.

THE PHYSICAL IMMUNE SYSTEM AND PANDEMICS

Consider a few of the physical pandemics that ravaged the human race discussed in the prior chapter. The Black Death occurred between 1347 and 1353. The virulence of the epidemic was entirely unexpected, killing close to 60 percent of the population of Europe but the disease retreated rather rapidly by 1353. What caused that deceleration and the end of one of the worst plagues that ever impacted the human race?[8]

Certainly "conscious" behavior played a role even though much of it was misplaced. For example, many ethnic groups were persecuted because they were thought to be carriers of the plague—Jews, lepers, pilgrims, and foreigners among them.[9] However, there were also rational and intelligent approaches to controlling the plague, even though no one knew what caused it. One of the more positive interventions was a forty-day quarantine known as "Cordon Sanitaire," which prevented people from leaving or entering infected areas.

The more involuntary immune system also played a role. The plague, caused by the *Yersinia pestis* bacterium, impacted those with already weakened immune systems, such as the elderly and those in poor health. Those who had healthier immune systems not only survived, but also "passed along stronger genes to their children, resulting in a hardier post-plague population."[10 11]

One gene called TLR2 (Toll-like receptor 2) caused a heightened immune response when exposed to plague bacteria.[12] A recent study of the gene CCR5 shows it may also have played a defensive role.

> The Black Death drove natural selection in the human population. Those with the mutation were more likely to survive the plague and pass on their genes than those without which caused an increase in the percentage of people with the mutation.[13]

The Spanish Flu

The Spanish flu occurred at a time (1918–1919) when viruses were unknown. Again, voluntary prophylactic measures that attempted to boost the immune system were undertaken such as using garlic. Other actions like initiating a quarantine were enormously effective. If one looks at the mortality curve of the Spanish flu, it looks very similar to the rise and fall of the Black Death with a rapid deceleration in the spread of the disease.

The Spanish flu quickly went into remission, but why did it do so? First, older people who were previously exposed to a variant of the virus, did not succumb to it as readily as younger people whose immune systems had no immunological memory of the disease. The sharp decline of infections occurred after exhausting the number of people who did not have immunity or any resistance. A 2014 study concluded:

> The explanation turns out to be surprisingly simple: People born after 1889 were not exposed as kids to the kind of flu that struck in 1918, leaving them uniquely vulnerable. Older people, meanwhile, had been exposed to flu strains more closely related to the 1918 flu, offering some immunity. Simply put, the Spanish flu owed its ferocity to a switch in dominant influenza varieties that had occurred a generation earlier. "All a matter of timing," says virologist Vincent Racaniello of Columbia University in New York.[14]

More Diseases and More Quasi Bell-Shaped Curves

An influenza epidemic in 1986 rises and then decelerates as older individuals with previously conferred immunities failed to fall victim to the disease. A measles epidemic appears and recedes into remission as a vaccine is introduced. The epidemic of polio similarly collapses into remission when a vaccine is introduced and as an environmental pollutant like DDT, which impacts the central nervous system, is halted. In "The Mathematics of Diseases," Cambridge scholar, Matthew Keeling, mathematically models two disease outbreaks. Both resemble bell-shaped curves (see figure 2.1). [15]

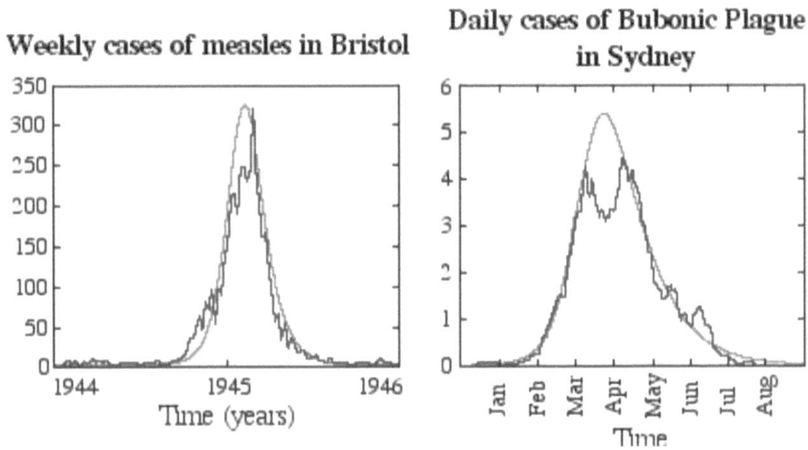

Figure 2.1 Mathematical Models of Epidemics. Graphics courtesy of Matthew Keeling

In fact, epidemiologists have identified a generalized curve of how any epidemic or pandemic proceeds. It rises to a peak, and then the immune system defenses (or interventions like vaccines that strengthen the immune system) are introduced as the disease tails off. [16]

VOLUNTARY (CONSCIOUS) AND INVOLUNTARY (UNCONSCIOUS) IMMUNITIES

Some epidemics come to a close almost entirely as a result of the autonomic operation of the immune system (i.e., without any serious conscious interventions). The Spanish flu would seem such an example.

Other epidemics retreat as a result of exceptional human intervention. SARS is a highly virulent disease that began in Guangdong, China, with no known cure. The coronavirus that causes SARS could survive for long periods on an inanimate object, and could infect "entire hospital wards if workers did not follow infection guidelines." [17]

About 10 percent of those infected died from the disease, so clearly there was a pre-existing autonomic immunity against it—or what can be called its "unconscious" dimension. However, disease remission was much more the result of careful and deliberate measures to quarantine those infected and strict adherence to infection protocols—or what can be called the "conscious" dimension.[18]

In either case, again we see the familiar bell-shaped curve and the happy news that the possible pandemic was decelerating and tumbling into remission by the intervention of the immune system in combination with voluntary, conscious, intelligent, and deliberate actions.[19] Without the quarantines and infection protocols, 10 percent of the human population, or seven hundred million people, could have died from relying on the involuntary immune system alone.

A more compelling example of the conscious side in human self-preservation is the situation with AIDS. This is a disease that directly attacks the human immune system. Almost 600,000 Americans have died from AIDS related complications since the pandemic started in the early 1980s.[20]

The HIV virus destroys immune cells called CD4 T cells, and the patient is left open to opportunistic infections that lead to death.[21] Normally, the immune system would fight off these infections, but when compromised by HIV, the disease ravages the body.

Early on, attempts were made to educate regarding safe sex practices, but such interventions did not turn the tide. Today, the majority of new infections come from the gay community. In 2014, about 20 percent of all gay men in the United States were HIV positive and about half unaware of their condition.[22] Untreated HIV will evolve into AIDS within five to ten years.

This pandemic would likely have continued its exponential rise if not for the advent and discovery of antiretroviral drugs. Taken in combination, these drug cocktails reduce the viral load and lower the mortality.

What is important is the remission of the pandemic was not solely due to operation of the immune system, but resulted from conscious, deliberate attempts to aid and abet, boost and enhance, the immune response through medical discoveries and willful adherence to treatment protocols.[23]

PSYCHOLOGICAL PANDEMICS AND THEIR REMISSION

It is at this point that we start to notice something strange. When looking at physical pandemics, there was a recurring bell-shaped curve decelerating into happy territory, recovery, and remission. However, when plotting psychic barbarities, whether they occurred recently or one thousand years ago, there is a repeating set of curves with uncanny similarities to physical pandemics.

If one plots the rate of violent death in the United States since 1776, there are two rising curves that decelerate about as rapidly as they ascend, one representing the Civil War and the other representing World War II.

How curious! If one looks at mortality in the Atlantic slave trade, mortality rises from 1700 forward and then sharply falls into remission with the Civil War and banning of slavery. Another happy denouement.

The genocides committed by the Ottomans against Armenians, Assyrians, and Greeks also exhibit this familiar pattern. The savagery rises to a peak, and then decelerates as the empire collapses and the modern, secular state of Turkey appears.

What counterforce pushed that rising curve down and into remission instead of accelerating and permitting those three pashas to succeed with their brutal campaign of murder and crucifixion so the Ottoman Empire could be saved and flourish for another six hundred years? Was a psychic immune system at play?

When Jung opined that war was a "psychic epidemic," perhaps he was not merely waxing poetic, but meant to be taken literally, as if there are "outbreaks" of evil, barbarity, and murder that are gradually brought under control by deep and unknown, self-preservative mechanisms within human psychology.

The insanity of Pol Pot's regime, once graphed, shows this same rapidly accelerating thrust of murder and mayhem reaching an apex and then retreating. It could have spiraled upwards. The regime could have metastasized and grown. More killing fields could have opened, but things did not turn out that way. Is there a counterforce that remediates pathogens, pathologies, and psychopathologies and can return the system to order, equilibrium, and tranquility? (See figure 2.2)[24]

The rapid-fire explosion of alliances in World War I, which engulfed sixteen million victims, ended just like a pandemic declines. Mortality returned to baseline. Ditto for the outbreak of collective insanity called World War II that consumed sixty million individuals and exterminated humans in a manner never before seen.

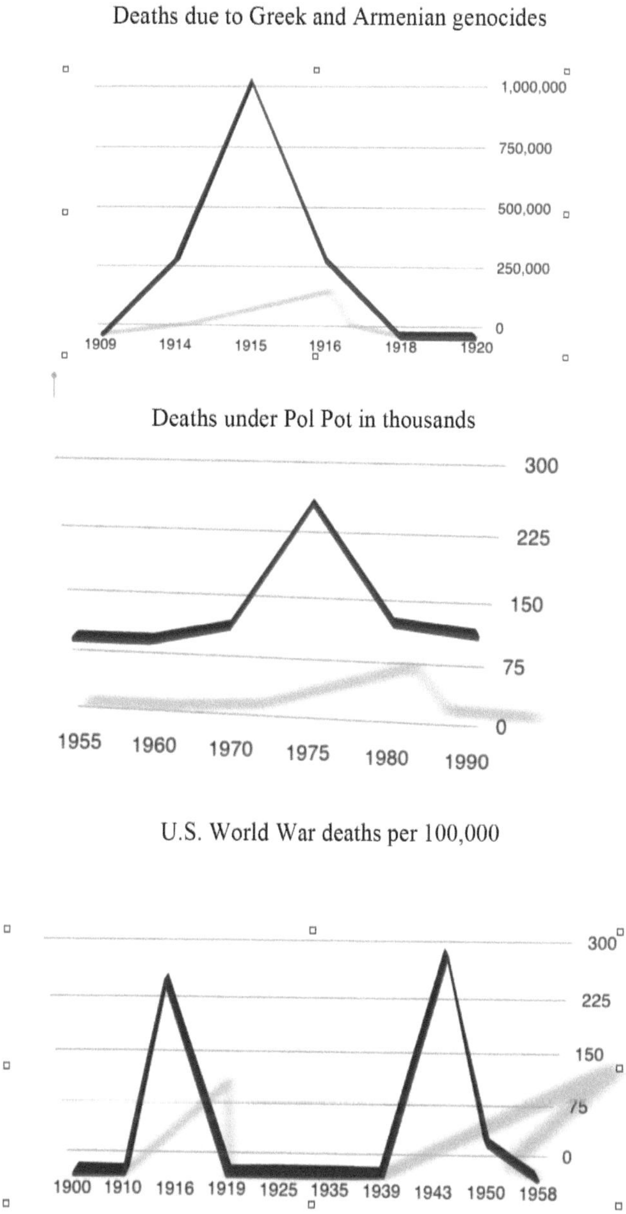

Figure 2.2 Psychic Epidemic Mortality Curves
Data that comprises these graphics is from from the following sources. Pol Pot graphic: http://www.anychart.com/blog/2012/03/13/how-to-choose-chartgraph-type-for-seeing-data-over-time/. World War graphic: Persuade Me Politics, accessed 2015, https://persuademepolitics.wordpress.com/2015/07/30/now-most-peaceful-time-in-world-history/. Greek and Armenian Genocide graphic: R. J. Rummel, Statistics of Democide. Charlottesville, Virginia, Center for National Security Law, Transaction Publishers, Rutgers, University.

Auschwitz, one 472-acre plot hosted the premeditated murders of a million people. Rather than witnessing these psychic outbreaks proliferate and grow, they too came to an end. Mortality retreated. The psychic disease falls into remission just as physical ailments do, and the curves returned to baseline.

With Stalinism, once again the same result: executions, paranoia, summary internal deportations, ideologically inspired famines, and the gulags, but rather than growing worse after Stalin, they mysteriously decline and retreat.

Compare the *physical* pandemic of the Spanish flu with the *psychic* pandemic of Stalin's labor camps (see figure 2.3). The curves are remarkably similar, except that one refers to a physical outbreak in which the immune system plays a dominant role, and the other refers to a psychological epidemic in which an unknown counterforce appears to play a dominant role.

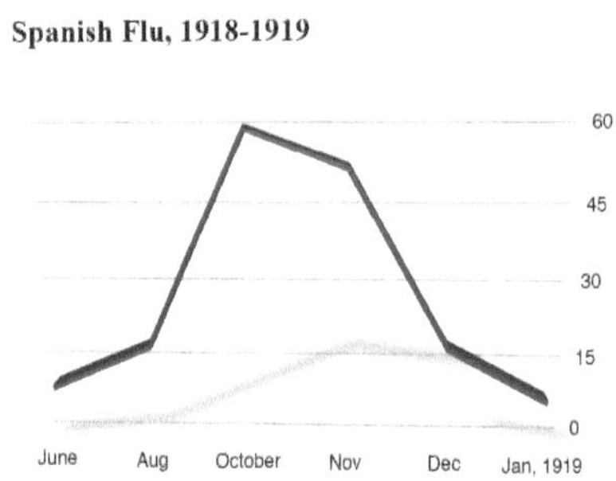

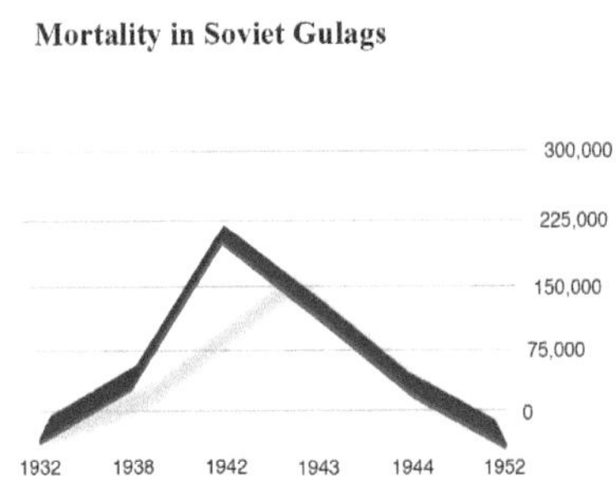

Figure 2.3 Comparing Physical and Psychic Epidemics
Graph of deaths in Soviet gulags developed from the following source: J. Otto Pohl, Ethnic Cleansing in the USSR, 1937–1949 (Santa Barbara, CA: Greenwood Press, 1999). Figures for Spanish flu developed from H. Nicholls, Plo Pandemic Influenza: The Inside Story. National Museum of Health and Medicine Biology, vol. 4 (2006).

Both diseases or epidemics retreat. The retreat of the physical pandemic is a result of the immune system. What do we call the retreat of Stalin's psychic pandemic? What is the name given for this counterforce that generates such an incredibly happy deceleration in human suffering? Is there a psychic immune system that operates like the physical immune system, or is this an extraneous and irrelevant comparison?

Every time one looks at another outbreak of evil, genocide, or collective murderousness, the same curve appears. It rises to a peak and then a counterforce—or resistance—pushes it back to baseline, to peace and quiescence. Consider the thirty-eight million who died under Maoism. That curve does not relentlessly push upward. Again we ask, why didn't the "Gang of Four" which included Mao's wife, Jiang Qing, succeed and prosecute an even more robust form of Maoism? To the contrary, the killings stopped, the Gang of Four was arrested for treason, and a generation of businessmen in suit and tie took the reins of power and moved China in an entirely different direction?[25]

There are no graphics on the deaths accumulated by Genghis Khan and the Mongols, but after his death the Mongol empire became significantly more peaceful. Khan's descendants failed to conquer the rest of the earth as he had hoped, and murderousness came to an end.

Timur's dynasty and its atrocities occur in the first thirty-five years of his reign, which roughly begins in 1370. Here the vast majority of the killings occur—close to twelve million souls. After his death, murderousness predictably recedes:

> The vast empire he carved proved to be difficult to keep; his son and successor, Shahrukh (r. 1405–47), barely managed to maintain the empire's boundaries, and subsequent Timurid princes sought to establish their own kingdoms, weakening the empire with internal strife.[26]

After Timur's death, atrocities retreat, the psychic epidemic eases into remission, and under descendant Shah Rukh a golden period of Persian art commences in place of the savagery preceding it. Shah Rukh died in 1447. As Charlie Chaplin opined: "The hate of men will pass, and dictators die, and the power they took from the people will return to the people."[27]

Seeing the Invisible

When physical epidemics retreat, we refer to it as the "remission of disease" and a return to some kind of homeostasis and equilibrium of the system. Computing how long it takes for that return is enormously variant, but in table 1.3 the length of all the many physical pandemics was calculated, and it took approximately ninety-nine years to bring the most formidable human *physical* epidemics and plagues back to baseline.

The same calculation for psychological epidemics, wars, and genocides was thirty-seven years, at least for the darkest moments of human history that were identified—eleven gloomy case histories from the Mongols to Pol Pot.

Admittedly, diseases and epidemics, whether physical or psychological, do not always conform to perfect normal curves, but they often approximate them. They ascend, reach a crest, and return to baseline. When it comes to physical diseases, the causal agent that brings them back is generally the immune system. It kicks in (involuntarily) or we facilitate its work by conscious and deliberate prophylactic measures (voluntary). However, there is no name for any process, entity, or counterforce in the psychological sphere that operates to bring humanity out of its darkest moments, to attenuate the conflict, and draw it back down to baseline and into the light.

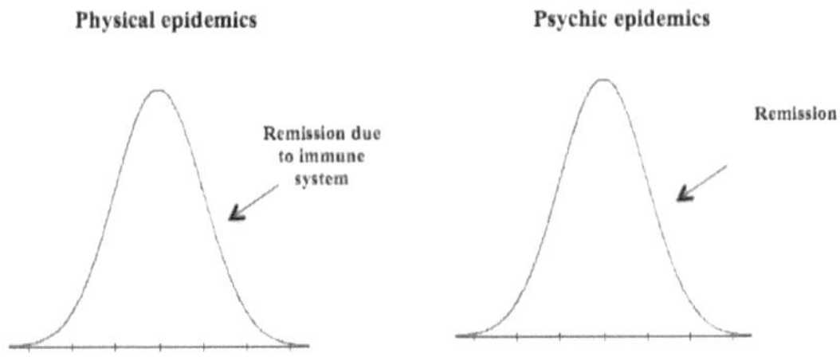

Figure 2.4 Physical and Psychic Epidemic Curves

Instead it is called "victory," "defeat," "surrender," "capitulation," "revolution," "counter-revolution," "thaw," "armistice"; it goes by many names. Whatever the name of this counterforce, it manages to re-establish homeostasis and return to nonviolence in roughly thirty-seven years. There are many instances where it is entirely logical to assume the atrocities would or could have continued, proliferated, and metastasized, but the pandemic failed and slid back into remission. The horrors came to an end. The evil turned away from its peak, retracted—and it did so regularly and predictably. As Ghandi reminded us, these outbreaks of murderousness always come to an end . . . *"Think of it. Always!"*

Confronting an Absurdity

It would be consummate absurdity to suggest that a mother who nurses her son back to health from a cold or flu by keeping him at home, giving him plenty of fluids, vitamin C, and Vicks Vaporub cured him of his illness. She certainly helped the immune system do its work, but the fever retreated, only in part, because of her efforts. More accurately, she aided the immune system through conscious and deliberate nursing. However, if her son had no immune system, nothing she did would have saved him. Without it, he would never survive, no matter how much care he was given.

David Vetter suffered from a genetic defect at birth that left him with no immune system. He lived inside a plastic bubble most of his life. Any infection or invasive agent would kill him. He died at the age of twelve in 1984. Other children with this disorder, called SCID, now can get bone marrow transplants or gene therapy to create the missing immune system.

So, it is farcical to say the mother who nursed her son back to health did so all on her own. Quite the contrary, she abetted her son's internal immune system, and without it he would have died unless he lived inside a germ-free plastic bubble like David Vetter.

PSYCHIC EPIDEMICS AND THE BIASES OF HISTORY

However logical, that is not how we view psychic epidemics, war, genocide, and our long list of barbarities. We make no mention of any immune system or any internal, autonomous, self-preservative process at all.

Instead, we habitually attribute the end of hostilities to human conscious interventions: Harry Truman defeated the Japanese. Roosevelt, Churchill, Stalin, and their generals Eisenhower, Patton, and Zhukov beat the Nazis. Pol Pot was vanquished by the invasion of the Vietnamese communists. The three pashas were replaced by Ataturk.

The form of this historical bias is best expressed as *General X defeated General Y at the Battle of ABC*. That is the algorithm; it is how we view the end of these dark moments of human history; and is how we conceptualize the progression of all human psychic epidemics.

The absurdity is that we completely ignore the possibility that some other force may be operating behind the scenes that we know nothing about. Our historical interpretations of events may be just as naive and ill-conceived as the mother who boasts that she cured her son of a cold without any knowledge that his immune system did most of the work, operating furiously behind the scenes to preserve his life.

Thucydides noticed something influenced a sick person's outcome, but couldn't name it. Two millennia passed before someone hypothesized there was some force inside every human being that fights off diseases. In psychology, we are still in the age of Thucydides, noticing that psychic epidemics always come to an end, and peace is restored. However, we are bereft of any name for the entity that might exist and operate inside, that is, within the human condition.

The fact that each of our major barbarities curve downward, looking suspiciously like the remission curves of physical disease, has not persuaded us to believe in a psychic immune system or, in more poetic language, a natural human instinct or revulsion against darkness, evil, and murder.

Ghandi felt it was love and goodness that invariably triumphed over evil. However, if one approaches this matter with a scientific attitude, there is no evidence to conclude that good conquers evil or that righteousness always destroys immorality.

One simply observes the obvious: collective murderousness generally ends and returns to a state of quiescence and peace. Nonviolence routinely prevails over violence in virtually each of the nightmarish moments we've reviewed in human psychological history. The question of this text is what system or counterforce is unleashed to bring about these positive outcomes?

It is rather easy to document an almost in-bred aversion to violence in human beings. Networks censor photographs of extreme violence and death precisely because of this reflexive abhorrence of seeing real-life atrocities. While some people do seek out violent stimuli, or have a morbid attraction to it in film or video games, it is invariably vicarious, safely viewed at a distance, and rarely enjoyed up close and personal.

One of mankind's notorious killers, Heinrich Himmler, the Nazi henchman charged with exterminating Jews, could not watch the atrocities he designed and ordered others to carry out. When he visited an SS execution field where Jews were shot in the back of the head and fell into a ditch where they were buried, Himmler fainted. He couldn't bear seeing the slaughter. Most people cannot cope with witnessing barbarity. There is a psychological *bias* in the human constitution that abhors violence and consistently prefers peace over war and life over death.

However, each time our histories of barbarity and genocide conclude with a happy ending—the war is over, battles are won, killing has stopped—we inevitably cite the actions of leaders, heroes, generals, kings, monarchs, lords, khans, sultans, and sundry potentates while remaining insistently blind to the fact that positive outcomes may instead result from an instinctive aversion to evil, cruelty, and barbarity that dwells inside the human heart.

The concept that is developing in this text, most properly stated, is that not only do we have a physical immune system and a complete set of self-preservative, autonomic reflexes and instincts to insure our survival. There may also be a *psychic* immune system that reflexively loathes violence and the extermination of one's own kind just as aggressively as the physical immune system abhors infection, disease, and other threats to survival.

NOTES

1. Philippa Lang, *Science: Antiquity and its legacy* (London, I.B. Tauris, 2015), 25
2. The Gallery of Natural Phenomena, accessed 2015, http://www.phenomena.org.uk/features/features/miasma.html.
3. Kendall Smith, "Louis Pasteur, the Father of Immunology?" PMC, US National Library of Medicine, 2012, http://www.ncbi.nlm.nih.gov/pmc/articles/PMC3342039/.
4. "Quotes by Eman Farouk," accessed 2015, http://www.goodreads.com/quotes/919058-break-a-bone-and-as-the-broken-part-heals-it-becomes.
5. Karen Rowan, "Why Baby's Hungry Cry Tugs at Women (But Not Men)," Live Science (2013), http://www.livescience.com/36964-baby-cries-women-men-brains.html.
6. Simon King, "Reflex Reactions, Our Body's Rapid Defence Mechanism," Positive Health, 2010, http://www.positivehealth.com/article/chiropractic/reflex-reactions-our-body-s-rapid-defence-mechanism.
7. Note that use of antibiotics can actually deplete the physical immune system; see Tina Hesman Saey, "Antibiotics may make fighting flu harder," *Science News*, 179, (2011), https://www.sciencenews.org/article/antibiotics-may-make-fighting-flu-harder.
8. Ole J. Benedictow, *The Black Death, 1346–1353: The Complete History* (Woodbridge, Suffolk, UK: Boydell Press, 2004).

9. David Nirenberg, *Communities of Violence,* (Princeton, NJ: Princeton University Press, 2015).

10. Stephanie Pappas, "Black Death Survivors and their Descendants Went on to Live Longer," *Scientific American,* May 2014, http://www.scientificamerican.com/article/black-death-survivors-and-their-descendants-went-on-to-live-longer/.

11. Sharon DeWitte, "Health in Post-Black Death London 1350–1538," *American Journal of Physical Anthropology*, April 17, 2014.

12. Stephanie Pappas, "Black Death Likely Altered European Genes," Live Science, (2014) http://news.discovery.com/human/evolution/black-death-likely-altered-european-genes-1402031.htm.

13. "Biologists Discover Why 10 Percent Of Europeans Are Safe From HIV Infection," *Science Daily*, April 3, 2005.

14. Dan Vergano, "Mystery of 1918 Flu that Killed 50 Million Solved," *National Geographic,* (2014), http://news.nationalgeographic.com/news/2014/04/140428-1918-flu-avian-swine-science-health-science/.

15. Matthew Keeling, "The Mathematics of Disease," accessed in 2015, https://plus.maths.org/content/mathematics-diseases?sa=X&ved=0CCYQ9QEwCGoVChMIt4LRoqH3xgIVT5aICh23Ngo_. Graphic courtesy of Matthew Keeling, Zoology Department, Cambridge University

16. "Epidemic Curves," *Society, the Individual and Medicine,* University of Ottawa, 2015, accessed at http://www.med.uottawa.ca/sim/data/Public_Health_Epidemic_Curves_e.htm.

17. "SARS Stopped Dead in its Tracks," *CNN.com/Health,* 2003, http://www.cnn.com/2003/HEALTH/06/17/sars.wrapup/.

18. Janice Hsueh-Ling, Samuel Ken-En Gan, et al., "Understanding the T Cell Immune Response in SARS Coronavirus Infection," *Emerging Microbes and Infections,* 2012, 1, doi:10.1038/emi.2012.26, http://www.nature.com/emi/journal/v1/n9/full/emi201226a.html.

19. Mead Over, "Five Steps to Reduce the Economic Impact of Ebola," Center for Global Development, 2014, http://www.cgdev.org/blog/five-steps-reduce-economic-impact-ebola.

20. "AIDS Statistics," New York City AIDS memorial, 2013, http://nycaidsmemorial.org/aids-statistics.

21. Dan Cossins, "How HIV Destroys Immune Cells," *The Scientist,* 2013, http://www.the-scientist.com/?articles.view/articleNo/38739/title/How-HIV-Destroys-Immune-Cells/.

22. Meredith Melnick, "CDC: 20% of Gay Men are HIV-positive, but Nearly Half Don't Know It," *Time,* September 26, 2010, http://healthland.time.com/2010/09/26/study-20-of-homosexual-men-are-hiv-positive-but-only-half-know-it/.

23. "Before You Start Drug Therapy," UCSF HIV In Site, (2012), http://hivinsite.ucsf.edu/insite?page=pb-treat-01-00.

24. Data for these graphs developed from the following sources: Pol Pot graphic, http://www.anychart.com/blog/2012/03/13/how-to-choose-chartgraph-type-for-seeing-data-over-time/. World War graphic: Graphic developed from data at Persuade Me Politics, accessed 2015, https://persuademepolitics.wordpress.com/2015/07/30/now-most-peaceful-time-in-world-history/. For Greek & Armenian Genocide: R. J. Rummel, Statistics of Democide. Charlottesville, Virginia, Center for National Security Law, Transaction Publishers, Rutgers, University.

25. Roderick MacFarquhar and Michael Schoenhals, Glossary of Names and Identities in *Mao's Last Revolution* (Cambridge, MA: Harvard University Press, 2006).

26. "The Art of the Timurid Period," Heilbrunn Timeline of Art History, accessed 2015 http://www.metmuseum.org/toah/hd/timu/hd_timu.htm.

27. Charlie Chaplin, *The Great Dictator,* https://www.youtube.com/watch?v=W2ftZ1g4FtE.

THREE

Nuclear Winter

Noam Chomsky said, "There are two problems for our species' survival, nuclear war and environmental catastrophe, and we're hurtling towards them, knowingly."[1] If there is a self-preservative system, which includes a psychic immune system, and its purpose is to ensure not just the survival of individuals but also the survival of our species, then certainly one might look for evidence of it when investigating the greatest existential threat to our survival, all-out nuclear war.

In the last seventy years, species *Homo sapiens* developed the capacity to destroy itself. In this chapter, we will review one of the greatest threats ever created by humankind and ask whether there is any "hidden psychological variable" or "counterforce" against the incredible armamentarium humanity's dark side has amassed.

HUMANKIND'S NUCLEAR HISTORY

The human race experimented with dropping nuclear weapons on civilian populations twice. In Hiroshima, upwards of 130,000 people were killed or injured in 1945 after exposure to a sixteen-kiloton bomb called "Little Boy." In Nagasaki, a twenty-kiloton bomb dubbed "Fat Man" killed or injured sixty-five thousand.[2]

Since the end of World War II, close to two thousand nuclear bombs have been detonated as part of atomic testing programs. The United States conducted one thousand such tests, three hundred of them in the atmosphere.[3] The Soviet Union was credited with seven hundred detonations; France, 210; Britain, 45; China, 45; India and Pakistan, six each.[4] No one knows if, how, when, or where Israel tested its weaponry.

Atmospheric testing of nuclear weapons exposed the human population to significant health issues from radiation fallout particularly between 1945 to 1980.

> Each nuclear test resulted in unrestrained release into the environment of substantial quantities of radioactive materials, which were widely dispersed in the atmosphere and deposited everywhere on the Earth's surface.[5]

Radiation from these tests caused 430,000 related cancer deaths with the ultimate long-term toll estimated at 2.3 million casualties, according to UN research.[6] The United States and former USSR agreed to ban atmospheric nuclear testing in 1963.

The Human Stockpile and a Nuclear Winter

There were once 65,000 nuclear weapons in the world, certainly enough to destroy the earth many times over. In 2013, those numbers winnowed down to roughly seventeen thousand, of which the United States possesses 7,700, Russia 8,500, Britain 225, France 300, China 240, India 100, Pakistan 100, and Israel 200 (estimated).[7]

A limited regional nuclear war, involving as few as fifty Hiroshima-size bombs detonated over population centers, would be enough to cross the threshold into a nuclear winter, says a 2006 report by the American Geophysical Union.[8] Even a relatively small-scale conflict would send five million tons of soot and smoke into the atmosphere, damaging the ozone layer and destroying most agricultural areas in North America and Eurasia.

The Journal of Geophysical Research noted that in a larger scale war—say a five-thousand-megaton exchange[9]—global surface cooling would be unprecedented. Survivors would be faced with freezing summers, a heavily-polluted atmosphere, 45 percent less rainfall, and the loss of most food crops,[10] *"enough to destroy civilization as we know it,"* at least in the Northern Hemisphere:[11] Millions of tons of soot would be wafted by west-to-east winds forming a band of particles across the entire Northern Hemisphere blocking out the sun for several weeks.

> The conditions of semidarkness, killing frosts, and subfreezing temperatures, combined with high doses of radiation from nuclear fallout, would interrupt plant photosynthesis and could thus destroy much of the Earth's vegetation and animal life. The extreme cold, high radiation levels, and the widespread destruction of industrial, medical, and transportation infrastructures along with food supplies and crops would trigger a massive death toll from starvation, exposure, and disease. A nuclear war could thus reduce the Earth's human population to a fraction of its previous numbers.[12]

A 2014 study revealed that even a more local nuclear confrontation, say between Pakistan and India, could presage a nuclear winter:

> Most people would be surprised to know that even a very small regional nuclear war on the other side of the planet could disrupt global climate for at least a decade and wipe out the ozone layer for a decade,[13]

ACCIDENTS WILL HAPPEN

There were over sixty accidents involving nuclear weapons.[14] For example, a plane crashed into a building housing nuclear weapons in England, and, in those days, there were unsophisticated fail-safe mechanisms on these bombs. The crash might have ignited one. It did not.

But these kinds of accidents are of no interest here. Such an accident would have a very small probability of starting a full-scale nuclear war. Our interest in this chapter is only with respect to incidents which could have caused humanity to incinerate itself or were genuine threats to human survival.

Instead of sixty accidents, there are instead far fewer. Here is a short review of humanity's *very* close calls with actual survival-threatening nuclear disaster and thus, nuclear winter. How many incidents were there? How did they come into being? How did they end? Who ended them? *What* ended them?

October 5, 1960

The Missile Warning group at Thule, Greenland, detected incoming nuclear missiles and a threat warning was relayed to NORAD, America's central data processing and control center tucked under a Colorado mountain. Preparations were made for nuclear retaliation. Before any missiles were launched, a computer glitch was detected that deducted two zeroes in the target-ranging data in Greenland. For example, the system reported the moon was only 2,500 miles away instead of 250,000 miles. The error was successfully identified before bombers were airborne.[15]

November 24, 1961

The Strategic Air Command early warning systems have triple-redundant telephone lines, so it was highly unlikely all three would fail at once, unless the United States was under some kind of terrorist or nuclear attack. On this date, all three warning system lines were cut. Consequently, all SAC bases in the United States went on alert and bombers were readied with engines running. It turned out the three so-called redundant communication lines were routed through the same relay station in Colorado, where an electrical fault caused them to all fail simultaneously.[16] The problem was discovered before the bombers took off.

October 1962

To defuse tensions during the Cuban Missile Crisis, British prime minister Harold Macmillan and NATO commander Gen. Lauris Norstad agreed not to put NATO on alert to avoid provocation of the USSR. A matching response by the Soviet Union would have brought the world closer to the threshold where mistakes or miscommunications could cause one side to act precipitously.

However, unknown to Norstad, NATO general Truman Landon decided *on his own* to order DEFCON 3, a substantial ratcheting up of preparedness at bases in West Germany, Italy, Turkey, and the United Kingdom. These alerts could have caused a Soviet counter-response, and accelerated the mounting tensions. However, the Soviets either failed to notice the rogue general's action or they ignored the escalation.[17] Regardless of the reason, the Soviets did not respond to Landon's provocation.

October 24, 1962

During the Cuban Missile Crisis, a Soviet satellite entered its orbit and shortly thereafter exploded. The blast led NORAD (North American Aerospace Defense Command) to believe the USSR was launching a massive ICBM (intercontinental ballistic missle) attack. Allegedly, this incident is still partly classified "possibly to conceal reaction to the event."[18] Not much more is known about it except the incident was quite serious and could have precipitated a nuclear outbreak.

October 25, 1962

Again, during the Cuban Missile Crisis, tensions were high, and the whole world was on edge because of the vast nuclear arsenals of the USSR and the United States. A bear was sniffing around the perimeter of the Duluth "Sector Direction Center," and triggered intruder alarms at all air bases in the area. The Volk Field alarm was incorrectly wired in Wisconsin, resulting in an order for nuclear-armed F-106 crews to scramble and prepare for takeoff.

> Dan Barry looked out his cockpit at the snow-swept runway. With his squadron assembled at Volk Field, he was second in line for takeoff. In the bay of his F106-A jet was an 812-pound Genie missile armed with a live nuclear warhead. The 27-year-old lieutenant believed a nuclear war had begun.[19]

A staff member drove to the runway, informed the pilots of the incorrect alarm and got them to stand down.

October 26, 1962

Yet another event happened during the Cuban Missile Crisis: there was a program of routine ICBM test flights out of Vandenberg Air Force Base. Despite the tensions over Cuba, Vandenberg continued the tests, and at 4:00 a.m. on October 26, an ICBM was launched. It must be assumed that Russian observers were monitoring U.S. missile activities as closely as the United States was watching Soviet rockets. Why there was no Russian response to this ICBM launch during the tense crisis remains a mystery.[20]

The president and his cabinet were completely unaware of the launch until after it occurred. President Kennedy was deeply disturbed—read furious—that such an event took place outside of his control at such a critical moment in history. Note that Vandenberg was a base that also was capable of launching nuclear missiles at Russia, and, thus, such a "test launch" might not have been taken lightly by them had it been noticed.[21]

October 28, 1962

Another incident occurred in Mooretown, New Jersey, at the height of the Cuban crisis when a radar station wasn't informed of a U.S. satellite flyby. Its sudden appearance on the horizon caused the radar operator to panic and alert NORAD the United States was under attack, adding to national paranoia that could have triggered a nuclear war. Actually a test tape which simulated a launch from Cuba was being run at the time while a satellite appeared over the horizon. The staff at NORAD became excited and thought impact would occur some eighteen miles west of Tampa, Florida, at 9:02 a.m.

The whole of NORAD was alerted, but before irrevocable action had taken place, it was reported that no detonation had taken place at the predicted time, and Moorestown operators reported the reason for the false alarm. During the incident, overlapping radars that should have confirmed or disagreed were not in operation. The radar post had not received routine information of satellite passage because the facility carrying out that task had been given other work for the duration of the crisis.[22]

November 2, 1962

The United States had a high-level Soviet spy operating in Moscow in 1962 named Col. Oleg Penkovsky. He was later caught and executed by the Soviets, but while operational, he had a code to warn the CIA if he was "convinced that a Soviet attack on the United States was imminent. He was to call twice, one minute apart, and only blow into the receiver." The CIA received that exact pre-arranged message on November 2, 1962.

Penkovsky had been arrested on October 22 and likely divulged his secret signal when interrogated. Thus, the caller who left the message for the CIA was not Penkovsky.[23] Nonetheless, a call was received following the secret protocol on November 2, 1962, and the caller blew into the receiver as instructed. U.S. officials did not respond even though it signaled a Soviet attack was imminent.

October 24, 1973

During the Arab-Israeli 1973 war, Israel was making gains in crossing the Sinai into the heart of Egypt. Russia, an ally of Egypt, warned the United States that if Israel advanced any further, it could provoke a nuclear response by the Soviet Union. The United States immediately went on nuclear alert and ordered DEFCON 3. "The consequent movements of aircraft and troops were of course observed by Soviet intelligence. The purpose of the alert was not to prepare for war but to warn the USSR not to intervene in the Sinai."[24]

The next day, October 25, as DEFCON 3 went into effect a mechanic in Michigan accidentally activated a military airbase alarm system. B-52 crews rushed to their aircraft and started their engines. The officer on duty recognized the alarm was false and recalled the bomber crews.

November, 1979

At NORAD's underground mountain complex, computers showed that a massive Soviet nuclear strike was underway. A "threat assessment" conference involving senior officers at all three command posts was convened. Launch control centers for America's fleet of Minuteman missiles received preliminary warnings the United States was under attack. The nation's air defense interceptor force was put on alert and ten fighter jets took off. The president's "doomsday plane" was airborne, but satellites failed to detect any Soviet launches and radar could not confirm an attack.

After the stand-down, a "training tape" was discovered inadvertently inserted into the computer that ran the nation's early warning programs. Thanks to the United States's early warning satellite system's accuracy in showing no Soviet invasion, the incident ended with a sigh of relief.[25]

June 30, 1980

In 1980, a curious and frightening event occurred in the continental United States:

> At 2:26 a.m. EDT, Secretary of Defense Brzezinski was alerted that early warning systems indicated 220 nuclear missiles were inbound to the U.S. A short time later, this figure was increased to 2,200. It had begun with a detection of just two SLBM launches, ending with an indicated all-out ICBM attack from the Soviet Union. Once again, bombers took off, the Pacific Command Airborne Command Post was launched, and the Minutemen ICBMs were warmed up. The alert was rescinded because again, radar readings from across the country did not agree with what was being displayed at NORAD. It took three days to isolate the problem. The fault was traced to a computer chip that cost 46 cents.[26]

September, 1983

The Soviets installed a new early warning system to detect missile launches against them. It followed a different kind of approach to the problem. Rather than scanning down on the Earth's surface, the Soviet satellites scanned the edge of the earth reducing the possibility that natural events would be seen as missile launches.

> Missiles, when they had risen five or ten miles, would appear silhouetted against the black background of space. Furthermore, when the edge of the Earth is viewed, light reflected from clouds or snow banks has to pass through a considerable amount of the atmosphere. A satellite has to be in a unique position to view a recently launched missile silhouetted against the black of space. To get that view, the Soviet Union picked a special type of orbit that it had used for its communications satellites. Those orbits, known as Molnyia orbits, come very close to the Earth in the Southern Hemisphere but extend nearly a tenth of the distance to the moon as the satellite passes over the Northern Hemisphere. From that position high above northern Europe, the Soviet Union's Oko (Eye) early-warning satellites spend a large fraction of their time viewing the continental U.S. missile fields at just the right glancing angle. However, shortly after midnight Moscow time on Sept. 26, 1983, the sun, the satellite, and U.S. missile fields all lined up in such a way as to maximize the sunlight reflected from high-altitude clouds.[27]

The Soviet officer in charge, Lt. Col. Stanislav Petrov, indicated that the new system reported the launch of several missiles from the United States. Petrov saw as many as five missiles launched but decided not to inform his superiors.

He knew if the United States launched a missile attack, it would be massive and designed to overwhelm Soviet forces in a single strike. A handful of missiles was insufficient. "When people start a war, they don't start it with only five missiles."[28]

Had he relayed information that five missiles were in the air, his superiors might have reacted far more aggressively. Petrov has been regaled as a man who prevented World War III. Petrov later commented on his decision: "It is nice of them to consider me a hero. I don't know that I am. Since I am the only one in this country who has found himself in this situation, it is difficult to know if others would have acted differently."[29]

January 25, 1995

Norway and the United States participated in a joint scientific expedition to launch a rocket to study atmospheric conditions and the northern lights. The rocket launch followed a 930-mile trajectory away from Russia. However, to a Russian radar technician, the flight appeared similar to the path a U.S. Trident missile would take to detonate a nuclear warhead high in the atmosphere and blind Soviet tracking instruments.

As a result, Russia was poised for a few minutes to launch a full-scale nuclear counterattack on the United States. President Boris Yeltsin said his "nuclear football," a device used to communicate with his missile command, was made active for the first time.

Fortunately, Russia's early warning system was functioning perfectly that day, and the display showed that no massive U.S. attack was lurking below the horizon. Another sigh of relief for a worried world.

MUCH CLOSER CALLS

Soviets Planned to Nuke China

In 1969, Moscow and Beijing had a border dispute. More than a thousand people died on both sides of this conflict. Chinese historian Lin Chenshan argues that China has faced five nuclear threats since 1949.

> Soviet diplomats warned Washington of Moscow's plans "to wipe out the Chinese threat and get rid of this modern adventurer," with a nuclear strike, asking the U.S. to remain neutral. However, Washington told Moscow the U.S. would not stand idly by. The threat worked, he added, and made Moscow think twice, while forcing the two countries to regulate their border dispute at the negotiating table. On October 15, 1969, he quotes Soviet premier Alexei Kosygin as telling Soviet leader Leonid Brezhnev that Washington has drawn up "detailed plans" for a nuclear war against the USSR if it attacked China.
>
> That same day, he says, Anatoly Dobrynin, the Soviet ambassador to Washington, told Brezhnev something similar after consultations with U.S. diplomats. "If China suffers a nuclear attack, they (the Americans) will deem it as the start of the third world war," Dobrynin said. "The Americans have betrayed us." The historian claims that

> Washington saw the USSR as a greater threat than China and wanted a strong China to counter-balance Soviet power.[30]

Clearly, the Soviet Union did not follow through on its nuclear threat.

A Closer Look at the Cuban Missile Crisis

There is a very chilling story about the Cuban Missile Crisis that was not told, or known, until the twenty-first century. As U.S. ships surrounded Cuba and faced off against the approaching Soviet convoy in a blockade of the island, three officers in a Russian submarine held the future of humanity in their hands. The true account of this tense event was revealed in 2002.

The way that most of the world heard the story was that Soviet ships stopped in their tracks and retreated without confrontation due to the U.S. naval blockade. It appeared that the United States had stared down the Soviets and won this round of gamesmanship. People around the world watched these tense events unfold on television and breathed a collective sigh of relief as Soviet ships retreated. President John F. Kennedy was seen as a hero who skillfully handled the crisis with reason, balance, and strength, and he was applauded for his intelligence and guile. Khrushchev, on the other hand, was seen as the loser and, in fact, removed from office the next year.

This popular perception of events, however, was quite untrue. What actually happened follows: The truth is that JFK made a secret deal with Khrushchev that was *kept* from the American people. The confidential agreement said once the Soviets removed their missiles from Cuba, the United States would pull its ICBMs from Turkey and promised, in turn, not to invade Cuba as a second concession. Quietly, discreetly, and a full six months after the Cuban standoff, JFK honored his pledge and quietly removed American missiles from Turkey.

However, the most frightening part of this story is that the world came much closer to nuclear war than anyone suspected, including defense secretary Robert McNamara. In 2002, McNamara attended a conference in Havana about the Cuban Missile Crisis. There he learned something he never knew earlier.[31] When Soviet vessels were approaching the American blockade—an aircraft carrier and eleven other ships—the United States did not believe they were carrying nuclear weapons. Unfortunately not true.

Soviet subs, in fact, had nuclear-tipped torpedoes McNamara knew nothing about. McNamara and the Joint Chiefs were similarly unaware of Soviet deployment of 160 nuclear weapons on Cuban soil that were readied for use. The United States did not know there were atomic weapons there either or that they were on standby and ready for use.

On a particular Soviet sub, B-59, batteries were running low and the air conditioning was spotty. It was cruising low and out of communication with Moscow. American ships began dropping depth charges to force the Soviet subs to surface and be identified. However, Soviet officers had standing orders to fire their torpedoes *if under attack.*

There were three officers aboard B-59, commander Valentin Savitsky, second in charge Vasili Arkhipov, and Ivan Maslennikov, a political officer. All three had to agree before launching a nuclear-tipped torpedo. Savitsky demanded they follow orders and retaliate for the depth charge attack by firing their nuke, which Maslennikov supported. Arkhipov opposed.

Had Savitsky prevailed, a nuclear blast would have destroyed the American fleet. A full-scale U.S. nuclear response would likely have followed, along with massive Soviet retaliation.

The sub had no contact with Moscow, so the crew did not know if war had broken out already. Arkhipov eventually persuaded Savitsky to surface and await orders from Moscow. Had Arkhipov failed, World War III would have ensued with a nuclear winter trailing behind it.

Here's a rendition of this event published in 2012 by the *New York Times*:

> The submarines, not hearing much from the Soviet high command, were trying to figure out what was going on by listening to American radio. . . . They were listening to Miami radio stations. On Miami radio the stories are about impending U.S. invasion of Cuba . . . the sense of panic on the submarine grows to the point that when the Navy spots B-59 and drops depth charges to try to get it to surface, the submarine's commander, Valentin Savitsky, orders that the nuclear torpedo be fired. The political officer agrees; only the refusal by Arkhipov, who died in 1998, prevents it.[32]

It is peculiar that neither in the United States nor present day Russia is there any movement to celebrate Vasilii Arkhipov Day.[33] His actions in persuading Savitsky against launching a nuclear torpedo was probably the single most heroic effort ever documented to save the world from destruction.

Golda Meir

The U.S. government, and to a lesser extent the American media, maintain a relative blackout on Israeli nuclear weapons. A majority of nuclear experts believe Israel possesses two hundred nuclear weapons, which are currently mounted on aircraft, underground Jupiter missiles, and cruise missiles, but no American president ever acknowledged this arsenal. The U.S. media generally plays up the nuclear dangers of other countries while maintaining a deafening silence on the Israeli stockpile.

Ron Rosenbaum in *How the End Begins,*[34] however, makes clear this formidable arsenal of nuclear weapons indeed exists. In 1973, during the Yom Kippur War, Israel was not doing well and was at a point where it feared being overrun. Prime Minister Golda Meir authorized a nuclear alert, ordering thirteen atomic bombs be prepared for missiles and aircraft.[35] A second source confirms this to be true.[36]

Nonproliferation expert, William Potter, alleges Meir gave her generals *discretion* to initiate a nuclear strike if the situation worsened.[37] This was perhaps the only time a nation's leader authorized the discretionary use of nuclear weapons and delegated that responsibility.

In one of the largest tank battles in modern military history, the tide turned for Israel.[38] The Israelis were victorious using conventional arms only, and their generals did not order, at their discretion, the use of nuclear weapons.

November 2, 1983: Able Archer

In the early 1980s, tensions with the Soviet Union were peaking. Ronald Reagan called the USSR "the evil empire" and spoke of "limited nuclear war." The Soviets believed Reagan was personally unstable, and that NATO might be planning a first strike, especially after America deployed new Pershing II and Tomahawk cruise missiles in Europe.

In 1983, NATO began an exercise called "Able Archer," which involved the *simulation of a first-strike* on the Soviet Union. The USSR had installed a new intelligence system called VRYAN that was focused on detecting any first strike activities. It is unlikely the United States or NATO knew anything about VRYAN at the time.

In May 1981, in a closed-session meeting of senior Soviet leaders, Leonid Brezhnev and KGB chairman Yuri Andropov said the United States was preparing a secret nuclear attack on the USSR and that it was not a war game, nor a simulation.[39] Project Able Archer involved coded communications, radio silences, actual participation by heads of governments, and simulated DEFCON alerts. The exercise was notable for its realism.

What planners failed to anticipate was the Soviet Union's reaction since it had suffered a surprise attack in the past when Hitler invaded. Many members of the Soviet Politburo believed the large military "exercise" by NATO was actually a ruse for a first strike:

> The Soviet Union, believing its only chance of surviving a NATO strike was to preempt it, readied its nuclear arsenal. The CIA reported activity in the Baltic Military District and Czechoslovakia; nuclear-capable aircraft in Poland and Germany were placed on high alert status with readying of nuclear strike forces. Former CIA analyst, Peter Vincent Pry, suspects that the aircraft were merely the tip of the iceberg; he hypothesizes that—in accordance with Soviet military procedure and

> history—ICBM silos, already at a high state of alert and difficult for the United States to detect, were also prepared for a launch. Commander Victor Tkachenko, stationed at a Soviet Missile Silo during Able Archer recounts, "When we reached the command bunker that night, we received a special order. We were told to immediately go to raised combat alert. It was so serious that there was a third man there with us, to maintain uninterrupted communications."[40]

Soviet forces in East Germany and Poland were also put on alert.

If Able Archer was not a simulation but a foil for an all-out attack, the USSR had only eight minutes to retaliate. Pershing missiles in Europe could hit Moscow within eight minutes of launch, so the Soviets had only an eight-minute window to make a retaliatory move. Over three hundred Soviet missiles were primed to fire.

To put it in slightly starker terms: the United States was eight minutes away from annihilation as the USSR was prepared to fire off over three hundred ICBMs. Defense secretary Robert Gates said that we came very close to causing World War III *"without even knowing it."*[41] The threat of nuclear war ended on November 11, because the exercise ended very much to the Soviet's surprise. Many historians believe this incident *"to be the closest the world has come to nuclear war since the Cuban Missile Crisis of 1962."*[42] It is also curious that most people in Russia and the United States know virtually nothing about this brush with annihilation.

When it turned out that Able Archer's decision to launch was merely an exercise and the launch only hypothetical, USSR missile batteries stood down, and everyone breathed easier. One moment's miscalculation, or one slightly over-anxious Soviet general during those critical eight minutes, was all that stood between humanity and a nuclear winter. In 2015 the United States released previously classified files on Able Archer. According to Klaas Voss from the Hamburg Institute for Social Research who reviewed these documents, "The war scare was as real as it gets."[43]

India and Pakistan, 1990

In 1990, insurgents occupied Indian-held Kashmir. In a surprise move, India ordered a huge build-up of troops along the border zone. The Pakistanis were caught off guard by the rapidity with which Indian troops were gathering on their frontier. They decided to pre-empt this with a possible nuclear strike on India.

An article, "On the Nuclear Edge," describes how in early 1990 American intelligence, observing via satellite, watched in real-time as the Pakistani military transported what were believed to be atom bombs from a suspected nuclear weapons facility to a nearby airport. Washington looked on with growing unease as the highways connecting the two sites were ominously closed to all traffic and the airport was locked down as Pakistani technicians began fitting the payload onto a squadron of F-16 fighter-bombers.

The White House hit the panic button and sent national security adviser Robert Gates to warn the Pakistanis to step back from the brink, while urging India to stay its forces on the border (if it knew what was good for them). Both Islamabad and Delhi relented in the face of American pressure and calm steadily returned. Gates admitted in the article that the crisis came perilously close to touching off a war. "Pakistan and India seemed to be caught in a cycle that they couldn't break out of," Gates says in the *New Yorker* piece. "I was convinced that if a war started, it would be nuclear." Others were even starker in their assessment: "It was the most dangerous nuclear situation we have ever faced since I've been in the U.S. government," remarked one U.S. official. "It may be as close as we've come to a nuclear exchange. It was far more frightening than the Cuban Missile Crisis."[44]

It is worth speculating what might have happened had American intelligence not been watching so carefully. If the satellite spy system had a glitch, or if rainstorms and heavy cloud cover made satellite snooping impossible, history might have turned out very differently, not just for India and Pakistan but for humankind as well.

A Summary of Close Calls

There may have been as many as 1,200 possible lethal incidents or nuclear accidents in toto. When a B-47 flying over Lakenheath Air Base crashed into a nuclear weapons storage facility in 1956, there were Mark 6 bombs stored there which did not have safety mechanisms. One officer remarked that it was a miracle there were no detonations. The entire crew of the B-47 perished in the incident.[45]

Another occurred in 1966 when a B-52 carrying four hydrogen bombs crashed, broke apart killing three of the seven-member crew off the coast of Spain. There were no detonations.[46] Such incidents were not our main concern. These events themselves could not have triggered a nuclear holocaust or a nuclear winter. Instead, in this chapter, only the most precipitous eighteen brushes with World War III and the possibility of all-out nuclear war were described.

Here is a table summarizing these encounters with nuclear Armageddon. In each incident—already described in detail—severity is rated subjectively on a scale of one to ten.

Date	Nature of disaster	Subjective rating of severity (1-10)	How resolved
Oct. 5, 1960	Computer error, Greenland	3	Human intervention
Nov. 24, 1961	Colorado; all three redundant communication lines severed	4	Human intervention
October 1962	Rogue NATO general bucks policy and issues readiness alert.	4	Soviets failed to notice or ignored the provocative action.
Oct. 24, 1962	Soviet satellite explodes in orbit during Cuban Missile Crisis, putting NORAD on alert	5	Details still may be classified on severity of U.S. response to this event
Oct. 25, 1962	Bear sets off alarm at Wisconsin base during Cuban Missile Crisis and planes readied for take off	3	Human intervention
Oct. 26, 1962	U.S. missile is launched at Vandenberg by mistake during Cuban Missile Crisis.	5	No data on why Soviets failed to respond to the perceived danger.
October 1962	Soviet sub crew prepares to launch nuclear torpedo at U.S. Navy ships in response to depth charges being dropped.	9.5	Human intervention; Russian officer convinces superiors not to follow standing orders.

Date	Nature of disaster	Subjective rating of severity (1-10)	How resolved
October 1962	Radar operators in New Jersey mistake a satellite for an ICBM and sound a nuclear alert.	9	Human intervention seems to have clarified the radar post was not informed of the satellite
Nov. 2, 1962	U.S. spy in Russia (Penkovsky) allegedly sends signal that nuclear attack from USSR is imminent	3	U.S. may have already known Penkovsky was arrested and signal likely sent by KGB
October 1969	USSR plans to attack China with nuclear weapons over continuing border dispute	5	U.S. learns of plans and informs USSR that it will respond if China is attacked.
October 1973	Golda Meir authorizes Generals to use nuclear weapons at their discretion if things get worse; weapons loaded and deployed.	9	Tide of six-day war turns in Israel's favor.
Oct. 24-25, 1973	Soviets warn U.S. of nuclear attack if Israel continues into Egypt. In Michigan, a base mechanic accidentally sets off alarm starting DEFCON 3. B-52s start engines.	4	Human intervention
November 1979	Colorado NORAD computer glitch shows U.S .under attack. Fighters scramble and President's "doomsday plane" launched	5	Human intervention

Date	Nature of disaster	Subjective rating of severity (1-10)	How resolved
June 30, 1980	Computer chip error shows 2,200 Soviet ICBMs launched toward U.S.	4	Human intervention; other systems unable to confirm launches.
September 1983	Soviet early warning system shows five U.S missiles launched at USSR	4	Human intervention; Soviet officer decides on his own that a system error occurred.
November 1983	NATO exercise Able Archer simulates first strike against USSR. Soviets view simulation as actual attack.	9	Exercise ends and defuses situation without U.S. knowing how close it came to starting World War III.
1990	Pakistan and India fight over Kashmir. Pakistan loads nuclear weapons on aircraft for possible launch	8	U.S. monitors movements and sharply warns Pakistan to halt any nuclear activity.
Jan 5, 1995	U.S and Norway launch missile for scientific mission. Soviets think it is a Trident in first stage of nuclear strike. Yeltsin is alerted.	6	Human intervention; Yeltsin has sufficient time to think and responds with caution.
Average rating		5.1	

Table 3.1 Major Nuclear Incidents

These eighteen events each had the capacity to trigger a deadly and full-scale missile attack and retaliation—in other words to spark World War III and a civilization-dooming nuclear winter.

Known Unknowns: A Conservative Assumption

Recall that scientists say an exchange of just fifty nuclear weapons on population centers would usher in a nuclear winter, and a large portion of the human race would perish. Before parsing this data in greater depth, let us make one additional and, hopefully, reasonable assumption.

The world, including its historians, did not know how close it came to a nuclear apocalypse during the Cuban crisis until 2002 when the Arkhipov story was revealed. Most stories of nuclear incidents moreover, are from Western sources with only a few originating in Russia or China.

Does this mean the Russians and Chinese had fewer close calls? More likely, it shows China and Russia have stricter standards of censorship and secrecy about their own episodes, failures, and computer glitches. Chinese historian, Lin Chenshan, believes there were at least five nuclear threats to China since 1949 that were not revealed.[47] Only one was listed in the prior table.

How many such incidents went unreported in the erstwhile USSR? Curiously, a leaked 2007 report shows that the Soviets planned to use 131 tactical nuclear weapons to attack Europe in 1964.[48] This incident also was not included in our table either.

Imagine, for example, a rogue Soviet general launching an ICBM against the United States that the Kremlin had to destroy in mid-air to avert war. The story would be put under deep cover in censored Russian archives, and we would know nothing about it today. Alternately, picture that a Chinese computer chip failure flashed an all-out U.S. attack was imminent and that it was only defused at the last moment by an officer who noticed a system malfunction. Again, we know nothing about that either.

For the sake of argument, then, add to that list of eighteen incidents two more which were undisclosed either by China or the USSR. That is, in fact, a very conservative assumption. That would give us twenty very close encounters with nuclear Armageddon.

The Luck Hypothesis

Many years after the event, Defense Secretary McNamara made a grim assessment of the Cuban Crisis and said, "In the end, it was luck. We were 'this' close to nuclear war, and luck prevented it."[49]

Really, Mr. Secretary? There are twenty events that threatened the human race with a nuclear winter. Did they all end up in our favor and not result in Armageddon because humanity just happened to be lucky? Think that one through. Luck implies chance. There were twenty nuclear incidents. All turned in our favor. How lucky is that? If one tossed a coin and heads stood for "no nuclear war this time," the odds of getting twenty heads in a row are a million to one.[50]

McNamara's "theory" to explain these close calls with a nuclear holocaust can be dismissed rather quickly. The chance of all these events falling in humanity's favor due to old-fashioned good luck is improbable to the extreme.

Another writer tackles this issue differently. In looking at twenty serious nuclear incidents, he opines: "If the risk in some of the events had been as high as one in ten, then the chance of surviving just seven such events would have been less than fifty/fifty."[51] The luck hypothesis is not going to cut it.

The "Rational" Actor Hypothesis

A more appealing approach is to say rational, sane, and balanced people *intervened* to defuse these threatening events. For example, someone noticed that all the data did not corroborate initial warnings in the Michigan, Greenland, and two Colorado alerts. That good luck was actually due to rational people taking action to find glitches and keep things under control.

When Soviet officer, Stanislav Petrov, was alerted by a computer that the United States launched five ICBMs, he questioned why a superpower would engage in a first strike with so few missiles. He made a sane deduction that it was a false alarm. He did not inform his superiors an attack was underway. He was confident it was a computer error, and he was right. Had he followed his orders and told his superior officer, a vastly different reaction on the part of the USSR might have been expected. Petrov prevented that from happening.

An officer in Michigan noticed a nuclear alert was accidentally triggered by a mechanic and personally drove to a runway to stop revved-up bombers from taking off. At first glance, the rational actor approach sounds like a reasonable theory. Maybe that is how to explain how humanity survived twenty serious nuclear events. Looking more closely, however, suggests other factors were involved:

- In the midst of the Cuban Missile Crisis, the United States fired a test rocket from Vandenberg Air Force Base. It seems the Russians did not detect the launch and thus failed to respond. There is no evidence a rational, sane Soviet actor intervened to save humanity by dismissing the rocket launched during the tense Cuban crisis as an American error. They just seemed to have missed the threat entirely. Not only was there U.S. stupidity in launching the missile, there was also stupidity by the Soviets in not noticing it. And this was a base from which nuclear missiles, not just test missiles, were launched. Thank God for human stupidity!
- When a rogue U.S. general put his command under DEFCON 3 despite orders not to do so, the Soviets did not escalate in kind. We

have no idea if sane Soviet minds intervened, or, once again, if they simply failed to notice American bases in Turkey went on nuclear alert. So, for the second time, while sane minds prevailed to save the world in some cases, stupidity and ignorance rescued the human race as well.

- During operation Able Archer, the Soviets panicked and thought a first strike was in progress. Americans were unaware the military exercise nearly triggered a nuclear war:

Intelligence official Douglas MacEachin recounted that when U.S. analysts first observed the Soviet Union's heightened alert status they wondered, "What's going on here?" The question later evolved to, "Are these people nuts?" The world was pushed toward the brink—and no American had known about it.[52]

The Able Archer exercise ended with Americans in a high state of ignorance of the Soviet Union's high alert status. There were no rational actors making informed decisions, on the American side, just inattention and rather grotesque stupidity. Darth Vaders and more known unknowns.

There is another factor to consider when mulling over this data, the role of Darth Vaders. Beyond computer glitches or clumsy bears, there are many generals, politicians, and allegedly "sane" actors who pushed, or tried to push humanity toward nuclear war. These advocates of the dark side are found in the shadows of power and pose an ominous threat to human survival.

For example, John F. Kennedy was America's youngest and most inexperienced president in 1960. No sooner had he been elected than his mettle tested in two areas: (1) The Soviets started to build the Berlin Wall, threatening wartime agreements not to divide the German city, and (2) in Asia, both Laos and Vietnam appeared to be falling to the communists.

Two of America's highest ranking generals held come-to-Jesus conferences with Kennedy in 1960, long before the Cuban Missile Crisis. Gen. Lyman Lemnitzer and Gen. Curtis Lemay sought authorization to use nuclear weapons in Berlin and in Southeast Asia. That is, they sought presidential permission to use nuclear weapons at their discretion.[53]

President Kennedy simply walked out of the first meeting. But there was a second conference which resulted in their making the same recommendation, this time with a renewed gravitas. They wanted presidential permission to go nuclear. Kennedy walked out again, threw his hands in the air, glanced back at the generals in the Cabinet Room, and said to an aide, "These people are crazy!"[54]

What if our inexperienced president acknowledged his lack of expertise in this area and said: "Well, generals, you have had much more knowledge on the battlefield than I, so I will defer to your assessments and recommendations. You have my permission to use nuclear weapons at your discretion."

General Douglas MacArthur tried to get President Truman to use nuclear weapons in Korea.[55] Admiral Arthur Radford and then Vice President Nixon urged Eisenhower to use nuclear weapons in support of the French in Vietnam.[56] Allen Dulles, the head of the CIA under President Kennedy, presented JFK with a plan for a nuclear, preemptive first strike against the Soviet Union.[57] President Nixon actively contemplated nuclear war against North Vietnam.[58]

Multiple Darth Vaders, Dr. Strangeloves, and people in positions of power have advocated the use of nuclear weapons to resolve conflicts. It would be foolish to argue America was the only country where influential people with such hawkish views were bending the ears of their leaders.

So, beyond twenty incidents, one might add myriad Strangeloves into the emerging equation. Who is to say that they are not still around? Vice President Dick Cheney monitored a study for using nuclear weapons against Iran as recently as 2005.[59] How many Soviet, Russian, and Chinese counterparts does he have, and how many times were they tempted to ring the doomsday bell since 1945?

As late as 2013, Indian officials advised residents of strife-torn Kashmir to prepare for possible nuclear war and urged them to build bombproof basements and stockpile food and water.[60]

When looking at how close the human race has come to self-destruction, there may have far more than twenty close calls to consider. Considering the scope of human irrationality, ignorance, insanity, and impulsivity, it is staggering that so many nuclear events took place without crossing that critical threshold.

So, pause for a moment and revisit the "rational actor hypothesis," and its relationship to the Cuban Missile Crisis. President Kennedy was one of the most intelligent presidents in American history, but he didn't know that over one hundred nuclear weapons were already deployed and ready for launch from Cuba when he ordered the blockade.

The total number of Soviet nuclear warheads on Cuba was 158. One hundred fifty-eight nukes. Now, "only" ninety-five to one hundred of those were ready to be used. "Only." But six to eight SS-4 medium-range ballistic missiles were also there, and also at "operational" status. Those SS-4s could have reached as far north as Washington, DC, with explosive yields of a little over a megaton each.

> Imagine that: the major cities of the South and the lower Eastern Seaboard subjected to at least eight megatons of yield, with no possibility of defense, with fallout going wherever it may. And that's just the "regional" problem—there's still those other ICBMs that Soviets had.
>
> Oh, and here's a fun thing: those Soviet nukes had no negative physical protection. Moscow vigorously asserted its authority in terms

> of actual nuclear use in the region, but if it had come down to it, there would have been little they could have done to stop a local commander from using one. What's shocking about this is that apparently the Americans had no clue. They didn't know there were strategic weapons there and ready to go.[61]

JFK also didn't know Soviet commanders on the ground were "delegated the authority to use these missiles on their own judgment."[62] Had he known these facts, he would never have engaged in this high level of brinkmanship to resolve the issues at all. But he didn't. He was in the dark. This sane, rational actor was ignorant.

McNamara was one of America's brightest defense secretaries, but despite a high IQ and "whiz kid" reputation, he was blind to the fact that he ordered the Navy to drop depth charges on a Soviet sub carrying nuclear torpedoes. Had he known what he was doing, he would *never* have been that reckless. He was in the dark. Another sane, rational actor blind and acting in ignorance.

Officers aboard the Soviet sub were debating whether to surface or fire their torpedo and destroy the U.S. fleet. They were intelligent men and well trained, but they did not know the United States was on DEFCON 2, the highest state of hair-trigger nuclear readiness in the nation's history.[63] Had they known that, they might not have been debating with each other at all, but immediately surfaced. They were in the dark, and they were also ignorant.

All these bright, rational, and sane men languished in dangerous states of ignorance. The truth of what occurred was not learned until forty years later. As the ships came closer to their confrontation off Cuba, philosopher Bertrand Russell penned an urgent telegram to President Kennedy: "Your action desperate. Threat to human survival. No conceivable justification. Civilized man condemns it. End this madness!"[64]

The matter did not end because smart, educated people made careful, deliberate, and informed decisions. This was how the media and historians tried to portray it at the time, but it simply was not true.[65] Blindness, ignorance, and stupidity *ruled the day,* not sanity or reason.

The crisis finally ended peacefully, but it wasn't because humanity had another lucky day, and it wasn't because intelligent, informed, rational people intervened to save the human race.

Reckless and Irrational Behavior during the Cuban Missile Crisis

Albert Einstein once said "Two things are infinite: the universe and human stupidity, and I'm not sure about the universe."[66] Since our existence today is very much a result of surviving these encounters—and at the risk of some redundancy—let us examine the specific instances of unalloyed awe-inspiring recklessness, stupidity, and ignorance.

The Cuban Missile Crisis happened over a period of thirteen days in October, 1962. It was certainly one of the most dangerous moments in the history of the human race. Unknown to most discussants of this conflict, and generally unmentioned, was that during this high intensity conflict, the United States continued detonating nuclear weapons in the atmosphere and so did the USSR. This is today almost impossible to believe, but true. On October 18, the United States detonated a 1.59-megaton bomb in the Pacific; it did so again two days later. On October, 22, the USSR exploded a three-hundred-kiloton weapon on its territory; one more for the United States on October 27, and an additional blast on October 28.

In other words six nuclear weapons were actually detonated right in the middle of the thirteen-day Cuban Missile Crisis.[67] On October 18, the United States detonated a 1.59 megaton bomb in the Pacific; on October 22, the USSR detonated a three-hundred-kiloton weapon in Kapustin Yar. Between the two, six nuclear weapons exploded right in the middle of the Cuban Missile Crisis.

Today, one would view atmospheric testing of nuclear weapons at such a critical time to be absolutely provocative, incredible grounds for misperception and miscalculation, and probably a symptom of consummate collective insanity, but at the time, it was just the way things were.

While "whiz kid" McNamara dropped depth charges on a Soviet sub carrying nuclear tipped torpedoes here is what was happening inside the Soviet sub:

> The Americans encircled us and began dropping grenades that were exploding right next to us. . . . "It felt like sitting in a metal barrel with someone hitting it with a sledgehammer. The crew was in shock." The bombardment went on for several hours and some sailors lost consciousness as oxygen ran low and temperatures inside the submarine soared above 122 degrees.[68]

That the United States was dropping explosives for hours on a Soviet sub where members of the crew had fallen unconscious and temperatures inside were 122 degrees without any knowledge that Soviet standing orders were to fire their nuclear weapons if under attack represents a second example of recklessness without parallel.

- Khrushchev sent Soviet nuclear-armed subs into the arena without sufficient command and control, particularly communication links with Moscow, so that submarine commanders were put in a position of detonating nuclear weapons at their discretion. This is clearly a third instance of egregious carelessness and stupidity.
- The Soviets did not have sufficient command and control over their nuclear weapons in Cuba either. There was a distinct possibility a rogue general or officer could have launched missiles against the United States without Moscow's approval.

> All this . . . convinced Mikoyan that "the Cuban tail was quite capable of wagging the Soviet dog." . . . What became clear to Mikoyan . . . is that the Soviets could not really control their Cuban ally . . . Mikoyan decided on his own that Castro could not be trusted and that the missiles must be removed from the island. . . . "So you have a law that prohibits transfer of tactical nuclear weapons to other countries? It's a pity. And when are you going to repeal that law?" Castro asked. "We will see," Mikoyan replied.[69]

This porous level of command and control the Soviets had over their nuclear weapons in Cuba represents a fourth symptom of flagrant thoughtlessness.

- As mentioned earlier, the United States had no knowledge that 158 nuclear weapons were already in Cuba at the time of the Cuban standoff and that close to one hundred were capable of being launched. Had Kennedy and McNamara known this, their strategy in the Cuban Missile Crisis would have been altogether different. This frightful intelligence failure represents the fifth symptom.
- Finally—and also mentioned earlier—a U.S. general launched a missile from Vandenberg Air Force Base in the middle of the crisis which could have set off a Soviet counter-reaction, and did so without knowledge of the president.

So this comprises a list of six instances of inestimable stupidity, negligence and recklessness. But still the human race miraculously survived what Bertrand Russell rightly called "madness."

After the crisis concluded, JFK and Khrushchev wrote to each other privately and in secret. Both were deeply shaken by this experience, and they quickly negotiated the nuclear test ban treaty banning atmospheric testing of nuclear weapons. JFK said about the treaty in his letter to Khrushchev,

> If it does represent a possibility of avoiding the kind of collision that we had last fall in Cuba, which was quite close and Berlin in 1961, we should seize the chance.[70]

Khrushchev replied, "It is important to reach an understanding . . . in order to make a good gift to the people, to let them rejoice in the news that a nuclear test ban agreement has also been reached and thus there will be no further contamination of the atmosphere."[71]

The following year the Kremlin and Washington agreed to establish a hotline, a direct communication link between presidents, all, we have to admit, quite rational, calm, and sane decisions.[72]

But when we return to this thirteen-day period of stupidity, hubris, brinkmanship, ignorance, and "madness," we still ask the question, what saved the human race? In view of all the irrational behavior that was occurring—not least of which was the detonation of six nuclear weapons during this period—what saved the day?

Had Savitsky and Maslennikov convinced junior officer Arkhipov to agree, the torpedo would have been launched and American ships surrounding Cuba annihilated. The nuclear reply by the United States would have been immediate and massive, and Soviet retaliation just as full-fisted. Within hours, the world as we know it would have ended. The wrong decision easily would have provoked a nuclear exchange that would have triggered a nuclear winter in the Northern Hemisphere.

Bertrand Russell's view was unassailable. Humanity stood at the threshold of sheer collective madness. Historian Arthur Schlesinger called the Cuban blockade drama "the most dangerous moment in human history."[73]

Sure, one can say the human race was "lucky," but that theory is improbable. One can say that rational actors and heroes intervened and saved the day, like Arkhipov and Petrov, but there are a handful of incidents where this theory doesn't work either. Sometimes a threat went unnoticed and unrecognized, and only unabated ignorance saved the day, not intelligence and sanity.

Is it possible that something else was governing and influencing events in the background? If it wasn't luck, nor the intervention of rational actors, was there some other factor or force that was in play? Was there some unknown, invisible, hidden, and unseen process operating during these tense—phylogenetically tense—precipitous moments in human history? The text is in search of exactly this extraordinary hidden variable. We cannot see it. We cannot measure it, but we are picking up on its scent.

The Doomsday Clock

Since 1947, *The Bulletin of Atomic Scientists* has published a "doomsday clock" showing how close humanity has come to the brink of nuclear disaster. If one calculated the times this group placed humanity at five minutes before midnight, it would encompass 1949–1960, 1981–1988, and 2007–2009, or roughly twenty of the last sixty-seven years. In other words, 30 percent of the time since 1947, humanity has hovered at five minutes before nuclear Armageddon.

Go back to the table of nuclear events and look at the ratings of "severity," and you will see they range between three and 9.5. For the sake of argument, consider any score above one as a human fever—and we can include in that table the two unknown and unreported events that were suggested needed to be added.

Scores above four would be a "severe fever," and those above eight would be classified as "severe fever, critical condition." If one adopted this taxonomy for one hypothetical moment, then humankind had twenty total fevers, thirteen of which were severe, and it was in critical condition four times since World War II. In the physical universe, fevers break because the immune system kicks in with accumulated or inherited resistances as it deploys its phalanx of antibodies.

This text has posited that some kind of internal, psychological immune system might also exist which is an expression of a collective self-preservative instinct. It kicks in, resists, defuses and tries to destroy negative eruptions—antigens—in the same way as the physical immune system does. What is proposed is that an elusive psychic immune system, operating as a positive counterforce, works to prevent threats to survival from reaching critical mass. It works in the background and often outside the realm of consciousness in the same way the physical immune system generally functions in the autonomic sphere.

If one presupposes that kind of positive force, it explains why in all the fevers we considered—and in the many we believe happened that we know nothing about—the patient did not die, and doomsday fears were averted. Despite all these serious episodes, the ignorance, irrationality, accidents, brinkmanship, miscalculations, and hubris, there was never a seizure, convulsion, or moment of flat lining. Not a single atomic bomb was used in war in the last seventy years.

In the Middle Ages, a time of alchemy when humans knew little about germs or viruses, good fortune was ascribed to luck or the intervention of divine spirits. Religions encased such magical views and superstitions in ritual. Through alchemy, astrology, or religion, humanity could explain sundry plagues and disasters to itself and then celebrate its good fortune.

However, as humankind increased in consciousness and expanded its knowledge base, it learned there was an internal world called the immune system which was a construction of brilliant and incredible complexity. The immune response has been the primary agent in saving the human race from diseases, pandemics, plagues, and extinction.

The question is whether a similar protective system exists in the psychological sphere, and if so, could it attack human psychological pandemics and antigens in the same way? What is proffered is not to think about this metaphorically "as if" a psychological immune system existed, but quite literally that there is such a system that we simply never noticed.

When insanity, self-destructiveness, war, depression, villainy, genocide, or maniacal Strangeloves appear—regardless of the source, reason, or nationality—the psychic immune system is activated, identifies the threat, and mobilizes against it. The theory is nuanced—and, perhaps still appearing preposterous to some— but the implications are enormous.

In other words, it wasn't that Arkhipov was unusually brilliant on that day. Or, on another day, it wasn't that Petrov, who saw five missiles coming and decided not to tell his superior—thereby saving the world—was some sort of ultra-conscious wizard or genius. And it wasn't the derring-do of another Wunderkind-hero in Duluth who ran out on the runway to stop bombers from taking off. And the officers who noticed a bear tripped an alarm or that a computer chip gave false readings which set B-52s in motion were not American heroes who single-handedly stopped World War III.

And during operation Able Archer, when the USSR was eight minutes away from unleashing three hundred nuclear weapons against the United States, it wasn't another heroic example of a cautious, highly intelligent Soviet wizard who made the decision not to press the button and, once again, gloriously saving the human race from annihilation. That is a comic book interpretation of human history.

Instead of asserting geniuses, wizards, gurus, and highly sane, heroic people to save the world, something else is put forward. Return to the mother who ministers to her child with a cold, keeps him at home, gives him plenty of fluids, and nurses him back to health. She is a devoted mother, and certainly his hero. But she is neither the genius nor the wizard who saved his life. His immune system is. She is only an adjunct, a helper. She did nothing more than aid and assist his immune system to bring the illness to an end.

So, too, with our long litany of nuclear events which could have threatened the survival of our species, our heroes, Arkhipov, Petrov, the Duluth technician, and whoever else intervened to save the day—and the human race—these people are like that mother. They are adjuncts to a deeper process, a collective instinct for survival that exists in all human beings and is not merely directed toward individual, group, or national survival, but is phylogenetic and intimately related to the survival of our species.

The psychic immune system runs parallel to our physical immune system; it is an epiphenomenon of the physical immune system, and it acts in the same way. Only we can't see it, and it is, so far, ineffably hidden and invisible.

Sometimes one can kick-start the physical immune system with deliberate efforts like nursing your child and intervening to augment his internal immunities with vitamins and appropriate care. Yes, but his immune system operates independently of these kind interventions anyway.

So too, you can kick-start the psychic immune system with conscious, deliberate, and, indeed, heroic efforts like arguing as best you can aboard that sub. Yes. But the human psychic immune system is also involved and operates independently of these deliberate interventions too. Think of it. Savitsky and Maslennikov say "Fire!" Arkhipov says "Surface!" The human race is outnumbered two to one in that conversation!

Noam Chomsky said the human race was "one word away" from nuclear annihilation.[74] If Savitsky and Maslennikov got Arkhipov to agree, you would not be reading this page. Do we merely think that this was a conversation between three men? Did the human race have no skin in this game, no dog in this hunt? Is it really so preposterous to suggest it might have?

The theory of the psychic immune system proposes that there was another hidden force inside that submarine, and it is the same force that exists inside every person which, like it or not, keeps us joined at the hip to our fellow man. In this view, Arkhipov is not merely a hero; he is also a "vessel" through which the human race—humanity—expresses itself. And indeed Savitsky and Maslennikov also were "connected" to this force.

They knew their children in Moscow would perish if they said "Fire!" They knew, somewhere in their hearts, that millions would be sacrificed by their decision. When they were debating with each other, yes, there were conscious thoughts crossing their minds: "Was it treasonous to surface and violate Soviet standing orders when being attacked? Would they be court-martialed if they did?"

But there were other thoughts too, and a deeper process occurring—which was a stronger force that was present in that 122 degree submarine. It is a collective force that keeps us from going over the edge. It keeps us safe, aligned, balanced, and works interminably toward safety, health, peace, longevity exactly the way the physical immune system does.

Arkhipov returned to Moscow. All three men never were applauded for their decision, and neither were they prosecuted. Arkhipov died in 1998 of radiation poisoning admired only by his family and a few fellow officers.[75] Today, he is recognized posthumously for saving the world by increasing numbers of people.

But it is just as naive for us to believe that the human race was saved by the actions of one man as it is to think that mom saved her child's life when she gave him Vitamin C and kept him home from school? There is another process that is present—hidden, unknown, unmeasured—but palpable. It offers a remarkably ubiquitous explanation for how humanity survives these threats.

It isn't just luck. It isn't because wizards, geniuses, and superheroes single-handedly won the day over barbarism, self-destructiveness, and madness. To the contrary, there is some other reason why the human race was rescued from the edge of nuclear annihilation twenty straight times in a row, and without incident, since 1945.

NOTES

1. Bridget York, "The Nuclear Age of Peace?" 2013, https://prezi.com/fmrrixfxj5na/the-nuclear-age-of-peace/.
2. Atomic Archive, National Science Digital Library, http://www.atomicarchive.com/Company/Company.shtml.
3. "Gallery of U.S. Nuclear Tests" (2001), Nuclearweaponarchive.org.

4. "Soviet Nuclear Test Summary"(2001), Nuclearweaponarchive.org.

5. "General Overview of the Effects of Nuclear Testing CTBTO," retrieved 2015, http://www.ctbto.org/nuclear-testing/the-effects-of-nuclear-testing/general-overview-of-theeffects-of-nuclear-testing/.

6. "General Overview of the Effects of Nuclear Testing CTBTO."

7. Robert S. Norris and Hans M. Kristensen, "Global nuclear stockpiles, 1945–2006," *Bulletin of the Atomic Scientists* 62, no. 4 (July/August 2006), 64–66.

8. Steven Starr, "Catastrophic Climatic Consequences of Nuclear Conflict, INESAP," accessed, 2015, http://inesap.org/node/11.

9. M. Fromm, B., Stocks, and R. Servranckx, et al. "Smoke in the Stratosphere: What Wildfires have Taught Us About Nuclear Winter", *Eos, Transactions, American Geophysical Union*,(Washington, DC: American Geophysical Union, 2006).

10. Alan Roboc, Luke Oman, and Georgiy Stenchikov, "Nuclear Winter Revisited," *Journal of Geophysical Research* (2007), http://onlinelibrary.wiley.com/doi/10.1029/2006JD008235/abstract.

11. Robert Ehrlich, *Waging Nuclear Peace* (New York: Suny Press, 1985), 272.

12. *Encyclopedia Brittanica,* accessed 2015, http://abyss.uoregon.edu/~js/glossary/nuclear_winter.html.

13. Charles Choi, "A Small Nuclear War Could Trigger Catastrophic Cooling," 2014 http://news.yahoo.com/small-nuclear-war-could-trigger-catastrophic-cooling-181056235.html .

14. Benjamin K. Sovacool, "A Preliminary Assessment of Major Energy Accidents, 1907–2007," *Energy Policy* 36 (2008).

15. Alan Borning, "Computer System Reliability and Nuclear War," 2001, http://www-ee.stanford.edu/~hellman/Breakthrough/book/chapters/borning.html.

16. Alan Philips, "20 Mishaps That Might Have Started Accidental Nuclear War," (1998) http://nuclearfiles.org/menu/key-issues/nuclear-weapons/issues/accidents/20-mishaps-maybe-caused-nuclear-war.htm.

17. Philips, "20 Mishaps."

18. Philips, "20 Mishaps."

19. Chris Hubbuch, "False Alarm: How a Bear Nearly Started a Nuclear War," LaCrosseTribune.com http://lacrossetribune.com/news/false-alarm-how-a-bear-nearly-started-a-nuclear-war/article_bc6f4da6-a89c-5d7d-bf0a-e41150753b62.ht.

20. Philips, "20 Mishaps."

21. Scott D. Sagan, *The Limits of Safety: Organizations, Accidents, and Nuclear Weapons* (Princeton, NJ: Princeton University Press, 1993), 79.

22. Philips, "20 Mishaps."

23. Philips, "20 Mishaps."

24. Philips, "20 Mishaps."

25. Geoffrey Forden, "False Alarms in the Nuclear Age," Nova, 2001, http://www.pbs.org/wgbh/nova/military/nuclear-false-alarms.html.

26. Archie Wood, 2004 http://everything2.com/title/accidental+nuclear+war.

27. Geoffrey Forden, "False Alarms in the Nuclear Age," Nova, 2001.

28. David Hoffman, Washington Post Foreign Service, (1999) http://www.washingtonpost.com/wp-srv/inatl/longterm/coldwar/shatter021099b.htm

29. Anastasiya Lebedev, MosNews, (2004) "The Man Who Saved the World Finally Recognized," http://web.archive.org/web/20110721000030/http://www.worldcitizens.org/petrov2.html

30. "USSR Planned Nuclear Attack on China in 1969," *The Telegraph* 2010, http://www.telegraph.co.uk/news/worldnews/asia/china/7720461/USSR-planned-nuclear-attack-on-China-in-1969.html.

31. Marion Lloyd, "Soviets Close to Using A-Bomb in 1962 Crisis, Forum is Told", Boston Globe 2002, A20.

32. Neil Genzlinger, "Same Cuba Crisis, Different Angles 50 Years Later." World News, 2012, http://article.wn.com/view/2012/10/22/Same_Cuba_Crisis_Different_Angles_50_Years_Later/.

33. Lloyd, "Soviets Close to Using A-Bomb."

34. Ron Rosenbaum, *How the End Begins*. (New York: Simon & Schuster, 2011).

35. Seymour Hersh, *The Third Temple:The Story Behind the Vanunu Revelation,* (New York: Amana Books, 1989), 147

36. Mitch Ginsberg, "Dayan Pushed PM Meir to Use Nuclear Weapons in 73 War," *The Times of Israel,* Oct 3, 2013.

37. A recent article by Avner Cohen challenges this. He asserts that Israel only prepared to fire a "demonstration" nuclear weapon at this time. See "When Israel Stepped Back from the Brink," *New York Times*, Oct 3, 2012.

38. Able Archer Escalation, Althistory, http://www.militaryeducation.org/10-most-epic-tank-battles-in-military-history/.

39. Able Archer Escalation, Althistory,

40. Nathan Jones, "One Misstep Could Trigger a Great War," 2009, http://gradworks.umi.com/1465450.pdf.

41. Tony Rennell, "September 26th, 1983: The Day the World Almost Died," Daily Mail, (2007) http://www.dailymail.co.uk/news/article-505009/September-26th-1983-The-day-world-died.html, based on the documentary, *1983 The Brink of Apocalypse, BBC.*

42. Benjamin B. Fischer (2007-03-17), "A Cold War Conundrum: The 1983 Soviet War Scare", Central Intelligence Agency, https://www.cia.gov/library/center-for-the-study-of-intelligence/csi-publications/books-and-monographs/a-cold-war-conundrum/source.htm#HEADING1-12.

43. Sam Roberts. "NATO War Games Unwittingly put Soviets and US on 'Hair Trigger' in 83 Analysis Suggests." *New York Times,* November 9, 2015.

44. Chagatai Khan, "On the Nuclear Edge by Seymour Hersh," (2009), http://chagataikhan.blogspot.ca/2009/05/on-nuclear-edge-by-seymour-m-hersh.html.

45. Eric Schollser, "Nuclear Weapons: An Accident Waiting to Happen," *The Guardian,* 2013.

46. Tony Long, "Jan. 17, 1966: H-Bombs Rain Down on a Spanish Fishing Village". *WIRED Magazine*(January 17, 2008).

47. "USSR Planned Nuclear Attack on China in 1969," *The Telegraph* 2010,http://www.telegraph.co.uk/news/worldnews/asia/china/7720461/USSR-planned-nuclear-attack-on-China-in-1969.html.

48. Henry Samuel, "Soviet Plan for nuclear attack unearthed," *The Telegraph,* 2007, http://www.telegraph.co.uk/news/uknews/1563692/Soviet-plan-for-WW3-nuclear-attack-unearthed.html.

49. James Blight and Janet Lang, *The Fog of War* (Lanham, MD: Rowman & Littlefield, 2005) 58.

50. David, "The numbers in 'Tails you Win,'" Understanding Uncertainty, http://understandinguncertainty.org/numbers-tails-you-win-science-chance.

51. Philips, "20 Mishaps."

52. Jones, "One Mishap."

53. James Douglass, *JFK and the Unspeakable* (New York: Orbis Books, 2010), 109

54. Douglass, *JFK and the Unspeakable*, 109

55. Korean War FAQ, http://www.zzwave.com/cmfweb/history/faq7.shtml.

56. "The U.S. Air Force's Indifference to Nuclear Weapons," *Bulletin of Atomic Scientists* 2008, http://thebulletin.org/us-air-forces-indifference-toward-nuclear-weapons-0.

57. Andrew Marshall, "The National Security State and the Assassination of JFK," Global Research, (2010) http://www.globalresearch.ca/the-national-security-state-and-the-assassination-of-jfk/22071.

58. Mike Schuster, "Nixon Considered Nuclear Option Against N. Korea" NPR, 2010 http://www.npr.org/templates/story/story.php?storyId=128337461.

59. Sherwood Ross, "US Plan to Attack Iran with Nuclear Weapons Devised under Bush," Global Research 2012, http://www.globalresearch.ca/obama-prepares-protracted-afghanistan-occupation/5308984.

60. Gardiner Harris, "India Warns Kashmiris to Prepare for Nuclear War," *New York Times*, January 22, 2013.
61. Alex Wellerstien, "About Those Nukes in Cuba," The Nuclear Secrecy Blog 2012 http://blog.nuclearsecrecy.com/2012/10/25/about-those-nukes-in-cuba/.
62. Tibor Toth "A Nuclear World," *Chicago Tribune*, Ocotber 26, 2012 http://articles.chicagotribune.com/2012-10-26/opinion/ct-perspec-1026-nuke-20121026_1_test-ban-nuclear-warheads-doomsday-clock. Graphic developed from CTBTO Preparatory Commission, Vienna International Center.
63. Eric Schlosser, *Command and Control* (New York, Penguin Press, 2013), 292.
64. Cited in Schlosser, *Command and Control*, 293.
65. Michael Dobbs, "Cuban Missile Crisis," *New York Times*, 2015, http://topics.nytimes.com/top/reference/timestopics/subjects/c/cuban_missile_crisis/index.html.
66. Albert Einstein: 10 of His Best Quotes, *The Telegraph* http://www.telegraph.co.uk/news/science/science-news/9176616/Albert-Einstein-10-of-his-best-quotes.html.
67. Tibor Toth, "The Cuban Missile Crisis and Nuclear Testing," CBTBO, 2012, http://www.ctbto.org/press-centre/highlights/2012/the-cuban-missile-crisis-and-nuclear-testing/
68. Vladimir Isachenov, Cultura Cubana, 2002, https://groups.yahoo.com/neo/groups/culturacubana/conversations/topics/7583.
69. "Cuban Missile Crisis' Untold Story: Castro Almost Kept Nuclear Warheads on the Island," *Huffington Post*, October 15, 2012. Original source *The Cuban Missile Crisis*, (1962) National Security Archive (New York: Norton, 2003).
70. "Cuban Missile Crisis' Untold Story."
71. "Cuban Missile Crisis' Untold Story."
72. Euronews, 2011, http://www.euronews.com/2011/06/17/back-in-the-day-united-states-and-soviet-union-create-a-hotline/.
73. Dobbs,"Cuban Missile Crisis"
74. Noam Chomsky interviewed by Tavis Smiley, NPR, 2003, http://www.chomsky.info/interviews/20031119.htm.
75. "The Men Who Saved the World" Military History, 2013, http://militaryhistorynow.com/2013/07/15/the-men-who-saved-the-world-meet-two-different-russians-who-prevented-ww3/.

Part II

Epiphenomenon

A Glimpse into the Hidden World of the Psychic Immune System

FOUR

An Overview of the Physical Immune System

The theory toward which this text has been moving is that there is a psychological immune system which operates much like our physical immune system. To pursue this more deeply, it is necessary to get a better feeling for what makes up the *physical* immune system first.

Earlier, it was shown that organs like the spleen, thymus, or lymph nodes and listed T cells, B cells, macrophages, lymphocytes, or dendritic cells are the army of foot-soldiers in the physical immune system that keeps us alive.[1] In this chapter, we explore a more comprehensive, albeit brief, view of that whole system.

Generally, the physical immune system is split into the innate and adaptive functions.

> Although the innate and adaptive immune systems both function to protect against invading organisms, they differ in a number of ways. The adaptive immune system requires some time to react to an invading organism, whereas the innate immune system includes defenses that, for the most part, are . . . present and ready to be mobilized upon infection.[2]

The Innate Immune System

The innate immune system, as the name implies, is present at birth and comes into play "immediately or within hours of an antigens appearance in our body."[3] The skin protects and makes us impervious to many infections. Sweating helps flush out toxins and intruders; so does saliva, or blinking, tearing, or coughing where infectious agents are removed or stopped before they enter the body.

The innate immune system also uses white blood cells to attack infectious agents, most often by creating an inflammatory response at the site of the invasive attack.[4]

> The long battle between humans and infectious microbes has left its marks all over us. . . . The thousands of species of bacteria that swarm over us cannot penetrate our multilayered skin. Entry points, such as the eyes and nose, are bathed in moisture to help flush out pathogens. The lining of our lungs releases bacteria-killing compounds.[5]

There are individual and ethnic differences in our innate immunity too. Blacks are susceptible to sickle cell anemia more than Whites, but less susceptible to malaria. There are twenty known diseases which particularly afflict Askhenazy Jews.[6] [7] Whites have twice the incidence of arthritis as Hispanics.[8] African-American males have less susceptibility to certain cholesterol issues than others, a resistance already present at birth.[9] There are many configurations of innate immunity.

The Adaptive Immune System

Adaptive immunity works more slowly. Here immunities develop as a result of exposure, or prior exposure, to toxins and pathogens. If you have had a particular flu, for example, you may be immune from catching it again, while another person without that contact, has no immunological memory and thus succumbs to the disease.

The adaptive immune system is "antigen-specific" which means it identifies pathogens and attacks them individually. The adaptive immune system uses white cells called lymphocytes that work to focus the immune response. "These include an incredibly elegant molecule, called the 'antibody,' that is produced in huge numbers during an adaptive response, and moves through the bloodstream during an infection, targeting germs with incredible accuracy."[10]

Another writer explains it further:

> The adaptive immune system has the advantage of being, well, adaptable. It's not just about reacting to things, but about trying to anticipate what we *might* be infected with, and remembering what has infected us in the past. Instead of inheriting our adaptive immune systems along with our innate systems, we just inherit the tools to make ours up as we go along.
>
> There are two main white blood cell types responsible for adaptive immunity, T-cells and B-cells, which do different roles, working together to keep invaders out. . . . B-cells are your ranged attackers, lurking in the lymph nodes attacking pathogens from afar, while T-cells are your melee troops, patrolling the tissues, looking for any cell that's showing signs of disease.[11]

The Artificial Immune System

The adaptive immune system has another component known as *artificial* immunity. In fact, it may be the most important part of the human immune response.

"Artificial" means it is outside our natural hard-wired immune system, and refers to conscious, deliberate interventions that boost our immunity. These aides give the immune system—pardon the pun—a shot in the arm, but they are not "natural" or part of our autonomic immunities.

Take the example of SARS: In 2002, the SARS epidemic began. SARS, Severe Acute Respiratory Syndrome, is a pneumonia-like syndrome that boasts a mortality rate of 10 percent of those infected. The virus transferred from animals to man, either from bats, civets, or both, and the leap from animal to man occurred in China.[12]

China initially withheld information on this disease, and, as a result, it spread more than it might have. Since this was a viral disease, treatment with antibiotics didn't work. The most effective treatment was isolation, quarantine, wearing protective gear, and hand washing—very similar to the approach made during the Ebola epidemic.

These strategies fall in the category of the "artificial," because they involve intentional and rational interventions to prevent disease.

Without artificial intervention, the fatality rate of SARS would have consumed 10 percent of the human population, roughly seven hundred million people. But only 775 people actually died from it worldwide,[13] quite a remarkable achievement for the artificial immune system.

There is, however, a downside to these interventions. Human behavior, conscious or otherwise, can also deplete the immune system, not just give it a boost. Lifestyle, smoking, drinking, lack of exercise, vitamin deficiency and other situations weaken it as can overuse of antibiotics which creates antibiotic resistance. There are some twenty-five thousand different antibiotic products which were remarkably successful with tuberculosis, Strep, Staph infections, etc. However,

> according to researchers today the constant use of antibiotics with humans and livestock is a leading factor in our growing inability to eradicate disease. The overuse of these "wonder drugs" has improved the strength of our ever-evolving bacterial population. Our efforts have pushed them to evolve. We shoot them with a big "gun"; they mutate, become stronger and elude that "gun" down the road. Then a new bigger "gun" is required.[14]

Eighty percent of antibiotics sold in the United States are used in animals.[15] This is done not only to mitigate unhygienic feedlot issues, but also to promote growth. Such widespread use predisposes the human population to antibiotic resistant pathogens. Despite efforts to control their use, sales of these drugs rose by 37 percent from 2009 to 2012.[16]

Paul Roberts, author of *The End of Food,* says there are new strains of bacteria that are immune to entire classes of antibiotics, and the process is escalating. A study by the National Antimicrobial Resistance Monitoring System reported in 2013 that half of the samples of ground turkey, pork chops, and ground beef collected from supermarkets contained "bacteria resistant to antibiotics."[17] Furthermore, it is estimated that antibiotic use in agriculture will increase by 67 percent in developing countries. China already leads the world in their use, and India currently does not even have regulations in place on their use or overuse.[18]

So, while the artificial immune system through vaccinations, quarantines, antibiotics, sanitation, and other strategies may be credited with significantly increasing human life expectancy, the approach carries foreboding downsides through excessive use and overuse both in agriculture and in treating human diseases.

This completes a short overview of the *physical* immune system in its innate, adaptive, and artificial dimensions. In the next chapter the journey into the constituents of the *psychic* immune system begins, but before doing that, it is necessary to mention what this text is not addressing before describing what it is.

What the Psychic Immune System is Not

As we are about to enter several mysterious rooms searching with a flashlight for our invisible psychic immune system, there is one door we are going to ignore. It is called "psychoneuroimmunology," an imposing field in academic psychology, but one that is not relevant to the odyssey upon which we embark.

This avant-garde specialty looks at whether psychological factors influence the physical immune system. There is a lot of evidence here, but it is the wrong kind. For example, there is strong empirical evidence that stress can deplete our physical immune system just as joy, optimism, and social support strengthens resistance to physical diseases.

Individuals who report more negative emotions and stress got the flu more frequently than those with more positive affective states.[19] Children who come from more cohesive families succumb to influenza less often and show a higher frequency of antibodies.[20] HIV infection progresses more rapidly in individuals who have higher levels of stress and less social support.[21] The lower the rate of psychological stress in women with breast cancer, the greater were their T-helper cells and cytokines[22] Both in humans and animals, higher rates of stress produce lower immunities.[23]

Indeed there is a long empirical legacy that convincingly shows that stress and negative emotions hurt our resistance to diseases,[24] but that is not the concern here, and neither is psychoneuroimmunology. We are not interested in whether psychological factors influence the *physical* immune system, but whether a psychological immune system exists which protects from *psychological* calamities.

The question posed is quite different: Do human beings have a standalone *psychic* immune system that protects from psychological outbreaks and psychic epidemics, and, if so, how does it work?

This is a thoroughly unpopulated area that has received almost no academic attention. As an indication of the rarity of the concept of the *psychic* immune system, there are only 98 titles of articles in the psychology database since 1975 that even come close to using the term, and few refer to the psychological immune system directly.[25]

Freud hinted at it with his concept of Eros. Jung did too with his notion of the collective unconscious and archetypes. Despite the fact that both were quite opaque on the issue, at least each should be credited for attempting to break new ground. Only a handful of psychologists have timidly ventured into these waters.

We thus begin an expansive field trip over virgin, unexplored, but hopefully not alien terrain.

NOTES

1. Paul Linnemeyer, "The Immune System, an Overview," 2008, http://www.thebody.com/content/art1788.html?getPage=2.
2. Kenneth Todar, *Online Textbook of Bacteriology*, accessed 2015, http://textbookofbacteriology.net/adaptive.html.
3. The biology project, Immunology, "Introduction to Immunology tutorial," University of Arizona, (2004),http://www.biology.arizona.edu/immunology/tutorials/immunology/page3.html.
4. Stuart Turvey and David Briode, "Innate Immunity," 2011, http://www.ncbi.nlm.nih.gov/pmc/articles/PMC2832725/.
5. Carl Zimmer, http:/discovermagazine.com/2009/mar/17.
6. Carmeli, Daphna Birenbaum "Prevalence of Jews as Subjects in Genetic Research: Figures, Explanation, and Potential Implications," *American Journal of Medical Genetics*, 2004, 130.
7. C. Clairborne Ray, "The Roots of BRCA1 Mutations for Ashkenazi Jews," *New York Times*, October 12, 2015.
8. Note that arthritis is a disease driven by both the innate and adaptive immune systems.
9. Stefano Romeo, Julia Kozlitina, Chao Xing, et al., "Genetic Variation in PNPLA3 Confers Susceptibility to Nonalcoholic Fatty Liver Disease," *Nature Genetics*, 40 (2008):1461–65.
10. "Innate Immunity," How it works, British Society for Immunology, accessed 2015, http://www.immunologyexplained.co.uk/HowItWorks.aspx.
11. Jamie Heather, "T-cell Receptors Part One," (2013) http://jamimmunology.blogspot.com/2013/02/TCR-part-1-the-immtroduction.html.
12. R. A/ Fouchier, T. Kuiken, M. Schutten, et al. "Aetiology: Koch's Postulates Fulfilled for SARS Virus," *Nature*, 2003, 423.
13. "Summary of Probable SARS Cases with Onset of Illness from 1 November 2002 to 31 July 2003", World Health Organization (WHO).
14. "Your Immune System, Antibiotic Overuse," Benjamin Associates LLC (2014), http://immunedisorders.homestead.com/antibiotics.html.

15. Gardiner Harris, "Steps Set for Livestock Antibiotic Ban," *New York Times,* March 24, 2012.
16. Sabrina Tavernise, "Antibiotics in Livestock: FDA Finds Use is Rising." *New York Times,* October 2, 2014.
17. Stepani Strom, "Report on U.S. Meat Sounds Alarm on Resistant Bacteria," *New York Times,* 2013.
18. Olga Kazan, "The Antibiotics Problem in Mean," *The Atlantic,* 2015, http://www.theatlantic.com/health/archive/2015/03/the-next-big-antibiotic-resistance-threat/388430/.
19. Maryann Gierloff, "Positive Emotions and Immune Response to Influenza in Medically Stable Older Adults," *Dissertation Abstracts International* 2013, 73.
20. R. Clover, T. Abell, L. Crawford, et al., "Family Functioning and Stress as Predictors of Influenza B Infection," *The Journal of Family Practice,* 1989, 28.
21. S. Kennedy, *The Prager Handbook on Stress and Coping,* (Santa Barbara, CA: Greenwood Publishing, 2007).
22. B. Bloomberg, "Psychosocial Adaptation and Cellular Immunity in Breast Cancer Patients," *Journal of Psychosomatic Research,* 2009, 67.
23. E. Tacoma and L. Huey, "Psychic Distress and the Immune Response," *Life Sciences,* 1985, 36.
24. J. D. Cacioppo, "Autonomic, Neuroendocrine, and Immune Responses to Psychological Stress," *Psychological Beitrage,* 2000, 42.
25. See Psych Info database 1975–2014 under "psychological immune system."

FIVE

The *Innate* Psychic Immune System

Fight-Flight, Competition, and Territoriality

We begin by admitting that no one knows if there is a psychological, or *psychic,* immune system, so the inquiry begins on thin ice from the start. Second, whatever psychological immune system may exist, the presumption made is that it sits on top of the physical immune system and mirrors it like an epiphenomenon.

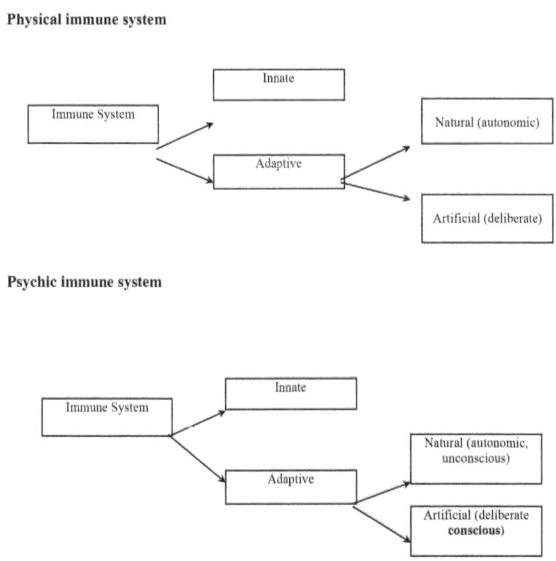

Figure 5.1 Overview of Physical Immune System and Psychic Immune System as an Epiphenomenon
Graphic of the physical immune system developed from The Biology Project, University of Arizona, May, 2000, http://www.biology.arizona.edu.

The third conjecture that bears on this inquiry is that whatever the psychic immune system might be, it is a positive force ultimately concerned with self-preservation and survival. Those are three incipient assumptions.

So, just as the physical immune system has an innate dimension, let us look for innate constituents of the hypothetical *psychic* immune system. We begin with the most pervasive survival mechanism throughout the animal kingdom and inside ourselves, fight and flight.

SURVIVAL: FIGHT AND FLIGHT

Certainly, the most basic survival process found in virtually all living creatures is the fight-flight reflex, and it is as innate as the knee-jerk. Fight and flight processes in humans and most primates involve a physiology worthy of attention.

The Adrenaline Rush

As soon as the nervous system detects a threat, activity in the hypothalamus signals the pituitary gland to release chemicals into the bloodstream. As this happens, nerve signals reach the adrenal gland, which releases substances called catecholamines like epinephrine. This primes the animal, or man, for fighting or fleeing.[1] From here cortisol, a stress hormone, is released increasing blood pressure and blood sugar. All of this provides an immediate energy boost to the entire system, an adrenaline rush in more common parlance.

Epinephrine then contracts certain muscle groups and beads of perspiration and raised hairs appear on the surface of the skin. This prepares the body for extreme activity. In short, the body is pumped and primed.[2]

The fight-flight reflex is a fundamental innate reflex. To psychologist, Ben Martin:

> While the fight or flight response clearly can be learned, it also involves an innate reaction that operates largely outside consciousness. This was first recognized in the 1920s by physiologist Walter Canon, whose research showed that a threat stimulates a sequence of activities in an organism's nerves and glands. We now know that the hypothalamus controls this response by initiating a cascade of events in the autonomic nervous system (ANS), in the endocrine system and in the immune system.[3]

Rats will try to escape when threatened, but, if cornered, they will fight. Some animals remain perfectly still, freeze, and play dead. In fact, Joseph LeDoux of The Emotional Brain Institute says "fight-flight-freeze" is a more apt descriptor than merely fight-flight.[4]

Cold-blooded animals can sometimes change color quickly to camouflage themselves. When a skunk lifts its tail, most nearby animals know it is prepared to fight. When a dog's tail hangs between its legs, it is backing off from a fight.

> This instinct is alive and well, and functioning in each and every one of us . . . in order to mobilise our bodies to meet the perceived threat, we prepare for either fight or flight. . . . Our body begins to close down all extraneous functions, blood is pumped to the main muscles and away from the skin (we go pale) sugar is metabolised by the adrenalin, pupils dilate, digestion stops, skin sweats, breathing becomes shallow. . . . In this state we are only fit for survival. We can't listen, we can't be creative, we are a victim of this mechanism.[5]

MORE ON THE INNATE NATURE OF FIGHT-FLIGHT

Psychologists use the term "neuroception" to indicate that the nervous system is continuously evaluating risk in our environment. It scans for danger and threat. Some of these scanning functions are learned, others hard-wired. Low-frequency sounds, for example, elicit a sense of danger in animals and an approaching predator. Reptiles and amphibians have similar reactions.

"In contrast, high-pitched screams from another mammal (not just our children, but also our dogs and cats) elicit a sense of urgent concern or empathy for another who may be feeling pain or being injured. With humans high frequency screams shift our attention to the specific individual who is screaming. Through exposure and associative learning, we can link these features with other events."[6]

Fight, Flight, War, and Instinct

The fight-flight response is highly autonomic and instinctive in man, and, as one theorist puts it, large-scale wars happen "for the same reason that most violence does." When threatened, we protect ourselves whether it is on an elementary school playground or confronting invaders from Kosovo to Kashmir:

> Deep in our neural architecture and chemistry, probably in our very genes, we have a powerful set of instinctive subconscious systems that help us detect and respond to danger, whether it's a direct physical threat, a threat to our resources, or even a challenge to our basic ideas about social structure. These precognitive systems have evolved to help us survive. They fire up before thinking and reason even have a chance to contribute to our response to risk.[7]

The process of fight, flight, or freeze occurs in virtually every animal including man.

> Before thinking even has a chance to get going, we respond to danger by instantly rearranging our bodily systems and metabolism to either fight, flee, or freeze. . . . One of the things those initial changes do is magnify the power of instinct over reason as our response to the risk continues. We not only use instincts first and thinking second, but in an ongoing risk response, we use emotions and instinct more than reason.[8]

Neuroscientist Joseph LeDoux concurs:

> emotions can flood consciousness. This is so because the wiring of the brain at this point in our evolutionary history is such that connections from the emotional systems to the cognitive systems are stronger than the connections from the cognitive systems to the emotional systems.[9]

How then does one deal with the issue of war when instinctive reactions are so much more powerful than conscious and rational faculties? Writer David Rolpelk offers a comment:

> Ending war would require that reason conquer these self-protective instincts. That's not entirely out of the question. We do have the capacity for thinking our way to a non-violent response to threat. And our powerful thinking cortex may yet evolve to become the more dominant contributor to our risk response system, developing smarter and more effective ways to respond to risk than our older hard-wired instincts which, so far, have worked pretty well. But for the foreseeable human future, when it comes to the perception of and response to danger, *thinking comes second and instinct comes first.*[10]

The Relaxation/Exhaustion Response

After fight-flight has commenced, there is a familiar graph. Adrenaline and cortisol, two important stress hormones are released. Both rapidly ascend and then immediately begin to taper down. The release of these two hormones is highly reminiscent of the bell-shaped curves examined at in earlier chapters on war and pandemics. They rise, crest, and then, just as rapidly retreat.

The decline of stress hormones is just as important as their increase, because should they not decline, exhaustion occurs and the entire physical immune system becomes compromised.[11] There are many psychophysiological consequences of prolonged or extended stress, or war.

First, during war, both male and female fertility suffer. Women who were exposed as prisoners of war or to bombardment had increased menstrual abnormalities. Males show a decline in semen viability. Long term stress, that is, long-term fight-flight mobilization, not only impacts human fertility,[12] but the same phenomenon is seen in numerous animal species.[13] [14] As fight-flight mobilization progresses, overall immune suppression happens too, but as the relaxation response commences, fertility returns and so does physical immune function.

A terse summary, then, of fight-flight and the relaxation polarity is provided by the Harvard Medical School:

> Fight-flight involves increased heart rate, blood pressure, respiration, higher pulse, increased muscle tension, production of cortisol, noradrenaline, and the response is unconsciously elicited. . . . The relaxation response is quite the opposite: decreased heart rate, blood pressure, respiration, pulse, oxygen consumption, and a reduction of cortisol and noradrenaline. It is stress releasing, allows an expansion or attention and involves an attitude of acceptance.[15]

So, it is quite necessary that fight-flight mobilization *ceases* and relaxation and homeostasis return. Otherwise, stress-induced diseases, loss of fertility, and compromised physical immune function occurs.[16]

The Conscious and Unconscious Sides of Fight-Flight

Certainly when one enters a business proposition, or buys a stock mutual fund, one takes on risk, and the approach is cautious, conscious, and rational. When we make a decision to buy a home, we try to do so in a safer neighborhood where risk and danger to ourselves and our children is minimal. There is obviously a conscious dimension to risk behavior and fight-flight human psychology.

At the same time, one cannot dismiss how deeply rooted the fight-flight response is—how autonomic, automatic, or instinctive—and how it rouses a person even before the conscious mind has even fully appreciated the danger.

In the earlier cited example of how women responded to the sound of a baby crying far more readily than men, a tomography study wanted to know just how rapid that response was. Their brain centers registered the crying within one hundred milliseconds—about the time needed to blink—and women who never had children showed the same response pattern.[17] It is hard to argue this is a learned response, since women who are not mothers also have the same reactivity. A great deal of fight-flight, in other words, is hard-wired and represents an undeniably unconscious substrate in human psychology. That it connects the child to its food supply quite clearly shows this to be an innate survival reflex.

Is There a Collective Fight-Flight Reflex?

In the prior discussion of wars and how they seem to come to an end in similar fashion to epidemics, one wonders if fight-flight mobilization in an individual ever happens collectively. Do societies or nations engage in fight-flight, or is this only confined to individual psychology?

Mobilization not only happens within an individual, but seems to have the capacity to elicit herd behavior and mass psychology too. In the stock market crash of 1987, known as Black Monday, panic selling was overwhelming with a 24 percent one-day drop occurring in a matter of hours.[18]

In August 2011, the stock market had another panic attack with $2.3 trillion in investor wealth evaporating in a single day.[19] Surely, panic-selling frenzies represent collective flight responses, and, inasmuch as they are often irrational, it can be assumed they may be, at least in part, instinctual.

MORE INNATE PSYCHIC IMMUNITIES: FEAR, HAPPINESS, AND INTELLIGENCE

If fight-flight is a partially innate process that protects from danger, are there other built-in, heritable traits which could be candidates for the innate psychic immune system? To get closer to this idea, return to the physical immune system for a moment. More seems to be known about genetic immune deficiencies than about inherited immunities.[20] There are inherited deficiencies, for example, which make a person prone to numerous invasive bacteria.[21] The Chinese have a missing variant of a particular gene which protects against influenza and are more vulnerable as a consequence.[22] Other inherited immune deficiencies are a form of ataxia, Wiskott-Aldrich Syndrome, and thymic aplasia.[23] But there are also inherited physical immunities too.[24] Some groups have stronger immunity to TB or hepatitis, and genetic, inherited differences are the likely explanation.[25] [26]

When speaking of *psychic* immunities and deficiencies, a few of each type can be found as well. Vulnerability to psychosis or depression may have genetic components.[27] Those who have a gene labeled 5-HTTLPR have a stronger probability of encountering problems with depression. The gene, appropriately, has been labeled the "depression gene."[28]

One study reports that 32 percent of stress vulnerabilities may be genetic, that is, may be due to inherited predispositions toward stress.[29] So, if heritability for psychological diseases and disorders exists, is it not logical to assume there might be heritable defenses against psychological illness as well, to wit, innate *psychic* immunities?

There is considerable evidence, for example, that many of our fears are inherited. Research points to fear of the dark, the unknown, great heights, or slithering snakes may be "left over from our ancestors."[30] John Hettema and colleagues in Sweden studied ninety pairs of identical twins and eighty-three pairs of fraternal twins. Identical twins have the same genes, but fraternal twins are "as different as children born separately from the same parents." In the study the sets of twins were shown different images. Some were frightening (spiders, snakes), others were neutral (triangles and circles).

> The twins were also given a mild electrical shock as they viewed some of the images. During the testing, researchers measured the subject's skin electrical conductivity, which usually increases in states of fear and anxiety due to increased output from the person's sweat glands. When the researchers analyzed the results, they found that the identical twins *had the same responses.* They also discovered the non-identical twins experienced differing responses. Traditionally, fear is something that has been thought of as a learned response. A person endures a frightening experience and then learns to be anxious and apprehensive when it happens, or the potential for it to happen again arises. The process is referred to as, "conditioning." Dr. Hettema said, "Now we can say that the fear conditioning process in humans is controlled, at least to some extent, by genetic factors. Between one-third and one-half of the fear conditioning process *appears to be inherited.*" Fear is a desirable and natural response to dangerous situations.[31]

Additional work with identical and fraternal twins shows correlations between identical twins are significantly greater than between fraternal twins leading psychologists to believe the trait as "heritable." The following phobias seem to have heritability scores of at least 20 percent or higher: animal phobias, blood injury phobias, and agoraphobia.[32] In other words, animal, blood-injury, and agoraphobia have a genetic or inherited component as well as a learned and cultural side to them. As Kendler and Prescott argue in *Genes, Environment and Psychology,* natural selection has created a predisposition to form phobias to snakes, spiders, rats, and high places than of

> objects that are considerably more dangerous in the modern world, such as handguns, electric outlets, and knives. This would occur, the theories predict, because only objects or situations that reflected true danger over the *tens of thousands of years of human evolution* would produce phobia-proneness. Guns, knives, and electric outlets are too new in evolutionary time to have yet produced enough selection for fears of them.[33]

Fear plays a role in survival, and specific fears which were historically prominent in protecting humans from danger appear heritable. Fears protect us. The psychic immune system protects us.

The Happiness Gene

If fear is adaptive, essential for our survival, and at least in part, innate, this represents a second building block of the so-called innate psychic immune system. But there is more. It is empirically well established that happiness and optimism provide defense against many psychological illnesses and, in turn, a significant body of research shows happiness has a genetic component.

For example, individuals who have two sets of the gene called 5-HTT "are almost twice as likely to say they are satisfied with life compared to those who lack a copy."[34] The study, from the *Journal of Human Genetics*, reports that "it has long been suspected that this gene plays a role in mental health."[35]

Another study reported that in a survey of one thousand identical and fraternal twins, genes control half the personality traits that make people happy while factors such as relationships, health, and career are responsible for the rest of our well-being. "We found that around half the differences in happiness were genetic," said Tim Bates, a researcher at the University of Edinburgh who led the study reported in the journal *Psychological Science*.[36]

Happiness and optimism are related to overall psychological health, so, if happiness has a genetic basis, it would certainly be fair to assert that the psychological immunities conferred on happier individuals have an innate basis.[37] [38] [39]

More on Inheritance and Identical Twins

Genetic factors extend far beyond fear proneness and happiness. Mental disorders have genetic components, in particular schizophrenia, major depression, alcoholism, anxiety disorders, and panic disorders. So do authoritarianism and religiosity appear "heritable."[40]

It is awe-inspiring just how much of a psychological nature we may inherit. Two identical twins, Jim Lewis and Jim Springer, were raised apart beginning at four weeks of age. They finally met in 1979 when they were thirty-nine years of age. They discovered they both were prone to nail biting; both smoked Salem cigarettes; both suffered from tension headaches, both drove the same type of car, and both took vacations in Florida and even stayed at the same beach. Genes seem to be involved in these unusual symmetries.

The well-known Minnesota Twin Family Study which was run from 1979 to 1999, followed identical and fraternal twins separated at an early age:

> "We were surprised by certain behaviors that showed a genetic influence, such as religiosity [and] social attitudes," said Nancy Segal, an evolutionary psychologist at California State University, Fullerton, "Those surprised us, because we thought those certainly must come from the family [environment]. . . ."
>
> Another study of four pairs of twins found that genetics had a stronger influence on sexual orientation in male twins than in female twins. . . . Another study, commissioned by the editor of the journal *Science*, looked at genetics and IQ. The Minnesota researchers found that about 70 percent of IQ variation across the twin population was due to genetic differences among people, and 30 percent was due to

> environmental differences. . . . Moreover, a study in 1990 found that genetics account for 50 percent of the religiosity among the population—in other words, both identical twins raised apart were more likely to be religious or to be not religious, compared with unrelated individuals. . . . Another study found that happiness and well-being had a 50 percent genetic influence.[41]

So fear proneness, happiness, intelligence, even religiosity have a genetic basis, and some of these heritable psychological traits are clearly correlated with health and mental health.

A few conclusions can be proffered from this pithy review of the literature:

- There appears to be a genetic, biological, or inherited basis for some psychological traits.
- Some of these traits are related to danger detection, survival, health, and mental health.
- Of these candidates for the innate psychic immune system we can include fight-flight reflexes, fear responsiveness, optimism, happiness, and intelligence—all of which have some innate basis, and all arguably related to security and survival.

INCEST AVOIDANCE

Another element of the innate psychic immune system is incest avoidance. Freud first alerted the world to the ubiquity of the incest taboo in the human species, but he saw the cause to be found in the Oedipal or Electra Complexes. A century after Freud's theories, a far more elegant explanation for incest avoidance has emerged from evolutionary biology and sociobiology. Sometimes referred to as the Westermark effect, it insinuates that incest avoidance helps protect the gene pool from the emergence of recessive genes or what is known as genetic homozygosity.

When mating with someone outside one's gene pool, the chance of passing on recessive genes is only 50 percent. But when individuals sharing a large number of genes reproduce, passing on recessive disorders increases exponentially. Examples include cystic fibrosis, sickle cell anemia, and albinism. Other side effects of inbreeding include increased risk of infertility, birth defects, cleft palates, heart conditions, facial asymmetry, and neonatal mortality. In one study some 40 percent of children who were the product of first-degree incest had recessive disorders, congenital physical malformations, and intellectual deficits: "When first-degree relatives mate, the risk of their child suffering from an early death, serious birth defect, or mental disability increases to almost 50 percent."[42]

Most unfortunate for Freudians, though, is that incest avoidance is not *sui generis* to the human population. It is common in the animal kingdom, too, from birds to primates. Numerous biologists—Bischof, 1976, van den

Berghe, 1982, and Durham, 2014—present reams of evidence for the aversion.[43] Over two hundred species from baboons to macaques to capuchins, have a built- in "inbreeding avoidance mechanism."[44]

> Nonhuman primates provide abundant evidence for an inhibition of sexual behavior among closely related adults. This finding is consistent with the idea that inbreeding avoidance behavior is a naturally selected behavior that was already present among animals before humans evolved. The primate data support Westermarck's theory that familiarity during immaturity is a major reason for this avoidance. Mating among adults is most inhibited among maternal relatives in species in which these have close associations.[45]

Anne Pusey of the Department of Ecology at the University of Minnesota reports that in twenty-eight studies of animals, breeding between parents and offspring was rare, and in only two species did these kinds of unions compose more than 5 percent of the total.[46]

With respect to human incest aversion, one telling study examined odor preferences among family members versus strangers. In blind tests, odors of family members were found *more noxious* than odors of strangers in mother-son and father-daughter configurations and, curiously, at puberty odor aversion between opposite-sexed siblings increased as well. Especially opposite-sexed siblings showed a pronounced dislike of each other's smells but the same phenomenon did not appear with same-sex siblings. According to Dustin Penn at the university of Utah, "the avoidance of inbreeding could definitely be at work."[47] In other words, close family members smell worse than strangers, a rather palpable symptom of innate incest aversion.[48]

So why, we might ask, is incest aversion part of the innate psychic immune system? The answer is that an instinctive aversion to inbreeding is a protective mechanism to promote viability of the gene pool and it is unambiguously an aspect of phylogenetic self-preservation.

There is additional and corroborating evidence too. In another olfactory experiment, college age men were asked to wear an undershirt for two days. The shirts were then given to women to determine to which scent they felt most attracted. The experimenters concluded women were most attracted to men with immune systems different from their own.[49]

Family members have more similar immune systems than more distant relatives or strangers—innately—and therefore attraction to opposite sexed persons outside the family unit supports the idea that incest aversion may be innate across the human species.[50]

COMPETITION, AGGRESSION, AND TERRITORIALITY

There are two major tendencies within the human condition, both related to our survival, both potential candidates for the innate psychic immune system, and yet both rather diametrically opposed to one another: aggression and territoriality on the one hand, cooperation and nonviolence on the other.

Let us first review the Rambo interpretation of evolution: territorial competition, dominance, and aggression, and Freud's remark that "The tendency to aggression is an innate, independent, instinctual disposition in man."[51]

Aggression, Territoriality, and Dominance: To the Victor Go the Spoils

There is a plethora of scholarly work on the nature of human aggression and competition, and both genetic and environmental factors are apparent. Further, there are clear prototypes in the animal kingdom. Probably the most significant contribution to this subject comes from Robert Ardrey's *Territorial Imperative* and much of what follows is influenced by his work.

Alpha males appear for good reason. They compete for genetic dominance in breeding, and thus enhance the hardiness and survivability of the group. In the vast majority of cases, competitions between dominant males for territory and reproductive rights is the primary behavioral motif.

In many species, only a few males may fertilize an entire herd. With the Uganda kob, males compete for a slice of territory on their breeding ground, called the "stamping ground." Estrous females have no response to males who have not succeeded in obtaining a slice of turf. These males congregate on the perimeter of the arena unable to copulate at all.

The dominant males are proudly regaled on their hard-won pieces of real estate, usually about fifty feet in diameter—and do virtually all of the breeding. One single doe required copulation ten times in a day, and the dominant male similarly had to defend his territory against challengers five times in an hour and a half.

In one Wyoming observation setting of sage grouse mating rituals, 355 cocks were assembled and 141 hens. The champion males fought for and defended five territories, and "*three quarters of all matings were accomplished by only four dominant males.*"[52] As power, dominance, and territory expand, so too do fertility and breeding rights. The patas monkey lives in fairly large groups but contains only a single large dominant male and his harem of females. The gorilla travels in bands ruled with total authority by a single chief. The will of the leader is rarely challenged.

> In the aggressive baboon on the other hand, we find the harshest of all primate authorities. The large baboon troop with numbers of up to a hundred occupies a huge permanent range which is exclusive in that none ever intrudes. . . . All cooperation rests on fear of an oligarchy of three, four or five powerful males . . . whose combined dominance none dares challenge.[53]

Japanese monkeys form similar unchallengeable oligarchies as does the African vervet. Dominance and subordination seem to characterize most animal societies with the possible exception of certain schooling fish. "We may deplore baboon tyranny, with its gang of thugs at the top, but the baboon is nevertheless an outrageous evolutionary success from the Sudan to the Cape of Good Hope, and the effectiveness of his society has made him the equal of the leopard and very nearly of man."[54]

In human society there are remarkable parallels: Harems of at least several hundred women have been the norm for the emperors of all major civilizations: Aztec, Babylonian, Chinese, Egyptian, Incan, Indian, and Roman.

It is probably fair to say that men with absolute power have routinely fathered several hundred children—rather in the manner of a successful bull elephant seal.[55] Not to forget Genghis Khan's 20,000 offspring.[56] As Khan proudly boasted: "The greatest pleasure is to vanquish your enemies and chase them before you, to rob them of their wealth and see those dear to them bathed in tears, to ride their horses and clasp to your bosom their wives and daughters."[57]

In the evolutionary descent of human history, one observes large doses of dominant males governing various social units, from the family, to the community, to the state. Territoriality constitutes the basis of political activity, while the "law" often represents the cumulative decision making and tradition of dominant males.[58]

Males fight for territory, for resources, and for breeding rights. But the violence emitted is particularly and peculiarly male-to-male, a pattern also found in primate and chimpanzee communities, that is same-sex violence.[59]

Adult male mortality rates in human communities, due to intergroup aggression, in New Guinea and Australia, ranged between 25 percent and 28 percent . . . similar in scope to chimpanzee mortality rates from violent male-to-male encounters.

Crime statistics from Australia, Botswana, Nigeria, Scotland, Uganda, and a dozen different locations in the United States, from thirteenth- and fourteenth-century England, nineteenth-century America—from hunger-gatherer communities, tribal societies, and medieval and modern nation-states—all uncover the same fundamental pattern. In all these societies . . . "the probability that a same sex murder has been committed by a man, not a woman, ranges from 92 percent to 100 percent."[60]

Rather ubiquitous on our planet, then, males engage in primate-flavored, dominant, aggressive, sexual, and territorial behavior: a man is nine times as likely as a woman to commit murder, seventy-eight times as likely to commit forcible rape, ten times as likely to commit armed-robbery, six and a half times as likely to commit aggravated assault, and American men are eight times more likely to commit violent crime than women.[61]

As for predation on another's territory and food supply, the archetypal male is thirteen and half times as likely to commit fraud, or be arrested for carrying a lethal weapon, ten times more likely to burgle, nine times more likely to steal a car, eight times more likely to vandalize, and seven times more likely to fence stolen property than a woman.[62] This behavioral "biogram," as one author calls it, may be an epiphenomenon of even deeper struggles too, that is, cellular competitions.

In a study of a female animal in heat, which had mated with two different males, the sperm from each mating was tracked in her vaginal tract. To the surprise of the investigators, sperm differentiated into "swimmers" and "defenders," and some of the sperm from one donor squared off to fight off the sperm of the other.

The fight for dominance is acted out not just outside in the arena of the breeding ground, but at the microscopic level where representatives of each dominant male fight the same battle going on outside. Opponent sperm tries to annihilate the sperm of the second donor, and the winner penetrates the ovum first, winning the evolutionary competition.[63] The title of the book is revealing as well, *Sperm Wars*.[64]

This male phenotype is found virtually everywhere. Even civilized and educated males often fall into grandiose delusions of omnipotence, wealth, property, and power—and the content of such fantasies often involve frequent and numerous sexual contacts, myriad numbers of partners from fantasies of harems to an afterlife spent with seventy-two virgins.[65] At least 30 percent of American males currently indulge in such atavistic, sexual fantasies.[66]

Whether all-male bands of orangutan thugs or primal hordes of *Homo sapiens*, the biogram propels males to assert dominance over women, over each other, over territory, over adversaries, all in hope—at least in the eye of evolutionary psychologists—of succeeding in securing unlimited breeding rights. Jealousy and possessiveness is an obvious by-product of this process, and recent studies show male sexual jealousy to be *ubiquitous* on this planet.[67] "Man and the monkey have more in common than mere anatomy. . . Our infant species is not as yet divorced from evolutionary processes."[68]

Territoriality, Sex, and the Innate Releasing Mechanism

A wasp and an antelope have not shared a common ancestor for five hundred million years, yet their territorial and mating behavior is virtually identical. An antelope comes to an arena where territory is defined and reproductive possibilities are aroused and pursued. A wasp will behave the same way even if his territory is not greater than a mere stone. Both will defend their terrain against all intruders, but only during the mating season. If the wasp is taken one thousand feet away, it will only be a matter of time before he is back on his perch and prepared for his ancient ritual.[69]

A deer mouse rarely leaves a range of more than fifty yards in diameter and one hundred yards is his lifetime limit. Yet taken a mile away from his home, he finds his way back with very little difficulty. Selecting a deer mouse only five weeks old, who has never left the immediate vicinity of the nest and taking her two miles away, she "reappeared contentedly in her home trap in exactly two days."[70]

The albatross pairs for life, a long life, and flies great distances. When it returns to its breeding grounds it will make its nest less than thirteen feet from last year's nest, despite the disappearance of all markings due to storms, tides, and so forth. Some birds were carted off to the Philippines, Japan, and Hawaii. One bird traveled 4,120 statute miles to return to his nest. Another traveled 3,120 miles from Hawaii without a single island to mark their journey.[71]

Alpha Fish and Archetype

Ethologist Nikolaas Tinbergen coined the term "innate releasing mechanism." By this he meant that certain stimuli will elicit a whole and massive innate response complex in an animal. In a classic experiment, a fish is introduced into a tank. Shortly thereafter it identifies a stone or a pebble which it then seems to call home. With that, the fish becomes a proprietor; he is now dubbed the alpha fish. That is when the trouble starts:

> The experiment was designed to test what effect *prior* residence would have on the outcome of the competition for dominance. At this time "intruders" are introduced into the tank. Half of the intruders were larger than the resident, half smaller. The experimenter found that size and strength would have some effect on the determination of which would be the alpha fish, *but not much.* It was residence that counted. Even when the resident was the smaller fish, he would be the first to challenge four times as often as the larger intruder. And when the struggle was resolved, the *intruder would be the loser four times as often if he was the smaller fish, three times as often even though he was the larger.*[72]

Intruders, whether robins or baboons, are long-shots in invading territories held by others of their own species. The endless tales of fights for dominance over territory—and the odds favoring proprietors over intruders, regardless of size—seems a classic law of territory, a law understood far more by animals that intruding man:[73] Ardrey opines, however, that the more sophisticated primate species (apes, baboons, vervet, rhesus, and Japanese monkeys, "no longer intrude but maintain each other's exclusive space by avoidance."[74]

Consider the idea of the innate releasing mechanism, instinct, or archetype and its relationship to the territorial imperative in the following anecdote: Ardrey recalls his youth in the 1930s was accompanied by a fashionable kind of intellectual cynicism, disbelief, with a smattering of existentialism and angst.[75] There was no strong cultural tradition of fealty much less militaristic fervor. On December 7, 1941, all that changed. When the Japanese bombed Pearl Harbor something massive, instinctive, and collective was "released." Was my response to Pearl Harbor innate or conditioned? This is the question we must ask. Was it something I had been born with or something I had been taught? Was it truly a command of genetic origin, an inheritance from the experience and natural selection of tens of thousands of generations of my human and hominid ancestors? Or was it a display of a cultural heritage to which I had been conditioned during my lifetime?

> We were conditioned, it is true. The generation that was to respond to the last man on Pearl Harbor's dawn had been conditioned to believe that wars accomplish nothing. Had America been an enormous laboratory and had we all been albino rats, no more elegant experiment could have been devised to test the powers of social conditioning . . . except in the unpopular anticipations of a far-sighted few, nothing in our sympathies, our fears, or our revulsions persuaded us that war could ever bring human solutions.
>
> To the very last moment we preserved like laboratory rats the perfect posture of our perfect conditioning. Then all in an hour, evolution took charge. . . . Towers of reason, of impeccable design, will topple in a dusty instant. . . . The intruder[76] will have knocked. . . . The territorial imperative is as blind as a cave fish, as consuming as a furnace, and it commands beyond logic, opposes all reason, suborns all moralities, strives for no goal more sublime than survival.[77]

The intruder indeed knocked. Draft boards were overwhelmed with volunteers. Students dropped out of college and joined the service.[78] In Britain, a million volunteers rushed to the aid of their country.[79] The invasion of the arena, or the nation, by an intruder "releases" an instinctual territorial reaction that Ardrey calls the "inspired lunacy" of the proprietor.

Over My Dead Body

Walter Stephens had a border dispute with his neighbor, Robert Hall, over a property line issue. The long-standing dispute finally erupted, and Stephens was charged with bludgeoning then shooting his neighbor and throwing his body in a bonfire. "Stephens was arrested in his back yard that afternoon when deputies found him next to the bonfire, with Hall's arm sticking out of it."[80]

This twenty-eight-year-old man will likely spend the majority of his adult life in prison over a few feet of disputed acreage. Was this act premeditated or was he so overcome with maniacally "released" emotion, that he was momentarily psychotic, possessed, and fully absent any higher faculties, just like the wasp, the antelope, or the alpha fish in response to a territorial intrusion.[81]

Territoriality has very much to do with males and alpha males in particular: "Just as chimpanzees have their high ranking alpha male and his partners, humans have their pharaohs, kings, nobles, emperors, sheiks, dictators, czars, chiefs, prime ministers and presidents."[82]

> Since human origin, individuals and groups have had continuous conflicts in search for the best economic resources, the most fertile land, and the most sustainable reproductive social group. For this reason, human history is full of aggressive conflicts and sanctioned aggressive behaviors. . . . It is widely agreed among evolutionary anthropologists and sociobiologists that aggression is a biologically universal human characteristic. . . .[83]
>
> All humans feel the need to eliminate competitors, or the offspring of competitors to protect reproductive capital such as territory and mates.[84]

So, as difficult as this is to admit, human aggression, territoriality, dominance, and violence must somehow be included as part of the psychic immune system in that such behavior enhances survival and the protection and defense of resources necessary for individual and group survival.

Some theorists strongly argue that human aggression is not inherited or heritable despite whatever parallels are seen with primate alpha-male dominance seeking.[85] Others believe there has been a selective breeding for aggression. After all, cattle have been bred for docility;[86] could humans have been bred to be more aggressive?

Serotonin 5HT is thought to play a role in suppressing inter-male aggression. Mice who were missing specific 5HT genes appeared more aggressive and violent in their attacks. Indeed some researchers believe they actually have found the "warrior gene." Studies of a mutation in the neurotransmitter metabolizing enzyme monoamine oxidase A (MAO-A) have been shown to cause a syndrome that includes violence and impulsivity in humans. . . . An American group studying monkeys called MAO-A a "warrior gene" in 2004."[87]

Another 2008 study found three genes (MAO-A, DAT1, and DRD2) associated with an elevated risk of violent and delinquent behavior, especially people who experienced stresses during childhood.[88]

Genes and inheritance, in other words, provide a *backdrop* for environmental conditions to elicit or release an aggressive response. There appears to between a strong relationship between nature and nurture here, or between innate or inherited aggression and environmental releasing stimuli.

The Collective Side of Territoriality and Dominance, the Male Fratriarchy

Anthropologist Lionel Tiger's *Men in Groups* proposes that rather than relying on a single alpha male, males form coalition or gangs of dominant males, which together made them unchallenged hunters especially in bringing down large game.

Human evolutionary success depended as mightily on cognitive skill but also on cooperative and united team behavior. Loyalty to the group is a legacy of man-the-hunter. Fealty and mutual interdependence ensures survival, and any failure to believe your brother will be there for you when you need him threatens the hunt and the viability of the hunting party, so argues Professor Tiger.

Semper Fidelis. One for all and all for one. From loyalty in the military, loyalty in the Mafia, obedience in the all-male priesthood of the church, all these inflection points underscore the survival of the group depends upon a functional, cohesive, brotherhood.

The army and the Mafia are but droplets in the history of fraternity and all-male groups that span the millennia: the Orangemen, Masons, Ku Klux Klan, Carbonari, The Terrorists of Bengal, Fenians, Nihilists, Mahdists, Troubadours, Camora of Naples, Communeros in Spain, Broederbund of South Africa not to mention the Bolsheviks, the Mensheviks or the Crips of Los Angeles. Male gangs to Lionel Tiger are

> exaggerated examples of human . . . bonding propensities. . . . The adoption of special dress, language, ritual, and moral structure by members of secret societies, and even by member of a men's hut, indicates the existence of a bonded group commitment and fellowship. . . . An initiation ceremony, with its attendant physical pain and isolation from parents, demonstrates to the youngster that his nuclear family is no longer his sole protector, refuge, and security. The strong emotion experienced by initiates generates identification with the group . . . but also produces an exceptionally strong bond among the initiates.[89]

In psychoanalytic terms, the contemporary urban gang is a sublimated hunting band, an exclusively all-male enterprise where commitment and devotion transcend all prior loyalties. Initiation rites are painful. Hazings, ordeals, tattoos, and incisions on initiates are ancient, prehistoric, and all quintessentially male. In military or mafia subcultures, male loyalty directly correlates with survivability. One weak link in the chain, the snitch, the stoolie, the Judas, defector, or deserter threatens the survival of the whole enterprise. As in animal societies, male loyalty is not merely prized, but the entire initiation-loyalty-membership process is related to rank, territory, aggression, and violence.

In "The Phylogeny of Gangs," David Davis points out that rank and territory are the goals of most animal fighting. He concludes a wide variety of observations suggests *that fighting for rank or territory is innate.*[90] According to another anthropologist: aggression is heavily dependent on genetics. "Probably only the means of fighting and the object of attack are learned."[91]

In a baboon troupe, when a dominant male is admitted into the fraternity—usually after a brawl where he has defeated other dominant males—the initiate gets into a supplicant position, extends his buttocks, and an older baboon, the elder, pats his bottom ceremoniously two or three times. This new dominant male then becomes a permanent member of the troupe.

The baboon initiation ritual is a close parallel to the hazings at American universities or how one becomes a knight in England—by kneeling in a supplicant position and being "tapped" on each shoulder by the more dominant knight.

Human male behavioral patterns and initiations can be viewed as less culturally conditioned and more archetypal and instinctive with parallels running deep into the primate world—all of it, apparently, having some adaptive significance.

Threat and Surrender Rituals in Animals and Humans

Consider the close parallel between human and animal threat and surrender rituals. When a wolf fights with another, the loser generally rolls on his back, exposes his belly, and the victor walks off without killing him. This is a noted surrender ritual in the animal kingdom.[92]

So, too, . . . with the gentoo species . . . where the male defending his four-foot territory will fight anybody including his mate, unless she makes the proper bow at the border.[93]

In Japan the depth of a bow is related to a person's social standing. When both persons bow to one another, the individual bowing deepest invariably bows to the higher status (more dominant) person.

Bowing and raising one's hands in surrender parallel animal rituals and have a specific function.[94] These are some ritual inhibitors of aggression, which, like assuming a begging-posture or bowing, may have some biological component.[95] Threat rituals function to inhibit aggression.

A military parade, for example, communicates how prepared the nation is for conflict, just like a baboon's wide-open mouth and chewing communicates determination, capacity and willingness to fight. This is usually sufficient enough to forestall any outbreaks of violence.

Parades of armaments on national days—the Fourth of July in the United States, May Day in the former Soviet Union—may be equivalent to the threat rituals of animals seeking to maintain or improve their status without engaging in actual violence.[96]

The function of these rituals is not merely to inhibit violence but simultaneously assert male dominance and supremacy. The Judge, the President, the Cardinal, the Fuhrer, His Holiness, Most Honorable Generallissimo . . . ladies and gentlemen, the dominant male is entering the room . . . all rise!

Sports, Male Bonding, Territoriality, and Reproduction

Curiously this male dominance-threat-aggression-territoriality "biogram" is acted out symbolically in sundry sporting matches. Here gangs of males compete for symbolic territory. In the process they identify themselves with totem and hunter symbolism—the braves, cubs, tigers, or lions. The flags, mascots, and identities of the teams are abjectly territorial and totemic. The Detroit *Lions*, New York *Giants*, Philadelphia *Eagles*, Chicago *Bears*, or the Arizona *Diamondbacks*,[97] all totemic images of strength, dominance, aggression, and territory. Furthermore, in sports, fertilization symbolism is legion. Males are cooperatively united against other males for the purposes of one horde implanting an object into the opponent's territory—symbolized usually as a female receptacle.

In basketball, the hoop is the incorporative symbol, and the struggle to place the ball through this ring is the object of the game. In hockey, a small object is passed between the brothers until it finally reaches the female holding pen. In football an egg-shaped oval reaches its ultimate destination between two goal-posts (legs?). To "score" is to achieve victory, dominance, status, but it is also measured by how many times you have penetrated the opposition's territory and placed the symbolic seed in the opposing horde's containers.

This psychoanalytic subtext points male psychology in the direction not merely of a defender of territory, but also of a collective predator, an intruder, where the primal horde of brothers attack other alien hordes to exploit, pillage, gain additional acreage—yardage—and gain consequent, albeit symbolic, reproductive rights, the spoils of war.

This theme is reenacted on a grand scale in every country of the world and televised weekly across the planet. More newspaper space is devoted to sports coverage than financial news. And, despite gains made by women in sport, this is primarily a vicarious and sublimated male ritual of territoriality and reproductive dominance; sports coverage favors males over females by a huge margin.[98]

To underscore the magnitude of the ritual and collective obsession, one in seven human beings on earth participated as spectators in watching the World Cup in 2014.[99] In sports, the rule of alpha-fish territoriality holds with a vengeance. Home teams (proprietors) *score more and win more* than visiting (intruder) teams. The phenomenon is well documented in hockey, baseball, and football with databases extending more than a century. Soccer seems to have the largest home team advantage ranging from 60 percent in Asia and Africa to 69 percent in the United States.

> In basketball, NBA teams win 62.7 percent of their home games. International cricket teams win 60.1 percent of home games. In the NHL, 59 percent of games are won by home teams. In rugby, the win rate for home teams is 58 percent, while in American football, it's 57.6 percent. In the United States, Major League Baseball home teams win 54.1 percent of the time. In Japan's Nippon League, that's 53.3 percent.[100]

The home team advantage is statistically well established in sports—just as proprietors in nature are more successful against intruders. But the unconscious nature of this drama is barely appreciated. Recent research, for example, has revealed that male competitors playing on home turf actually generate higher levels of testosterone before the game than does the visiting team, again underscoring how deeply autonomic this entire process is.[101]

Territoriality Update and the Causes of War

The exceptional work of Ardrey's *Territorial Imperative* has stood the test of time, but his research is now over fifty years old. Dominc Johnson and Monica Duffy Toft in the *Journal International Security* update the thesis under the title "Grounds for War: the evolution of territorial conflict." Their review brings us also closer to understanding the nature of warfare and territoriality, how territoriality is related to survival, and how innate and instinctive it is:

- "Territory is central to some of the most vexing cases of conflict, especially where different groups lay claim to the same ground. Jerusalem, for example has momentous significance for Christian, Jews, and Muslims alike. Each group is equally unwilling to yield control. Osama bin Laden referenced the foreign occupation of 'Muslim' *territory* as a primary basis for his holy war against the West.
- Territoriality is prevalent not only among humans but across the animal kingdom. . . . Territorial behavior facilitates effective competition for resources such as food, mates, shelter, breeding sites, and security from predators.
- Historically, the desire for territory has been a predominant cause of war. In a study of wars from 1648 to 1989, Kalevi Holsti found that 79 percent involved territorial issues . . . of seventy-nine interstate wars between 1816 and 1997, 54 percent should be classified as territorial. . . . From 1940 to 2000, 73 percent of all ethnic wars centered on the control of territory.
- Humans have a built-in propensity, one that is not wholly subject to standard conceptions of rational calculation, to privilege territory as all-important and indivisible.

- Territorial behavior has two distinct components: attack and avoidance. Residents tend to attack in defense of their territory (fight), intruders tend to withdraw (flight).
- In general, males establish and defend territory; they are also more likely than females to fight over it. . . . Across animal species territorial behavior . . . is most developed in adult males.
- When male elephants are in the reproductive state of Musth, "they have fifty times their normal level of testosterone. They become extremely aggressive and dangerous, systematically defeating much larger elephants. . . . This phenomenon has been found across a wide range of taxonomic groups including butterflies, damselflies, spiders, fish, salamanders, and birds . . . *residents are more likely to win fights to wrest their territories back from interlopers.* . . . On home ground, therefore, residents may be more effective fighters than nonresidents . . . concordant with widespread empirical observation that territory residents tend to win.
- Elsewhere in the world, interstate conflict over territory continues, from Kashmir and Israel/Palestine to the Falklands and the South China Sea . . . States are engaged in new conflicts over political and commercial control and use of land, ownership for the Antarctic, the Arctic Ocean floor, outer space, and near-Earth orbits, mobile phone frequency bands, undersea cables, and internet domains.
- If an evolutionary history of competition . . . led humans to develop a tendency to pursue violent strategies over territory, these tendencies may persist today. . . . Who can deny that a strong attachment to homeland helped Vietnamese nationalists to persist and ultimately defeat both France and the United States . . . or helped poorly armed Afghan insurgents defeat the might of the Soviet Union. . . ." (emphasis added)[102]

Unfortunately, therefore, we must welcome another candidate into the innate psychic immune system. However dark it may be, it is still concerned intimately with survival and self-preservation: competition, dominance, and territoriality.

With respect to the nature-nurture debate, certainly learning and culture influence its development and expression, but this male evolutionary biogram also has a clear, unambiguous, innate dimension to it as well.

The Autonomic Basis of Territoriality

Before leaving this controversial constituent of the innate psychic immune system, there is one important caveat: the role of consciousness in this discussion. Take sports: Obviously, when someone goes to a game, they consciously decide to invite friends. They save their money to finance season tickets; they examine upcoming schedules to see which games they will attend; they study and accumulate statistics on their favorite players. One cannot deny conscious foresight, rationality, and premeditation is involved.

At the same time, it is important to reflect how deep the entire evolutionary drama of alpha males, dominance-seeking, and territoriality extends into the animal kingdom, and how much of sports fascination is grounded on these powerful innate, instinctive, and unconscious predispositions.

Joseph Bargh and Ezequiel Morsella, cognitive psychologists from Yale, wrote an intriguing article entitled "The Unconscious Mind." They do not come from a psychoanalytic tradition at all. Instead, they reviewed cognitive psychology and evolutionary biology's take on the Freudian idea of the unconscious mind and came to some surprising conclusions. Psychology generally suffers, they say, from a "consciouscentric" bias, and

> actions of an unconscious mind *precede* the arrival of a conscious mind—that action precedes reflection. . . . Freud's historic importance in championing the powers of the unconscious mind is beyond any doubt . . . the unconscious mind is a pervasive, powerful influence over . . . higher mental processes . . . when placed in the broader context of the natural sciences, especially evolutionary biology, the widespread discoveries of sophisticated unconscious behavior guidance systems . . . make sense . . . unconscious processes are smart and adaptive throughout the living world, and the psychological research evidence that has emerged . . . has confirmed . . . in nature, *the unconscious mind is the rule not the exception. (emphasis added)*[103]

So, while fantasy football team members may be chosen with consciously mediated rationality and deliberateness, the underlying substrate, the "magic" of sport, the "participation mystique" that fans have—the etymology of the word fan, by the way, comes from fanatic—is a great vicarious drama of territoriality, dominance, totemism, and war ritualizing; and re-enacting millions of years of animal behavior that is both incredibly male and deeply unconscious in origin.

In sum, these darker and deeply innate predispositions of aggression, territoriality, and competition are related to human survival, and, to that extent, they are clearly nominees for admission to the psychic immune system whose essential function is the protection and survival of the species. However, there is a lighter side to this discussion which we will explore in the next chapter.

NOTES

1. U.S. National Library of Medicine, (2013), http://www.nlm.nih.gov/medlineplus/ency/article/003561.htm.

2. "How Cells Communicate During Fight or Flight," Genetic Science Learning Center, accessed 2015, http://learn.genetics.utah.edu/content/cells/fight_flight/.

3. Ben Martin, "Fight or Flight," Psyche Central (2013), http://psychcentral.com/lib/fight-or-flight/00030.

4. Joseph LeDoux, "'Run, Hide, Fight' is not How Our Brains Work," *New York Times*, December 18, 2015.

5. Kim Middleton, "Fight or Flight or Just Chill," Birds and More Birds, (2012), http://kimmiddleton.com/blog/45597/fight-or-flight-or-just-chill .

6. In D. Fosha, D. J. Siegel, & M. F. Solomon, eds. *The Healing Power of Emotion: Affective Neuroscience, Development, Clinical Practice,* (New York: Norton, 2009)https://lifespanlearn.org/documents/Reciprocal%20influences%20between%20body%20and%20brain%20-%20in%20press.pdf.

7. David Ropelk, "An End to War vs. the Animal Instinct to Survive," *Huffington Post,* (2010) http://www.huffingtonpost.com/david-ropeik/an-end-to-war-vs-the-anim_b_595282.html. Original Source: Joseph LeDeux, *The Emotional Brain* (1996) New York: Simon & Schuster.

8. Ropelk, "An End to War vs. the Animal Instinct to Survive."

9. Ropelk, "An End to War vs. the Animal Instinct to Survive."

10. Ropelk, "An End to War vs. the Animal Instinct to Survive."

11. James Wilson, "What is Adrenal Fatigue?" accessed 2015, https://www.adrenalfatigue.org/who-is-dr-wilson.

12. A. Abu-Musa, L. Kobeissi, A. Hannoun, et al., "Effect of War on Fertility: A Review of the Literature," (2008) PMID: 18644222 [PubMed - indexed for MEDLINE].

13. H. Hartmann, W. Bruere, et al., "General Adaptation Syndrome(Seyle) in Cattle," (1976), http://www.ncbi.nlm.nih.gov/pubmed/793558.

14. Nicholas Bakalar, "Stress May Affect Fertility, *Well*, (2014). http://well.blogs.nytimes.com/2014/03/24/stress-may-affect-fertility/?_r=2.

15. Neil Neimark, "Fight or Flight vs. Relaxation Response," accessed 2015 http://www.relaxationresponse.org/fightorflight.htm.

16. Martin, "Fight or Flight."

17. Fiona Macrae, "Why You Can't Ignore a Baby's Cry," November 1, 2012, Lifestyle/family/baby-toddler http://www.iol.co.za/lifestyle/family/baby-toddler/why-you-cant-ignore-a-babys-cry-1415929.

18. E. S. Browning, "Exorcising Ghosts of October Past," *Wall Street Journal,* October 15, 2007.

19. Amy Bingham, "Stock Market History: The 10 Worst Days," *ABC News* August 9, 2011, http://abcnews.go.com/Politics/stock-market-history-10-worst-days/story?id=14259116#1.

20. "What is Common Variable Immune Deficiency?" Genetics Home Reference (2015), http://ghr.nlm.nih.gov/condition/common-variable-immune-deficiency.

21. "Genetics and Immune Disorders," *Health Encyclopedia,* University of Rochester Medical Center, accessed 2015, http://www.urmc.rochester.edu/Encyclopedia/Content.aspx?ContentTypeID=134&ContentID=122.

22. "Genetics May Explain Why Some Chinese Hit Harder by the Flue," CBS News, January 29, 2013,http://www.cbsnews.com/news/genetics-may-explain-why-some-chinese-hit-harder-by-flu/.

23. C. Janeway, P. Travers, M. Walport, et al., *Inherited Immunodeficiency Diseases.* New York: Garland Science, 2001.

24. Janet Clay, "The Inheritance of Acquired Immunity," accessed 2015, http://jeb.biologists.org/content/12/1/49.full.pdf.

25. "Scientists Discover Ethnic Differences in Immune Response to TB Bacterium," Queen Mary University of London, (2015), http://www.qmul.ac.uk/media/news/items/smd/103133.html.

26. Hsu Li-Ching, Lin Sheue-Rong, et al. "Ethnic Differences in Immune Responses to Hepatitis B Vaccine," *American Journal of Epidemiology*, 143 (1996).

27. K. Hodgson and P. McGuffin, "The Genetic Basis of Depression," *Current Topics in Behavioral Neuroscience*, 2013, http://www.researchgate.net/publication/230733447_The_Genetic_Basis_of_Depression.

28. Romeo Vitelli, "Can Happiness be Genetic," *Media Spotlight*, February 25, 2013.

29. Amanda Gardner, "Genes May Play a Key Role in Stress." Health.com, September 19, 2012.

30. Harman Kagan, *The Psychological Immune System*. (Bloomington, IN: Author House, 2006), 20.

31. http://www.disabled-world.com/health/neurology/phobias/tei.php#sthash.ebj5X8PI.dpuf.

32. K. Kendler and C. Prescott, *Genes, Environment, and Psychology*. (New York: Guilford Press, 2007), 71.

33. Kendler and Prescott, *Genes, Environment, and Psychology*.

34. Stephen Adams, "Happiness Gene Discovered," *The Telegraph*, December 20, 2013.

35. Adams, "Happiness Gene Discovered."

36. Casey Kazan, "The Happiness Gene—Is It Inherited," (2008),http://www.dailygalaxy.com/my_weblog/2008/11/the-happiness-i.html.

37. See also. Arthur Brooks, "A Formula for Happiness," *New York Times*, December 14, 2013.

38. A second genetic mutation which produces anandamide is also related to happiness; it is often called the "bliss molecule," and is a mutation in the FAAH gene. Richard Friedman, "The Feel-Good Gene," *New York Times*, March 6, 2015.

39. A recent study in *The Lancet* takes issue with happiness data and alleges it is not correlated with good health or longevity. Denise Grady, "Happiness Doesn't Bring Good Health, Study Finds." *New York Times*, December 9, 2015.

40. Thomas Bouchard, "Genetic Influence on Human Psychological Traits," Current Directions in Psychological Science, (2004); Kazan, "The Happiness Gene—Is It Inherited," (2008),http://www.dailygalaxy.com/my_weblog/2008/11/the-happiness-i.html.

41. Tanya Lewis, "Twins Separated at Birth Reveal Staggering Influence of Genetics," Yahoo News, August 11, 2014, http://news.yahoo.com/twins-separated-birth-reveal-staggering-influence-genetics-182019977.html.

42. "Thinking About Incest 8: Primate Evidence and Anthropology," Living archives on eugenics blog, 2009 http://whatsortsofpeople.wordpress.com/2009/05/21/thinking-about-incest-8-primate-evidence-and-anthropology/.

43. Anne Pusey, "Mechanisms of Inbreeding Avoidance in Nonhuman Primates," *Pedophilia*, (1990), http://link.springer.com/chapter/10.1007%2F978-1-4613-9682-6_8#close.

44. "Thinking About Incest 8: Primate Evidence and Anthropology" Living archives on eugenics blog, 2009 http://whatsortsofpeople.wordpress.com/2009/05/21/thinking-about-incest-8-primate-evidence-and-anthropology/.

45. "Thinking About Incest 8"

46. Pusey, "Mechanisms of Inbreeding Avoidance in Nonhuman Primates."

47. Alison Motluk, "Close Family Smells Worse than a Stranger," *Daily News*, August 22, 2002, http://www.newscientist.com/article/dn2705-close-family-smells-worse-than-a-stranger.html#.VKMWBSgzfTI.

48. Motluk, "Close Family Smells Worse than a Stranger."

49. Randy Thornhill, Steven Gangestad, et al. "Major Histocompatibility Complex Genes, Symmetry, and Body Scent Attractiveness in Men and Women," *Behavioral Ecology* 14 (2003): 668–78.

50. It was necessary for me to clarify if intrafamilial immune systems are in fact more similar. I posed the question to Stanford professor, Paul Bollyky. His email reply follows: "Yes, genetically coded variation in immune responses exists and is heritable. You probably have an immune system that is more similar to your sibling's immune systems than it is to your cousins'. This is best understood in the context of the genes involved in organ transplantation rejection, the MHC (major histo-compatability complex) genes. You're much more likely to be able to accept a kidney from a brother than from a cousin. However, the kidney from your cousin is still likely to be a better immunologic "fit" than the one from a stranger.I hope this helps. All the best, Paul."

51. Roly Fletcher and Martin Milton, "Being Aggressive: An Existential Phenomenological Critique on the Psychological Literature on Human Aggression," accessed 2015, http://www.academia.edu/1108345/Being_Aggressive_An_existential-phenomenological_critique_of_the_psychological_literature_on_Human_Aggression.

52. Cited in J. Kroth, *Psychology Underground,* (2001) Columbus, OH: Academic Renewal Press.

53. Robert Ardrey, *The Territorial Imperative,* (New York: Atheneum, 1966), 224.

54. Ardrey, *The Territorial Imperative,* 222.

55. Kroth, *Psychology Underground,* (2001) Columbus, OH: Academic Renewal Press, 141–222.

56. Ewen Callaway, "Genghis Khan's Genetic Legacy Has Competition," *Nature,* January 23, 2015.

57. Callaway, "Genghis Khan's Genetic Legacy Has Competition."

58. Carl Jung, *Psychological Reflections.* (Princeton, NJ: Princeton University Press, 1977), 60.

59. Dale Peterson and Richard Wrangham, *Demonic Males: Apes, and the Origin of Human Violence* (New York: Mariner Books, 1997), 115.

60. Peterson and Wrangham, *Demonic Males,* 115.

61. Peterson and Wrangham, *Demonic Males,* 114.

62. Peterson and Wrangham, *Demonic Males,* 114.

63. Peterson and Wrangham, *Demonic Males,* 114.

64. Robin Baker, *Sperm Wars,* (London: Fourth Estate, 1996), http://www.robin-baker.com/books/sperm-wars/.

65. "Poll, American Sex Survey," October 21, 2004, ABC Newshttp://abcnews.go.com/Primetime/PollVault/story?id=156921&page=8.

66. "Poll, American Sex Survey."

67. "Who Says only Sperm Gets the Prize," *Science News,* January 30, 1999, 155.

68. Robert Ardrey, *The Territorial Imperative,* (New York: Atheneum, 1966), 224.

69. Lionel Tiger, *Men in Groups,* (1971) New York: Transaction, 63–65.

70. Tiger, *Men in Groups,* 63–65.

71. Tiger,*Men in Groups,* 152.

72. Robert Ardrey, *The Territorial Imperative,* (New York: Atheneum, 1966), 107.

73. Kroth, *Psychology Underground,* 182.

74. Ardrey, *The Territorial Imperative,* 107.

75. Kroth, *Psychology Underground,* 80.

76. Kroth, *Psychology Underground,* 181.

77. Tiger, *Men in Groups,* 232.

78. Stan Cohen, *America's Home Front During World War II,* 1991, http://www.ameshistory.org/exhibits/events/rationing.htm.

79. "Civil Defence During World War II," BBC History, accessed 2015http://www.bbc.co.uk/history/topics/civil_defence_ww2.

80. Kroth, *Psychology Underground,* 183.

81. "Murder Suspect in Court," *San Jose Mercury News,* November 25, 1998.

82. Kagan, *The Psychological Immune System,* 85.

83. J. Dennen and V. Falger, eds., *Sociobiology and Conflict: Evolutionary Perspectives on Competition, Cooperation, Violence and Warfare* London: Chapman and Hall, 1990,

accessedhttp://www.ukessays.com/essays/anthropology/anthropology-of-power-and-conflict.php#ixzz3FxSOnchb.

84. Bobbi Low, *Why Sex Matters: A Darwinian Look at Human Behavior,* (Princeton, NJ: Princeton University Press, 2000).

85. J. Gorebel and R. Hinde, *Aggression and War: Their Biological and Social Bases.* (London: Cambridge University Press, 2012).

86. D. Norris, J.W. Ngambi, et al., "Genetic Selection for Docility," *Journal of Animal and Plant Sciences*, 24 (2014): 13–18.

87. Randy Nelson, ed., *Biology of Aggression* (Oxford: Oxford University Press, 2006). See also: Randy Nelson and Silvana Chiavegatto, "Molecular Basis of Aggression," *Trends in Neurosciences* 24, no. 12 (2001): 713–19

88. Nelson, ed., *Biology of Aggression*.

89. Tiger, *Men in Groups*, 134–35.

90. Tiger, *Men in Groups*, 134–35.

91. Tiger, *Men in Groups*, 298.

92. Ardrey, *The Territorial Imperative*, 340.

93. Ardrey, *The Territorial Imperative*, 344.

94. Kroth, *Psychology Underground*, 174.

95. Ardrey, *The Territorial Imperative*, 340.

96. Ardrey, *The Territorial Imperative*, 345.

97. "On the Naming of Sports Teams I: Animals and Birds," accessed 2015 http://onscreen-scientist.com/?p=670.

98. "Media Coverage of Women in Sport," NSW Sport and Recreation, accessed 2015http://www.dsr.nsw.gov.au/assets/pubs/industry/info_mediawomen.pdf.

99. Thomas Campbell, "World Cup Final Breaks Records Worldwide for TV Broadcasters, July 14, 2014, http://www.iptv-news.com/2014/07/world-cup-final-breaks-records-worldwide-for-tv-broadcasters/.

100. Nathan Pinger, "Home Field Advantage: The Facts and the Figures," *Business*. March 4, 2014.

101. N. Neave and S. Wolfson, "Testosterone, Territoriality, and the 'Home Advantage," *Physiological Behavior*, 2 (2003): 169–75

102. Dominic Johnson and Monica Duffy Toft, "Grounds for War: The Evolution of Territorial Conflict, *Journal of International Security* 38 (2014): 7–38.

103. John Bargh and Ezequiel Morsella, "The Unconscious Mind," *Perspectives in Psychological Science*, 3 (2008): 73–79.

SIX

The *Innate* Psychic Immune System

Cooperation, Nonviolence, and Reciprocal Altruism

The next "hard-wired," innate constituent of the psychic immune system is quite the opposite of territoriality and dominance, namely cooperation, altruism, and even compassion.

COOPERATION, NONVIOLENCE, AND ALTRUISM

Human beings are organized in ways which enhance survival beyond dominance and predation. Husbands protect wives. Families protect children. Police protect neighborhoods. Armies protect nations. All of these social inventions work toward the preservation of the individual, the group, the nation, and the species.

Self-preservation through the survival-of-the-fittest Rambo paradigm is certainly one model most are familiar with, but it is not the only strategy species develop. Cooperation, non-violence, altruism, and peace-making is quite another and may be just as instinctive as the dominant male-aggressive predisposition—striking parallels of which can also be found in the animal kingdom.

Author David Rakoff says "Altruism is innate, but it's not instinctual. Everybody's wired for it, but a switch has to be flipped."[1] Physician Lewis Thomas stretches that argument to include wide swaths of the animal kingdom: "Animal have genes for altruism, and those genes have selected in the evolution of many creatures because of the advantage they confer for the continuing survival of the species."[2]

Strength in Numbers

Numerous animal species behave in collective and cooperative ways which augment and insure survival, red deer, chimpanzees, honeybees, African buffalos, baboons, and even cockroaches, to name a few.[3]

> A team of researchers presented 50 roaches with three shelters, each of which could hold 50 individuals. Since roaches prefer dark to light, they quickly divided into groups and fled into shelters. But rather than behaving chaotically, the roaches split into groups of 25, half filling two shelters and leaving the third empty. When larger shelters were introduced, the roaches formed a single group in just one of them.[4]

Cockroaches aggregate for a reason. Red monkeys group together collectively in a process called "mobbing" in which they form a large cluster and place themselves between predators in order to ward off attacks by chimpanzees. When goshawks try to attack pigeons, pigeons quickly morph into coveys which discourage the predator. This same rationale holds true for schools of fish, birds, even ant colonies.[5] Cooperation, in fact, may be an even more dominant trait in the animal kingdom than dominance and predation.

When bats fail to find sufficient blood on an evening's hunt, other bats, which were more successful, regurgitate blood and donate to other members of their troop. In bird species, other "helper" birds often protect the nest and help feed the youngsters while the parents are elsewhere.

Among primates, the bonobos are less hierarchically organized, and among the muriqui, the largest monkey in South America, there is no alpha male, no social rank, no dominance relationships, not even status seeking. Cooperative behavior in the animal kingdom is far more widespread than generally believed.[6]

Experimental Studies of Altruism

An interesting experiment on female chimpanzees presented seven chimps with a bucket containing thirty tokens. The tokens were color-coded and one color resulted in a "selfish outcome" while the other benefitted another chimp in a nearby compartment. The rewards were made up of banana slices wrapped in butcher paper that made a very loud sound when unwrapped.

> The chimp participants *nearly always chose the tokens that would yield food rewards for both the selector and the nearby observing chimp.* They would do this with or without solicitation from the chimp bystander, who could smell the bananas and hear the tantalizing paper unwrapping.[7]

Christophe Boesch, director of Primatology at the Max Planck Institute of Evolutionary Anthropology argues. . . .

> All studies with wild chimpanzees have amply documented that they share meat and other food abundantly, that they help one another in highly risky situations, like when facing predators or neighboring communities, and adopt needing orphans.[8]
>
> . . . all mammals, at least to some extent, can show empathy-based concern for others. Associated traits must have therefore emerged very early in mammalian evolution. . . . Cooperation—where individuals work together in order to create a benefit for an entire group—seems at odds with what many people assume are the basic forces of evolution. After all, it's a jungle out there, only the strongest survive, humans are selfish, etc.[9]

Primate studies confirm chimpanzees, which experience the death of a loved one, often preen the corpse and sometimes howl a long distress call. Mothers will hold a dead child and groom it for more than a week, and when attendants attempt to remove it, vigilant fights break out to prevent the removal of the dead animal.[10]

A more recent study reported by Japanese professor Michio Nakamura reveals a mother chimp carrying her disabled child who had the equivalent of Downs Syndrome. Not only was the child carried everywhere by her mother, since it couldn't walk, but the mother's sister also cared for it.[11]

Increasingly scientists are turning away from this single-minded view of evolution. Danny Grunbaum, an oceanographer at the University of Washington believes the role of violence and aggression in evolution is overestimated. Often we view documentaries, he opines, that show animals like elephant seals fighting each other, but "we're really seeing only a very small sliver of time. Much more of the time they're accommodating each other and respecting where the boundaries are—and that's cooperation. There is a tremendous amount of cooperation in nature."[12]

In the human gut there are colonies of *E. coli*, and when the colony is attacked by a virus, a "protective layer of cells forms which takes the brunt or attack while the cells beneath it survive."[13] The strategy is clearly an organized effort to immunize and protect some segments of the colony while sacrificing others. In effect this is a form of bacterial altruism.

Honeybees act similarly when a bee whose assigned job is to detect and ward off intruders. It actually stings the intruder; it protects the hive and the community, but the downside is that the stinging bee dies after attacking the intruder. So to add to bacterial altruism we note honeybee martyrdom.[14]

The South Dakota prairie dog and the Asian gerbil are remarkable in social structure and communication systems. When a predator approaches, rapid thumping goes on underground, a thumping which changes into whistles and alters frequencies as the predator closes in. When one prairie dog signals, so do others similarly alert the entire community. In one season of fifty-eight prairie dog offspring born, only one lost its life to a predator, a remarkable success story for social communication in the prairie dog city-state.[15]

Vervet monkeys shout out alarm calls to warn fellow members of the troop of an approaching predator, even though the monkey doing the screeching attracts attention and increases the risk of being attacked.

> In social insect colonies (ants, wasps, bees and termites), sterile workers devote their whole lives to caring for the queen, constructing and protecting the nest, foraging for food, and tending the larvae. Such behaviour is maximally altruistic: sterile workers obviously do not leave any offspring of their own—so have personal fitness of zero—but their actions greatly assist the reproductive efforts of the queen.[16]

Altruistic behavior, particularly warnings that attract predators, ought to reduce the chances of survival for the altruistic individual. But altruistic behavior reveals that group survival is very much part of the equation and indeed a phylogenetic self-preservative instinct can be found throughout the animal kingdom:

> To see this, imagine that some members of a group of vervet monkeys give alarm calls when they see predators, but others do not. Other things being equal, the latter will have an advantage. By selfishly refusing to give an alarm call, a monkey can reduce the chance that it will itself be attacked, while at the same time benefiting from the alarm calls of others. So, we should expect natural selection to favour those monkeys that *do not give alarm calls* over those that do. But this raises an immediate puzzle. How did the alarm-calling behaviour evolve in the first place, and why has it not been eliminated by natural selection? How can the existence of altruism be reconciled with basic Darwinian principles?[17]

The answer seems clear. The warning may risk the life of the individual, but it enhances the survival of the group, and even Darwin argued natural selection favors this heroic phylogenetic trait.

Studies on social communication, empathy, altruism, nonviolence, and cooperation in the animal kingdom may be recent, but the findings add a whole new light to the understanding of how nature works. Evolutionary biologists suggest that cooperation may be the most beneficial behavior evidenced on the planet.

> We literally would not be here without it. . . . Ants that march to the same drummer move faster. Fish rid other fish of harmful bacteria for a free meal. Small birds protect each other from predators. . . . If and when you're looking for it, you will never see an ant stuck in traffic. . . . As many as 200,000 ants a day pour out of their nest in search of food, splitting into two groups to form two outgoing lanes; they return in a single center lane, sometimes carrying more than 30,000 edible grasshoppers or other insects . . . the ultra-cooperative ability of these sim-

> plistic organisms arises from living in large groups for millions of years.[18]

When a predator enters the territory of a bird known as a flycatcher, the flycatcher will screech loudly. This is a risky move because it attracts the predator's attention; however, with that call, flycatchers then mob and the large conglomeration of birds scares the predator away.

Biologist Gerald Wilkinson from the University of Maryland reports that bats have a unique system of food sharing. If a bat goes two nights without finding blood, it presents a risky circumstance:

> Adult bats fail to find blood eight percent of the time. Younger bats fail one night out of every three. But hunger is rare because bats that find blood share it with bats that don't. But they do this only as long as the favor is someday returned. *If a colony didn't share food, four out of every five bats would die each year. But by cooperating, the death rate is slashed to one in four.*[19]

Physicist Fritjof Capra summarizes this line of thinking, "Nature nurtures life through communities. . . . This is a process that started with the first single-celled organisms. Life, from its beginning more than three billion years ago, took over the planet by networking, not combat."[20] [21]

Fish school, or shoal, in massive fields of activity. The purpose of operating in a synchronized field has numerous advantages: it has a hydrodynamic efficiency, in the same way that geese flying in a V-formation provides for better flow through the atmosphere. Second, schooling fish are protected against predators in this manner, and often confuse the senses of predators by the sheer magnitude of the school. Additional advantages are that the school provides increased access to potential mates.[22]

The behavior of fish in a school has a marvelous sociology. A shoal of sardines can be as long as four miles long and one mile wide moving at a depth of one hundred feet. When threatened, sardines will instinctively group in massive balls up to twenty meters in diameter.

Likewise, herring swim in schools at impressive speeds. Sometimes the field makes startling changes in shape and speed, as if its motions were choreographed. When individual fish are removed from the school, they appear agitated and their respiration rates change markedly. The herring have been taken out of context and separated from the field to which they are organically connected. One recent study of herring found that a single school in the Atlantic Ocean consisted of *over a billion individual fish* occupying an area the size of Manhattan.

Fire ants actually create such a mass that they can behave together either like a fluid or a solid depending on the situation. Scientists at the American Physical Society showed a video of ants which poured out of a funnel like a thick syrup. Ants under stress can also form themselves into a rough ball which can change its shape as it is being pressed down.

> When the aggregation struggled to keep its shape, the ants clung to each other acting like an elastic solid, rubber for example. In bridge construction, for instance, interest is great in materials that automatically repair cracks. The ants are experts at this kind of repair. When they turn themselves into a bridge for other ants, which they do, they scramble to quickly repair breaks in any damage to the structure.[23]

The shoal of a billion herring moves according to a certain algorithm; it is also able to calculate ocean temperatures, to sense the ebb and flow of existing currents in the Gulf Stream, and to adapt *in the present* to hydrodynamic conditions. Sometimes the entire school speeds off with a velocity up to forty-three inches per second.[24] [25]

Sociobiology of Cooperation

One can clearly see the vast and incredible social organization of numerous animal species from ants, flycatchers, bats, chimpanzees, honeybees, prairie dogs, and herring; in each case, there is an instinctive basis for their altruistic and cooperative behavior.

The study of cooperation and altruism as related to species survival began about 1975 with the work of E. O. Wilson, a Harvard biologist. Many felt this work was

> the most important evolutionary theory since *On the Origin of Species.* Darwin's theory of Natural Selection and the "survival of the fittest" implied a Machiavellian world in which individuals clawed their way to the top. Wilson offered a new perspective, which was that certain types of social behaviors—including altruism—are often genetically programmed into a species to help them survive. In the context of Darwin's theory of "*every man for himself*" Natural Selection, this kind of selflessness or altruism did not compute. E.O. Wilson resolved the paradox with a "*one for all and all for one*" theory called "kin selection." According to the kin selection theory, altruistic individuals would prevail because the genes that they shared with kin would be passed on. . . . By the 1990s this had become a core concept of biology, sociology, even pop psychology.[26]

The Biology of Compassion and Empathy

A number of studies point to empathy, altruism, cooperation, and compassion equally as instinctive as territoriality and dominance. Jack Nitschke, a psychologist from the University of Wisconsin, reported an experiment where mothers were given pictures of their babies to look at. Their brains lit up in the place that pleasurable, reward centers usually light up. Conversely, two Princeton researchers measured brain activity when subjects contemplated *harm being done to others,* and, quite to their surprise, similar regions lit up. In other words, one's children and victims of violence represent two quite different categories of individuals, but they are quite "united by the similar neurological reactions they provoke. This consistency strongly suggests that compassion isn't simply a fickle or irrational emotion, but rather *an innate human response embedded into the folds of our brains. . . .*" (emphasis added)[27]

Neuroscientists James Rilling and Gregory Berns corroborate that in an interesting way. In an experiment participants were given an opportunity to help someone else while their brain activity was being recorded. When helping others, the caudate nucleus and anterior cingulate showed activity. These are the same regions that light up when people receive rewards or pleasure.

> This is a rather remarkable finding: *helping others brings the same pleasure we get from the gratification of personal desire.* The brain, then, seems wired up to respond to others' suffering—indeed, it makes us feel good when we can alleviate that suffering.
>
> . . . When we feel threatened, our heart and breathing rates usually increase, preparing us either to confront or flee from the threat—the so-called "fight or flight" response. What is the ANS (autonomic nervous system) profile of compassion? As it turns out, when young children and adults feel compassion for others, this emotion is reflected in very real physiological changes: Their heart rate goes *down* from baseline levels, which prepares them not to fight or flee, but to approach and soothe. . . . Then there's oxytocin, a hormone that floats through the bloodstream. Research performed on the small, stocky rodents known as prairie voles indicates that oxytocin promotes long-term bonds and commitments, as well as the kind of nurturing behavior—like care for offspring—that lies at the heart of compassion. It may account for that overwhelming feeling of warmth and connection we feel toward our offspring or loved ones.[28]

Two more neuroscientists, Philip Cohen and Ewen Callaway, corroborate these conclusions asserting that the anterior cingulate cortex and the anterior insula are "active not only when we are in pain *but when others are.*" Using imaging studies, they found a positive relationship between a subject's empathy for a person in pain and neurological activity in the pain processing areas of the brain of the volunteer. Philip Cohen asserts "Humans are hardwired to feel empathy."[29]

Shihui Han and colleagues took seventeen Chinese and sixteen Caucasian volunteers from the United States, Europe, and Israel. They were shown videos of strangers who were in pain. The strangers were both Chinese and Caucasian. While viewing the videos brain scans using fMRI were made and results showed that these subjects responded more empathically to the strangers of the same ethnicity or the same country.

> Their responses actually indicated they "[felt] each other's pain about equally. . . . Interestingly, our brains seem to be 'hardwired' to feel more for certain groups over others, whether we notice or not. These

> groups appear to consist of people we can identify more with, whether through ethnicity, age, gender, or any other in-group. . . .
>
> Empathy is more pronounced the more similar you are to someone, the more close, socially close, you are to someone." He continues to say that empathy "evolved . . . for members of any species that is cooperative and social . . . it's important to take care of others in the group because you depend on [them], you survive by [them].
>
> While we seem to be hardwired to empathize more with certain groups over others, we're still united as a species to empathize with one another. . ."[30]

Studies of infants as old as seventy-two hours following birth were exposed to the sound of another infant crying. Reflexive crying—known as emotional contagion—predictably occurred.[31]

A subsequent study exposed newborns to another infant crying versus a variety of other stimuli (white noise or non-human cry sounds). The infants showed distress reactions to the cries of another infant more than any other stimuli.[32]

With respect to nurturance, breastfeeding and massage elevate oxytocin levels in humans. So does eating chocolate. When people engage in compassionate activities, (warm smiles and friendly gestures, they actually produce more oxytocin.

> Being compassionate causes a chemical reaction in the body that motivates us to be even more compassionate. . . . Primates such as great apes spend hours a day grooming each other, even when there are no lice in their physical environment. They use grooming to resolve conflicts, to reward each other's generosity, and to form alliances. . . . Certain touches can trigger the release of oxytocin, bringing feelings of warmth and pleasure. The handling of neglected rat pups can reverse the effects of their previous social isolation, going as far as enhancing their immune systems.[33]

One experiment injected subjects with oxytocin while controls got no such infusion. Those with ocytocin were 80 percent more likely to be generous than those not receiving the trust boost.[34]

Contagious yawning is still another symptom which flavors the debate on empathy. Chimpanzees show evidence of contagious yawning, indicating that they are aware of other's feelings. Dogs engage in contagious yawning far more if their owners yawn than when a stranger does, suggesting that "empathy and emotional proximity were the more likely factors."[35] Humans evidence this trait too, but it is seen less in autistic children and schizophrenics, both of whom have impaired empathic skills.

Social psychologists refer to empathy as "resonance," which they define as the mirroring of emotional expressions of another person. Contagious yawning and laughing are both examples. In schizophrenics, as you might expect, resonance is diminished and shows lower contagion rates.[36]

Oxytocin, Fight-Flight and Cortisol

Earlier, we discussed how stress hormones, cortisol and adrenaline flow during fight-flight, but the opposite process occurs with the "cooperation" hormone oxytocin. It is released liberally during childbirth and

> overflows as we look into the eyes of our newborn. It is also released in abundance with orgasm, laughter, play, hugging and giving. It's the twinkle in your eyes and the smile on your face hormone! Yes! The peace, love and granola anti-aging hormone! . . . Not surprisingly, oxytocin and cortisol have a love-hate relationship. Oxytocin and cortisol oppose each other. They are the two boxers in a ring, or the two kids on a seesaw. When one goes up, the other is forced to go down.[37]

The emerging field of "peace ethology" argues that competition and violence are not the trademarks of the animal kingdom, but cooperation is. As one author argues, animals fight and occasionally serious harm or kill one another, but the dominant paradigm is "predominantly prosocial . . . for many nonhuman primates, more than 90 percent of their interactions are affiliative rather than competitive or divisive."[38]

A recent study from behavioral genetics echoes that there is an innate basis for altruism and cooperation. Researchers focused on the COMT gene which is alleged to influence neurotransmitters in the brain. Participants were required to memorize a set of numbers and then try to repeat them correctly. When they completed the memory test, they received five Euros. After the test, the real experiment began rather surreptitiously. The subjects were shown an ad for a charity, the picture of a child named Lina from Peru who was holding a bracelet she had knitted.

> The experimenters left the room and told the participants they could anonymously donate to the charity some or all of the money they'd earned, though the experimenters were actually able to keep track of how much money each person gave . . . people with either of two of the variations of the COMT gene . . . *donated twice as much money to the charity as people with the other variation (called Met/Met), regardless of their gender*. . . . In fact, more than 20 percent of the people with the altruistic variations donated all of their money.[39]

However unexpected that may seem, a genetic or heritable basis for altruism seems a plausible conclusion.

A recent scientific text in evolutionary biology titled *Survival of the Nicest* suggests also that altruism is heritable.

> Humans are innately driven to cooperate, right down to the oxytocin that pours into the bloodstream when people witness acts of generosity. Oxytocin in turn promotes trust and good will, essential ingre-

> dients for sharing. We also come equipped with mirror neurons, brain cells that allow us to grasp and emulate other's emotions, laying the foundation for group responses aimed at the greater good.[40]

Cooperative and Altruistic Genes in Animals and Man

In an article from another avant-garde academic specialty, sociogenomics, researchers identified genetic contributions to how cooperative behavior is founded in both honeybees and fire ant colonies.[41] A specific gene, *Gp-9* plays a major role in social behavior and the nature of ant social organization.[42] *Amfor,* a foraging gene, regulates which bees will remain in the hive and which will become foragers. Within a hive there are genetic subpopulations, and of these, some cooperatively aggregate to protect the others.[43]

In a bee colony, when a single hornet enters the hive, it can kill up to forty bees a minute and can wipe out an entire colony of bees in about three hours. When this intruder enters the hive, five hundred worker bees will cooperatively surround it in a dense ball and vibrate their wings so that the temperature inside the hive rises to 116 degrees Fahrenheit. Hornets die at 114 degrees, so the frenzy of cooperative activity in the hive actually kills the intruder.[44] Behavioral geneticists show convincingly that cooperative behavior is not only related to survival but genetically influenced.[45]

Humans have these mechanisms too which are not only cooperative and affiliative but which provide a defensive immunity from threat.

> Families, clans, tribes, and nations also depend on this safety net when they are under attack and need to be defended by lots of group members. . . . We are not the only species that displays this characteristic . . . bears are most dangerous when their cubs are around; wolf packs act almost as one entity; lion prides defend their territory and each other; and the leader of a troop of chimpanzees depends on his coalition buddies to help him out when the going gets tough.[46]

Harman Kagan writes about Indians from New York State who spoke various dialects of Iroquois. They formed a union called the "league of the Five Nations," including the Mohaw, Oneida, Onondaga, Cayuga and Seneca. Each individual was part of a nuclear family that, in turn, belonged to a household, "which lived with other households in a longhouse, which constituted part of a clan, which belonged to a moiety, which made up a tribe, which in turn was part of the League of the Iroquois."[47]

Human social organization often exists for protection and defense, and thus the psychic immune system has distinct prosocial, cooperative, collective, and altruistic features.

Human Altruism, Jung, and the Archetype of the Hero

Long before the revolution in genetics, Carl Jung put forward the concept of the collective unconscious which was populated by archetypes or universal collective psychic traits. Most relevant to our discussion of altruism is the archetype of the hero.

Joseph Campbell, a Jungian and a mythologist, in *A Hero with a Thousand Faces* showed that every culture has a concept of a hero, either real, mythical, or both. Despite many variations on this cross-cultural theme, one central aspect is that the hero is prepared to sacrifice himself or herself for the benefit of the group, the community, the nation, or even mankind. "A hero," says Campbell, "is someone who has given his life to something bigger than oneself."[48]

Hero figures can be quite real—Miguel Hidalgo, Joan of Arc, Alexander Nevsky, Guiseppe Garibaldi—or mythic (Superman, Luke Skywalker, Captain Marvel, Red Star, Aquaman, Goku, Batman, James Bond, or Dr. Light). All cultures have a psychic imprint of a figure who rescues them from danger. And sometimes heroes are not just dedicated to saving a family or similar kin, but humanity itself. Jesus Christ is an archetypal example of the latter.

What is central to Jung's concept is that the archetype is an *instinctual imprint*, which is to say that it is found in every human being. It is a collective, yet unconscious, trait, so, while many of us individually may not be up to the task, the impulse of altruistic giving, self-sacrifice, and heroism resides in each of us and can be thought of as autonomic and innate.

Some contemporary examples of this innate altruism reflex follow:

- An eight-year-old boy repeatedly ran into a burning trailer to save the life of six people while losing his own life in the process.[49]
- A Texas mother saw a car speeding toward her child; she shoved her child out of danger, but was hit by the vehicle.[50]
- A forty-year-old man saw a young boy struggling in the Hudson River. He dove in to save the six-year-old child and drowned. Thelma Martin experienced a heartbreaking mix of emotions, grateful her son was alive, but mourning her friend who died saving him.[51]
- A thirty-year-old mother in St. Louis saw an SUV speed up and jump a curve in front of a drugstore. The driver had pressed the gas instead of the brakes, and the vehicle was headed straight for the woman and her daughter. The mother pushed her ten-year-old daughter to safety, but in so doing was hit and died at the scene.[52]

Such stories are commonplace, and the actions appear more reflexive and instinctive than premeditated, similar to when a soldier, seeing a grenade, throws himself on it to spare his comrades the fate he must now endure.

These observations are not merely anecdotal. A group of Yale researchers found three hundred volunteers to read commentary by over fifty contemporary "heroes."

> These men and women had all received the Carnegie Hero Medal for "civilians who risk their lives to save strangers"; the experimenters wanted to know *whether they had acted without thinking* or after exerting "conscious self-control" in order "to override negative emotions like fear." . . . The volunteers . . . analyzed the medal winners' statements for evidence of careful thought, or of unpremeditated action. Overwhelmingly, they found that day-savers rescue first and reflect second. As Christine Marty, a 21-year-old student who wrested a trapped senior citizen from her car during a flash flood said, "I'm thankful I was able to act and not think about it." (emphasis added)[53]

To recall, this entire discussion actually started back on a submarine approaching the shores of Cuba in 1962. Three Soviet officers debated whether to fire their nuclear tipped torpedoes as they were being attacked by American depth charges. Their standing orders to fire the torpedoes were left standing.

Instead, Arkhipov, a junior officer, argued against acting as they were required. His stance saved the world, making him a hero in the most profound Jungian sense.

The question is whether Arkhipov was simply brilliant and articulate on that day—in convincing his superior officers not to fire—or whether some invisible altruistic force was operating. This is the central question this text is posing.

Is it possible all three Soviet officers had an innate connection to some positive force that coursed through their hearts and souls and pointed them in the proper direction of survival and peace. This force, moreover, *overruled* and over-rode their conscious obedience to the naval service, their training, their officer status, and their mental conditioning.

Is it possible in moments of the gravest threat, the psychic immune system plays a role in human behavior with the same autonomic action as the mother, who without thinking, throws herself in front of a speeding car to save her child's life?

THE INNATE AVERSION TO INTRASPECIES KILLING

The final candidate, or nominee, to consider for inclusion in the innate psychic immune system is, for lack of a better term, the innate aversion to killing one another. Certainly, there is a biological basis for engaging in war, aggression, territoriality, and dominance, and it is easily seen how similar conflicts flare up in the animal kingdom. The general public, however, tends to generally reject any possibility there may be a biological—read *instinctive*—basis for peace, nonviolence, compassion, cooperation, and altruism. These are generally considered virtues and manifestations of education, culture, and consciously-guided moral sensitivities, rather than some innate or genetically influenced predisposition.

However, in a review of literature on cooperation, altruism, and compassion, we recognized the genetic and innate basis for these virtues may be quite substantial.

But one can go further and posit an actual innate aversion to killing one's own kind? Recall Heinrich Himmler fainting at the site of the execution ditches he oversaw and designed. Is there a biological, physical, instinctive revulsion against murder and killing that is pre-programmed or hard-wired into every human being?

Perhaps that is too much for any empiricist to tackle, but a few military observers are willing to stand at attention on this issue. Dave Grossman, a psychologist and professor of military science, in his book, *On Killing: The psychological cost of learning to kill in war,* writes: "the vast majority of soldiers are loath to kill in battle. Unfortunately, modern armies . . . have developed sophisticated ways of overcoming this instinctive aversion."[54]

Military historian S. L. A. Marshall says about 75 percent of soldiers *never fired their weapon during combat*:

> they will not return fire during combat if left to their own devices . . . the man who can endure the mental and physical stresses of combat still has such an inner and usually unrealized resistance towards killing a fellow man . . . that he will not of his own volition take life if it is possible to turn away from that responsibility.[55]

This phenomenon did not go unnoticed by other scholars. Ardant de Picq wrote of it in 1946; John Keegan and Richard Holmes in the film *Soldiers* discussed the reluctance to fire. Paddy Griffith provides similar data in his analysis of extraordinarily low firing rates by soldiers in Napoleonic and American Civil War regiments.

> The FBI's studies of nonfiring rates among law enforcement officers in the 1950s and 1960s, and countless other individual and anecdotal observations, all confirm Marshall's fundamental conclusion that *human beings are not, by nature, killers.* Indeed, from a psychological perspective, the history of warfare can be viewed as a series of successively more effective tactical and mechanical mechanisms to enable or force combatants *to overcome* their resistance to killing other human beings, even when defined as the enemy.[56]

Perhaps this is why states have invented long-range artillery, drones, rockets, aerial bombing, and more effective ways of keeping at a safe distance from the killing so as not to emotionally confront the instinctual revulsion first hand.

The question that pops up is when faced with a life-or-death situation, why not use your weapon? In Gettysburg, over 27,574 abandoned muskets were recovered; 90 percent of them were still loaded.[57]

> So why didn't these soldiers use their weapons? Lt. Col. Dave Grossman . . . looked at this evidence and concluded "that there is within most men an intense resistance to killing their fellow man. A resistance so strong that, in many circumstances, soldiers on the battlefield will die before they can overcome it." In some ways this isn't all that surprising. Very few people would seek out an opportunity to kill others. At the same time, you may find it hard to believe that it is sometimes impossible for soldiers to kill others even when their own lives are at risk.[58]

Military mavens say basic training is really an attempt to benumb and decondition young men to act against this innate aversion to killing. They are placed into aggressive and stressful conditions in basic training.

> Their egos are broken down and rebuilt within the context of group unity and loyalty. The verbal abuse of the drill instructor, the firing drills, the hand-to-hand combat—all are intended to get them accustomed to violence. The shift in training has vastly improved the willingness of U.S. soldiers to fire their weapons in battle, from 55 percent in the Korean War to approximately 90 percent in Vietnam.[59]

Grossman believes the aversion to killing is deeply rooted in our minds "Intra-species killing or murder generally does not come naturally or easily . . . this is a well and reliably known fact, not merely a theorist's hopeful assuming."[60]

Anthropologist Paul Roscoe studying tribal behavior in New Guinea came to the same conclusion: humans have an "innate aversion to killing."[61]

Social psychologists in *Emotion* asked subjects to pull the trigger of an unloaded gun pointed at another person's face. Participants were also asked to "view" other simulations of aggression. Measures of blood pressure and heart rate, known measures of disgust and aversion, were taken. Heart rates and blood pressures during and after the harmful tasks were the highest. The notion of physically injuring someone directly in front of you creates a substantial moral dilemma: "And because our species thrived from cooperation, it's no wonder that we're programmed to avoid directly harming others. . . . People are averse to performing harmful actions and often consider it morally wrong to harm a person even when it would save many more lives."[62] Commentators outside of social psychology proffer the same hypothesis:

> Every species, with a few exceptions, has a hardwired resistance to killing its own kind in territorial and mating battles. When animals with antlers and horns fight one another, they head butt in a harmless fashion. But when they fight any other species, they go to the side to

> gut and gore. Piranhas will turn their fangs on anything, but they fight one another with flicks of the tail. Rattlesnakes will bite anything, but they wrestle one another. Almost every species has this hardwired resistance to killing its own kind.[63]

In view of the high level of gun ownership in the United States—270 million guns,[64] and the apparent addiction of adolescents to violent video games, the idea that human beings have an innate aversion to killing seems immensely counterintuitive, but data supporting this notion comes from several sources.

Currently, more than one hundred thousand Vietnam veterans have committed suicide, almost twice the number of combat casualties.[65] The rate of suicide among servicemen and women in 2015—in all wars, not just Vietnam—is twice that of the general population.[66]

There is also concern about high rates of post-traumatic stress disorder (PTSD) in the military. It is estimated that 30 percent of Vietnam vets, 10 percent of Gulf War veterans and 20 percent of troops serving in Afghanistan and Iraq suffered from PTSD, while others believe as many as 50 percent of Afghan and Iraqi veterans may have such emotional overlay.

The causes of at least some of this mental trauma may be a natural aversion to killing or maiming others.

> injuries are primarily the consequence of late adolescents/young adults having undergone the sophisticated psychological and emotional conditioning regimen of basic training/boot camp—being programmed to kill—and then, upon experiencing the horror and insanity—the reality—of war, suffering the realization of the moral gravity of their actions on the battlefield.[67]

It is well known in the media that exposure to seeing another person being killed is more than a mere traumatic event. There is both an empathic response and an almost vicarious PTSD reaction. Art Markman, a psychologist from the University of Texas, said that viewing shocking traumatic events visually, creates "a tear in the fabric of the viewer's life similar to what happens when that person is the victim of a crime or experiences a death in the family."

> Yesterday, we were faced with the decision of whether to watch the horrific burning death of Lt. Muath al-Kaseasbeh, the Jordanian pilot captured by ISIS. . . . I interned in NBC's Breaking News department during the summer of 2004—a summer that saw some of the earliest beheading videos, which Iraqi militants began to release at regular intervals as a warning to the Western forces fighting against them. I will never forget the day the first beheading video was released. I did not see it, but one of the senior producers in our unit, giving a casual glance at the wires—a routine part of any newsperson's job—had, and he bolted out of his office, his face an unearthly shade that fluctuated

> between white and green. . . . Minutes later, the executive director of News . . . told us he wanted us off the wires immediately. He said that we were all adults and clearly he couldn't tell us what to do, but he did not want us seeing these kinds of images and then having to live with their effects for the rest of our lives. "These kinds of things can't be unseen," he told us, "They will be a part of you always, and I can't let myself know I did that to you. . . . People who do not give themselves the time and space to heal from seeing traumatic images can suffer from symptoms of post-traumatic stress disorder," notes Markman, noting the often permanent effects that these kind of traumatic images can have on their viewers.[68]

A question has been raised: Is there a fundamental counterforce in primates and in human psychology that operates to avoid violence and bestows an instinctive revulsion to witness destruction of members of our own species? It turns out the innate reluctance to kill other humans may be as biologically rooted and important to survival as are collective tendencies toward dominance, aggression, territoriality, and war.

Indeed, there is remarkable evidence suggesting a biological predisposition for our species to collaborate on peaceful solutions to conflicts, and to work collectively to improve survival for ourselves and our progeny.

CONCLUSIONS ABOUT THE INNATE PSYCHIC IMMUNE SYSTEM

So far, we examined only the innate aspect of the psychic immune system. As a review here are the six basic elements or constituents of this powerful force:

1. Heritable predispositions to fight and flight
2. Genetic predispositions toward fear, happiness, optimism, and intelligence
3. Incest avoidance
4. Dominance, aggression, and territoriality
5. Cooperation, altruism, empathy
6. The aversion to intraspecies killing

These six innate building blocks constitute a formidable array of protective defense mechanisms, shields, and layers of insulation against danger and threat faced by ourselves as individuals and our species—all of them to some degree hard-wired by nature to accompany us throughout life.

Moreover, two systems appear to operate against each other in reciprocal fashion. While one innate predisposition fights for territory, dominance, and resources, we have an opposite, but similarly innate, inclination toward cooperation, altruism, and nonviolence. The curve goes up and goes down with a hidden rhythm that courses through the timeline of human history.

Nature and Nurture

When using the word "innate," the old nature-nurture debate resurfaces. How can it be asserted that empathy or altruism may be innate and biologically rooted when it is well known both are conditioned by education, culture, and training? It is also easy to observe how absent and empty these qualities are without proper parenting and nurturing.

Harvard psychologist, Steven Pinker, in *The Blank Slate* puts a new twist on the nature-nurture debate. Rather than seeing it as an either-or proposition, he argues that innate tendencies are shaped and grown through education and learning, and separating the two introduces a false dichotomy. His discussion on the innate nature of language is illustrative:

> Obviously no language is innate. Take any kid from any race, bring them up in any culture and they will learn the language equally quickly. So no particular language is in the genes, but what might be in the genes is the ability to acquire language. . . . Humans are so innately hardwired for language that they can no more suppress their ability to learn and use language than they can suppress the instinct to pull a hand back from a hot surface. . . . There has to be innate circuitry that does the learning, that creates the culture, that acquires the culture, and that responds to socialization.[69]

In this chapter, we outlined some hard-wired circuitry—programmed for protection and survival—that has been named the *innate* psychic immune system. However, this is only one part of the entire system.

The physical immune system also has an innate side, but it has other features and functions too. So if the psychic immune system mirrors the physical immune system—or is an epiphenomenon of it—it should be expected that the psychic immune system has other dimensions to it as well. In other words, the journey is not finished. There is more data to collect on this inscrutable, and so far invisible, hidden world.

NOTES

1. Brett Leveridge, "David Rakoff," Salon.com (2001) http://www.brettnews.com/clips/rakoff.html.
2. "Lewis Thomas Quotes on Gene," Today in Science History, accessed 2015http://todayinsci.com/T/Thomas_Lewis/ThomasLewis-Gene-Quotations.htm.
3. Russell McLendon, "7 Examples of Animal Democracy," Mother Nature Network, November 4, 2012, http://www.mnn.com/earth-matters/animals/photos/7-examples-of-animal-democracy/cockroaches.
4. McLendon, "7 Examples of Animal Democracy."
5. H. Ronald Pulliam, "On the Advantages of Flocking," *Journal of Theoretical Biology*, 38, February 1973.
6. Kroth, *Psychology Underground* (Columbus, OH: Academic Press, 2001).
7. "Chimpanzees Not as Selfish as We Thought," *Discovery News*, August 8, 2011, http://news.discovery.com/animals/chimps-share-110808.htm.

8. "Chimpanzees Not as Selfish as We Thought."
9. "Chimpanzees Not as Selfish as We Thought."
10. Maggie Koerth-Baker, "Want to Understand Mortality? Look to the Chimps." *New York Times*, June 25, 2013.
11. "Japan Researchers Find Chimps Caring for Disabled Infant," Phys.Org, November 11, 2015, http://phys.org/news/2015-11-japan-chimps-disabled-infant.html.
12. Jeremy Smith and Alex Dixon, "Birds Do It. Bats Do It." The Greater Good (2009), http://greatergood.berkeley.edu/article/item/birds_do_it_bats_do_it.
13. Harman Kagan, *The Psychological Immune System* (Bloomington, IN: Author House, 2006), 20.
14. "Honey Bee Facts That You Probably Never Knew," accessed 2015, http://www.benefits-of-honey.com/honey-bee.html.
15. Kroth,*Psychology Underground.*
16. "Biological Altruism," Stanford Encyclopedia of Philosophy, 2013, http://plato.stanford.edu/entries/altruism-biological/.
17. "Biological Altruism."
18. Jeremy Smith and Alex Dixon, "Birds do it. Bats do it." *The Greater Good* (2009). http://greatergood.berkeley.edu/article/item/birds_do_it_bats_do_it.
19. Ibid.
20. Ibid.
21. A 2015 study by Erick Greene, a professor of biology at the University of Montana argues that species also "recognize the alarm signals of other species. Some can even eavesdrop on one another across classes." This expanded social network improves survival. Christopher Solomon, "When Birds Squawk, Other Species Seem to Listen," *New York Times*, May 18, 2015.
22. U. Kils, (1992). "The ecoSCOPE and dynIMAGE: Microscale Tools for in situ Studies of Predator-prey Interactions," *Arch Hydrobiol Beih* 36: 83–96.
23. James Gorman, "Ants that Can Flow like a Fluid or Move like a Solid," *New York Times*, December 16, 2013.
24. D. V. Radkov, *Schooling in the Ecology of Fish* (New York: Halstead Press, 1973).
25. This same phenomenon has recently been detected in bacteria. See Tany Lewis, "Bacterial Vortex: Microbes' Odd Swimming Behavior Explained," (2014), http://news.yahoo.com/bacterial-vortex-microbes-odd-swimming-behavior-explained-130929149.html.
26. Christopher Bergland, "Evolutionary Biology of Altruism," *Psychology Today*, December 25, 2012.
27. Dacher Keltner, "The Compassionate Instinct," Greater Good, March 1, 2004 http://greatergood.berkeley.edu/article/item/the_compassionate_instinct#sthash.Uy8hyZ4H.dpuf.
28. Keltner, "The Compassionate Instinct."
29. "All About Empathy," The Nerve blog, (2010), http://sites.bu.edu/ombs/2010/07/24/all-about-empathy/ .
30. "All About Empathy."
31. Nicole McDonald and Danial Messinger, "The Development of Empathy," accessed 2015 http://www.psy.miami.edu/faculty/dmessinger/c_c/rsrcs/rdgs/emot/McDonald-Messinger_Empathy%20Development.pdf.
32. McDonald and Messinger, "The Development of Empathy."
33. Keltner, "The Compassionate Instinct."
34. Anne Moir, "Brainsexmatters," (2015), http://www.brainsexmatters.com.
35. Anahad O'Connor, "The Claim: Yawning is Contagious Between Dogs and their Owners," *New York Times*, August 21, 2013.
36. H. Haker and W. Rossler, "Empathy in Schizophrenia: Impaired Resonance," *Eur Arch Psychiatry Clin Neurosci*, September 6, 2009.
37. Anna Cabneca, "Why Do I Feel Disconnected? The Cortisol-oxytocin Connection," accessed 2015, http://www.saragottfriedmd.com/why-do-i-feel-disconnected-the-cortisol-oxytocin-connection/.

38. Mark Bekoff, "Give Peace a Chance: We Do Not Have to Go to War," *Psychology Today*, March 14, 2013, http://www.psychologytoday.com/em/120246.

39. Graham Thompson, Peter Hurd, et al., "Genes Underlying Altruism," *Biology Letters*, October, 2013, http://rsbl.royalsocietypublishing.org/content/9/6/20130395.

40. "Stefan Klein, "Survival of the Nicest," *Science News*, January 10, 2015.

41. Fabio Manfredini, Oksana Rba-Grognuz, et al, "Sociogenomics of Cooperation and Conflict During Colony Founding in the Fire Ant Solenopsis Invicta," Plos, August 8 2013, DOI: 10.1371/journal.pgen.1003633.

42. Manfredini, Rba-Grognuz, et. al, "Sociogenomics of Cooperation and Conflict."

43. Warren Leary, "In Defense of the Hive," *New York Times*, May 21, 1991.

44. Harman Kagan, *The Psychological Immune System*, (Bloomington, IN: Author House, 2006).

45. Greg Hunt, Gro Amdan, et al, "Behavioral Genomics of Honeybee Foraging," April, 2007, http://www.ncbi.nlm.nih.gov/pmc/articles/PMC1829419/.

46. Kagan, *The Psychological Immune System*, 133

47. Kagan, *The Psychological Immune System*, 134.

48. Joseph Campbell, accessed 2015, http://www.brainyquote.com/quotes/keywords/hero.html#MEraYqXVdHriSCO6.99.

49. "NY Town Mourns Brave 8-year-old Who Died Saving Six People from Trailer Fire," NBC News, January 22, 2014, http://usnews.nbcnews.com/_news/2014/01/22/22404421-ny-town-mourns-brave-8-year-old-who-died-saving-six-people-from-trailer-fire?lite .

50. KHOU staff, "Texan Mom Jumps in Front of Car to Save Child," KHOU.com, February 1, 2013, http://www.khou.com/story/news/local/texas/2014/07/22/11954144/ .

51. Marcus Solis, "Woman who Saved Man in Hudson River Speaks Out," WABC-TV, September 9, 2014, http://7online.com/news/woman-who-saved-child-in-hudson-river-speaks-out/298690/.

52. "Mother Gives Own Life to Save Daughter in Freak SUV Accident," Fox 8, September 23, 2014,http://myfox8.com/2014/09/23/mother-gives-own-life-to-save-daughter-in-freak-suv-accident/ .

53. Katy Waldman, "Is Anybody Watching my Do-Gooding," Slate, October 20, 2014, http://www.slate.com/articles/health_and_science/medical_examiner/2014/10/psychology_of_heroism_and_altruism_what_makes_people_do_good_deeds.html .

54. Dave Grossman, *On Killing: The Psychological Cost of Learning to Kill in War and Society*, 2009, http://www.amazon.com/On-Killing-Psychological-Learning-Society/dp/0316040932 .

55. S. L. A. Marshall, *Men Against Fire: The Problem of Battle Command*, 2000 http://www.amazon.com/Men-Against-Fire-Problem-Command/dp/0806132809 .

56. Dave Grossman, "Aggression and Violence," Killology research group, 2000, http://www.killology.com/article_agress&viol.htm.

57. David Barsh, "Is There a War Instinct?" *Aeon*, October 15 2012, http://aeon.co/magazine/society/human-beings-do-not-have-an-instinct-for-war/ .

58. "The Psychology of Killing and the Origins of War," Smells Like Science, accessed 2015, http://smellslikescience.com/the-psychology-of-killing-and-the-origins-of-war/ .

59. Matthew Atkins, "The US Army's Ambitious Fight Against PTSD," *Science*, March 13, 2013, http://www.popsci.com/technology/article/2013-02/us-armys-ambitious-fight-against-ptsd .

60. P. Roscoe, (2007). "Intelligence, Coalitional Killing, and the Antecedents of War," *American Anthropologist*, 109, no. 3 (2007): 485–95.

61. Tom Weber, "Faulty Intelligence," *UMaine Today Magazine*, October, 2007, http://www.magarchive.umaine.edu/issues/v7i5/intelligence.html .

62. Sam Mcdougal, "Humans are Nicer than We Think," Motherboard, March 8, 2012, http://motherboard.vice.com/blog/humans-are-nicer-than-we-think .

63. "Killing is Unnatural," Killology Research Group, 2000, http://www.killology.com/art_trained_killing.htm .

64. Madeleine Morgenstern, "How Many People Own Guns and is Gun Ownership Declining?" *The Blaze*, March 19, 2013, http://www.theblaze.com/stories/2013/03/19/how-many-people-own-guns-in-america-and-is-gun-ownership-actually-declining/ .

65. "Over 100,000 US Vietnam Suicides to Date!" Renze.com, 2007 http://rense.com/general77/hdtage.htm .

66. Military Suicides 50% Higher than the General Population (CBS news, June 16, 2015).

67. Philos1, "Beyond PTSD: The Moral Casualties of War,"Daily Kos, June 15, 2007,http://www.dailykos.com/story/2007/06/15/346934/-Beyond-PTSD-the-Moral-Casualties-of-War-Part-2 .

68. Jennifer Uffalussy, "ISIS Beheadings, Plane Crashes: Why We Should Avoid Images That Can't Be Unseen," *Yahoo Health*, February 4, 2015, https://www.yahoo.com/health/isis-beheadings-plane-crashes-why-we-should-110078169512.html .

69. Steven Pinker cited on "Its' a Kids World, " PBS, Scientific American Frontiers, episode 505, http://www.pbs.org/saf/transcripts/transcript505.htm.

SEVEN

The *Adaptive* Psychic Immune System

In 1918, the Spanish flu pandemic spread throughout the United States killing more people than were lost in World War I, yet older people did surprisingly well. They previously encountered a milder version of the virus and thus had a stronger immune response. Prior exposure to a physical illness confers immunity, and thus it is called *adaptive* immunity. Does experience, learning, or prior exposure to a psychological threat or trauma confer a similar adaptive *psychological* immunity? This is an area psychologists call "resilience" or "hardiness," and the field is quite new.

RESILIENCE: "BEEN THERE, DONE THAT"

For example, one might assume that older individuals have been through dozens of hoops, while younger persons are still cutting their teeth. The senior, therefore, may benefit from a lower incidence of depression, mental illness, or stress because they have experienced it, learned to cope, and thus have a higher level of resilience.

There is empirical evidence to support this belief. One study found less anxiety in older adults compared to younger persons;[1] another showed older adults had lower levels of depression, despite the fact that they are far more prone to pain, debilitating illness, and the prospect of death.[2] A National Health Survey reports males over the age of sixty have lower rates of depression than younger men.[3] "Despite losses and physical decline, older adults report feeling content and have less psychopathology than the remainder of the population. This is thought to be due to resilience, the successful adaptation to adversity."[4]

This is very close to a concrete example of the clear and effective operation of the *adaptive* psychic immune system. However, other studies dispute the survey's conclusions and report high levels of suicide, depression, PTSD-proneness, and anxiety in older adults.[5] [6] The most recent study on the subject (2016) reveals that suicide rates in the United States have reached their highest levels in thirty years across all demographics save one, seniors over the age of sevent-five.[7]

Despite detractors, polls consistently reveal a U-shaped curve with those at the very youngest and oldest ages (eighty-two to eighty-five) reporting the highest levels of happiness.[8] A 2014 *Scientific American* article may have resolved the dilemma. It reports that after controlling for health, ethnicity, education, and relationship success, researchers found a feeling of well-being indeed increases with age, suggesting that resilience and the adaptive psychic immune system play a strong role.[9] In other words, learning how to survive tough life experiences seems to inoculate people to a variety of mental illnesses and increase their feeling of well-being.

Resilience and Psychological Immunity

The term "resilience" is easily intelligible and closely related to "immunity." It refers to an individual's ability to withstand trauma, stress, and myriad other psychological challenges. One study on resilience showed that younger adolescents reacted more to stressors than older children.[10] A second study looked at adults over the age of sixty-four and compared them to those under the age of twenty-six. Once again, older adults showed superior skills in problem solving and emotional regulation.[11]

People past the age of sixty-five have experienced significant personal losses with 14 percent of men and 45 percent of women surviving the death of a spouse.[12] Precisely because of these negative life events, their level of resilience—one might even call it "acquired immunity"—increases.

Clinical psychologist G. A. Bonnano of Columbia University is perhaps the nation's leading expert on human resilience. His work shows resilience is a clear outcome following a person's recovery from trauma and loss, and such acquired immunity "is more common than is often believed."[13]

Bereaved parents, spouses, and caregivers of a chronically ill life-partner were compared to a sample of non-bereaved counterparts. The exposed individuals were found to be significantly better adjusted than nonexposed caregivers. In short, one group had much better "psychological immunity."[14]

In correspondence with Professor Bonnano, I asked if he believed a psychic immune system existed for an individual,[15] and if his concept of "resilience" fit the paradigm. His email reply is instructive:

> People who are trained about what to expect when engaged in highly stressful events (e.g., firefighters, EMTs) have less PTSD as a group, so wouldn't prior experience confer the same benefit on people in general? The evidence seems to suggest that prior experience with a stressor does in fact help people next time they confront a stress, but *only if it's the same kind of event.*[16]

Bonnano asserts a psychic immunity exists, but does not generalize, contending it remains peculiar to the type of stressor previously encountered. Two authors advance his point of view in an article in *Molecular Psychiatry*:

> A mildly stressful episode may immunize the individual, thereby strengthening resistance to subsequent stressors. This phenomenon is often viewed as a form of behavioral immunization . . . based on accumulated new data, we suggest that the immunological memory does have a significant role in developing coping responses to stress. Therefore, we propose . . . an immunological mechanism which establishes stress resilience to a later challenge.[17]

Bonnano cautions that our adaptive psychic immunity is *specific*. If we receive a flu shot, we have an acquired immunity to a *particular variety* of influenza, but not to pneumonia or poison oak. Immunity appears to work the same way in the psychic immune system. If one has an acquired resilience to a certain type of traumatic event, like the loss of a loved one, that experience confers resistance to a subsequent bereavement. However, such immunity to loss doesn't help them cope with surviving a rape, an assault, a robbery, or other new traumas.

As we know, the physical adaptive immune system possesses "immunological memory." Antibodies developed to fight off a prior illness still protect if the infection returns. The parallel example with the psychic immune system involves learning and experience. One learns from prior traumatic experiences and becomes resilient to subsequent traumas in the psychic sphere just as there is an immunological memory of a prior antigen in the physical arena.

An addendum to this adventure requires a caveat that research of the topic we're investigating is very much in its infancy. Most of the studies cited on the psychological immune system and resilience are less than fifteen years old.

EPIGENES: ADAPTIVE PSYCHIC IMMUNITY AND INHERITANCE?

Carl Jung made a curious remark, "Who has realized that history is not contained in thick books, but lives in our very blood."[18] Is it possible that our parent's psychological suffering left them with some acquired resistances, and these could be passed on to us? Or, to the contrary, do we have to learn by trial and error all over again and all by ourselves? In other words, for those hard-fought battles parents faced and got through, is anything ever passed on *naturally or biologically,* or is it just through learning, and dad warning us not to make the same mistakes he made, that we make the appropriate adaptations? Prepare for a deeply counter-intuitive adventure.

A curious experiment was performed recently on mice that shook the academic world to its foundations. Researchers took an odor, acetophenone, a scent compared to cherries and almonds, and exposed male mice to it while giving them small electric shocks. He conditioned the animals to associate the scent with pain.

In an article published in *Nature Neuroscience,* the authors show that the aversion to this scent was passed on to their pups. They "shuddered" in the presence of acetophenone, even without a shock.

> Despite never having encountered acetophenone in their lives, the offspring exhibited increased sensitivity when introduced to its smell, shuddering more markedly in its presence compared with the descendants of mice that had been conditioned to be startled by a different smell or that had gone through no such conditioning. A third generation of mice—the "grandchildren"—*also inherited this reaction,* as did mice conceived through *in vitro* fertilization with sperm from males sensitized to acetophenone. Similar experiments showed that the response can also be transmitted down from the mother.[19]

How is that Possible?

This insinuation that inheritance of acquired characteristics is genetic, is evolutionary blasphemy. In days of old, the inheritance of acquired characteristics, an approach to evolution espoused by Lamarck, was utterly discredited. If one's parents were accomplished pianists, it did not mean that the offspring inherited any genetically transmitted musical aptitude. Well, say hello to the new kid on the block, epigenetics.

To our surprise, there are numerous studies that imply *adaptive traits* can be passed to subsequent generations.

> For plenty of obvious reasons, modern biological science has never been big on the idea of "genetic or ancestral" memories . . . e.g., the Jungian collective unconscious . . . and yet . . . epigenetic modifications . . . do seem to suggest that our ancestors' experiences can affect the biological development, and thus the minds of future generations . . . for more than a century, the whole Lamarck debate . . . seemed to be settled, but lately, it looks like some elements of Lamarckism may be making a surprise comeback in the new field of epigenetics, the study of gene changes caused by chemical factors other than modification to the DNA sequence itself.
>
> Epigenetic memory comes in various guises, but one important form involves histones, the proteins around which DNA is wrapped. Particular chemical modifications can be attached to histones and these

> modifications can then affect the expression of nearby genes, turning them on or off. . . . This has been shown in subsequent generations of plants which were exposed to extended periods of cold, and also demonstrated in how a mouse's environment can "affect the memory capacity it passes on to its descendants."[20]

Epigenetics proffers that experience or learning does not change DNA, but that learning influences how genetic information is expressed, turned on or turned off. Described further in *Advances in International Psychology*, the environment impacts cellular modifications that can be transmitted inter-generationally, the outcomes of which appear to last. The common belief was that environment and learning only impacted the current generation, but it now appears that strong environmental events can

> leave an imprint on the genetic material in both egg and sperm and thereby short circuit evolution and pass the trait to the next generation. . . . The change *does not occur in the genetic material,* but rather on the cellular material placed on top of the gene that tells the gene to switch on or off. These epigenetic changes represent the biological reactions to extreme environmental events.[21] A growing body of evidence suggests that environmental stresses can cause changes in gene expression that are transmitted from parents to their offspring, making "epigenetics" a hot topic. (emphasis added)[22]

The consummately important discovery seems to be that one generation can produce reverberations and echoes in a subsequent generation, contradictory to virtually everything biologists have taken as gospel for more than a century.[23] Epigenetics is the rock star of neuroscience today as highlighted in a flurry of new publications. There has been a tenfold increase only in the last decade of publications using the term "epigenetic" in their title. "Only in 2011 the figure of publications in the field had reached the astonishing amount of several thousands, possibly up to twenty thousand depending on the search criteria and at any rate has continued to increase since then."[24]

Evidence from Fat, Cancer-Prone, Yellow Mice

In 2006, two professors of radiation oncology, Drs. Jirtle and Waterland, performed a revolutionary genetic experiment. They took pairs of fat yellow mice which are named "agouti mice" because they carry the agouti gene which makes them ravenous, yellow, and prone to cancer and diabetes. They wanted to change the genetic legacy of these animals, and they succeeded. When the mice bred, they were not yellow like their parents, nor prone to these diseases, and they were also brown.

> *The effects of the agouti gene had been virtually erased.* Remarkably, the researchers effected this transformation *without altering a single letter of the mouse's DNA.* Their approach instead was radically straightfor-

> ward—they changed the moms' diet. Starting just before conception, Jirtle and Waterland fed a test group of mother mice a diet rich in methyl donors, small chemical clusters that *can attach to a gene and turn it off*. These molecules are common in the environment and are found in many foods, including onions, garlic, beets, and in the food supplements often given to pregnant women. After being consumed by the mothers, the methyl donors worked their way into the developing embryos' chromosomes and onto the critical agouti gene. The mothers *passed along the agouti gene to their children intact*, but thanks to their methyl-rich pregnancy diet, they had added to the gene a chemical switch that dimmed the gene's deleterious effects. "It was a little eerie and a little scary to see how something as subtle as a nutritional change in the pregnant mother rat could have such a dramatic impact on the gene expression of the baby," Jirtle says. "The results showed how important epigenetic changes could be." (emphasis added)[25]

The Jirtle-Waterland experiment represented a milestone because it demonstrated that the epigenome is responsive to environmental cues. "More and more, researchers are finding that an extra bit of a vitamin, a brief exposure to a toxin, even an added dose of mothering can tweak the epigenome—and thereby alter the software of our genes—in ways that affect an individual's body and brain for life." [26]

Lessons from the Father Passed to the Son, Epigenetically

Christopher Pierce from the University of Pennsylvania reports that male rats whose fathers were exposed to cocaine chose to ingest less of the drug than rats whose fathers never took cocaine. Pierce believes this is an adaptive effect since cocaine is a toxin. In other words, the fathers passed down information to their pups that would help them survive and avoid the substance, and they did so biologically or, to be precise, epigenetically.[27]

> The fact that epigenetic changes happen in mammals is just amazing. Does this mean we as humans have also inherited generations of fears and experiences? Quite possibly, say scientists. Studies on humans suggest that children and grandchildren may have felt the epigenetic impact of such traumatic events such as famine, the Holocaust and the Sept. 11, 2001, terrorist attacks. Those are really powerful studies—unfortunately so, since the effects have been detrimental to subsequent generations. But because environmental factors for human subjects can't be controlled, it is difficult to parse out the effects of epigenetics alone. . . . We're still scratching the surface.[28]

Toxins and Epigenetics

Another dramatic study comes from a laboratory at Washington State University where Professor Michael Skinner exposed pregnant rats to an endocrine disruptor. They used a chemical which was an agricultural fungicide, vincozolin. However, the chemical did not impact sexual differentiation, but it did lower sperm counts and decreased fertility in male offspring.

> The study seemed like a bust. . . . By accident, though, Skinner's colleague had bred the *grandchildren* of those exposed rats, creating a fourth generation, *or the great-grandchildren of the original subjects.* . . . "It's OK," Skinner told her. "You might as well analyze them. . . ." If nothing else, he thought, the exercise might take her mind off her mistake. So she went ahead and studied the rats' testes under a microscope. . . . What they found would not only change the direction of Skinner's research but also challenge a bedrock principle of modern biology. And Skinner would become the forerunner of a new way of thinking about the possible long-term health consequences of exposure to environmental chemicals. . . .
>
> The strange thing about Skinner's lab rats was that three generations after the pregnant mothers were exposed to the fungicide, the animals had abnormally low sperm counts—*but not because of a change in their inherited DNA sequence*. Puzzled, Skinner and his team repeated the experiments—once, twice, 15 times—and found the same sperm defects.(emphasis added)[29]

The team bred more rats, tested more chemicals, including substances that were correlated with diseases of the prostate, kidney, ovaries, and immune system. "Again and again, these diseases also showed up in the fourth- and fifth-generation offspring of mothers exposed to a chemical. 'In essence,' Skinner explains, 'what your great-grandmother was exposed to could cause disease in you and your grandchildren.'"[30] This is not only revolutionary, it is actually quite scary. Transgenerational epigenetics may still be in its infancy, but its implications have huge relevance for our discussion of the adaptive psychic immune system.

> Traumatic events to modern behavioral epigenetics ". . . leave molecular scars adhering to our DNA. Jews whose great-grandparents were chased from their Russian shtetls; Chinese whose grandparents lived through the ravages of the Cultural Revolution; young immigrants from Africa whose parents survived massacres; adults of every ethnicity who grew up with alcoholic or abusive parents—all carry with them more than just memories. Like silt deposited on the cogs of a finely tuned machine after the seawater of a tsunami recedes, our experiences, and those of our forebears, are never gone, even if they have been forgotten. They become a part of us, a molecular residue holding fast to our genetic scaffolding. The DNA remains the same, but psychological and behavioral tendencies are inherited. You might have inherited not just your grandmother's knobby knees, but also her predisposition toward depression caused by the neglect she suffered as a newborn."[31]

Survival, Fitness, and Epigenes

Studies on animals show that positive parental nurturance leaves epigenetic tags that enhance survival. This has been observed in three-spined sticklebacks[32] and mouse pups,[33] but data on humans is still thin. Can it be assumed that epigenes might be related to psychological immunity and survival? Writer Angela Miller examined epigenetic research in *Violence and Abuse in Society* and says, "Data so far tend to suggest that violent patterns of behavior perpetuate in generations to follow; peaceful nonviolent patterns of behaviors *will also perpetuate in generations to follow.*"[34]

HUMAN EPIGENETIC STUDIES

Although transferring these new insights to humans has only begun, some recent evidence is intriguing. An obese man went to have his stomach stapled in an ordinary bariatric surgery operation. A week before the operation he had donated a sample of sperm to Danish scientists. A year after the surgery he did so again. Using thirteen other similar cases, scientists found numerous genes that were methylated differently a year after the surgery. In other words, a surgical experience epigenetically altered gene expression.

A Belgian study also showed epigenetic differences between children with obese fathers and those with lean ones. Again the notion that one can epigenetically inherit the effects of behavioral characteristics of one's parents are gaining momentum, and these studies have graduated from rat pups to humans.[35]

A SPECULATION ABOUT EPIGENES

Following Miller's prior observations on violence, it might be conjectured that if epigenetic memories can be transferred generationally, and if they are adaptive, experience with conflicts and war might result in an epigenetic *aversion to violence and killing* in subsequent generations in the same way cocaine use in the father's generation of mouse pups was avoided in the second generation.

Europe saw two wars in the twentieth century. Has it learned anything from those experiences? Surely! However, has it epigenetically encoded anything that might create a natural, adaptive immunological resistance to further outbreaks of mass murder? That is quite a different question. Europeans speak over 234 different languages;[36] it is a diverse land with plenty of opportunities for conflict, misunderstanding, and violence. If epigenetic memories of hurtful odors can be passed on transgenerationally, perhaps peoples' memories of war and holocausts can build up a resistance to killing in their descendants.

Science is not even close to answering such a question, but observe one curious factoid. The Nobel Peace Prize in 2012, for the first time, was not awarded to an individual. It was given to the European Union for the advancement of peace and reconciliation that lowered the violence level of the region over a seventy-year period, an achievement worthy of the prize.[37]

Wars leave scars. Parents tell their children about bad experiences and horrors. This violent legacy becomes part of their learning, folklore, and heritage. However, beyond scars, stories, and cultural histories, it is possible epigenetic memories also form that are transferred to new generations, resulting in a stronger collective aversion to killing than previously existed. And when talking about a collective aversion to killing, are we not also talking about the impact of the psychic immune system?

CONTRARIAN OPINION

While these speculations are interesting, to provide time and space for contrarian opinion is also necessary. A counterpoint comes from Professor Jerry Coyne at the Department of Ecology and Evolution at the University of Chicago who notes:

> Athletes don't tend to produce muscular children, nor amputees legless ones. Translation: These epigenetic changes in the DNA aren't all that stable, folks, so we need to be really careful before touting them as important aspects of evolution. My conclusion: Though the results are intriguing . . . there's still no reason to see this type of heritable change as presaging the overturning or drastic revision of the current neo-Darwinian view of evolution.[38]

An important caveat from Professor Coyne

US VERSUS THEM IN THE ADAPTIVE PSYCHIC IMMUNE SYSTEM

It has long been known that in heart, liver, or bone marrow transplants, it is important to "match" the donor to the recipient. The physical immune system automatically reacts to that which is "nonself" and attacks foreign cells with vigor. Getting cells to be akin is essential to prevent a transplant from being rejected.

> The key to a healthy immune system is its remarkable ability to distinguish between the body's own cells, recognized as "self," and foreign cells, or "nonself." The body's immune defenses normally coexist peacefully with cells that carry distinctive "self" marker molecules. But when immune defenders encounter foreign cells or organisms carrying

> markers that say "nonself," they quickly launch an attack. Anything that can trigger this immune response is called an antigen. An antigen can be a microbe such as a virus, or a part of a microbe such as a molecule. Tissues or cells from another person (except an identical twin) also carry nonself markers and act as foreign antigens. This explains why tissue transplants may be rejected.[39]

The physical immune system is essentially xenophobic and constantly on guard for foreign intruders (pathogens).

In the epiphenomenal psychological plane of existence, one can see an amazing array of self-nonself or *us versus them* iterations ranging from Irish Catholics warring against Irish Protestants, to Southern Whites hanging Southern Blacks. There is a surfeit of *us versus them* battles throughout the millennia.

Is this psychological battle of self-nonself a curious epiphenomenon of the how the physical immune system actually works, or is this a false similarity coming to an errant, unsupportable conclusion?

> Bacteria, ants, bees, lions, chimpanzees and humans are all watchful for intruders who do not belong in their colony, hive, pride, group, or social organization. Bacteria have antigens and recognition sites, ants have soldiers; bees have workers, lions have adult pride members, chimpanzees have the alpha and beta coalition, and human have all these and more, including border guards and the Immigration and Naturalization Service.
>
> When invaded, bacteria have toxins, ants have pincers and armor coating, bees have stingers, lions have claws and teeth, chimpanzees have trees and strong arms, and humans have everything from guns to tanks to nerve gas. . . .[40] Considerable resources, wealth and energy go into the security and protection of a nation or a society because of its built-in predilection to stay alive and protect its physical well-being. So we see, among a vast array of possibilities, the creation and maintenance of defense departments and armed forces, the development of education systems and spy networks. . . . Like the biological immune system, which is programmed to keep out unwelcome intruders and keep the body safe, the psychological immune system directs governments and government leaders to keep out unwelcome intruders so that a nation or society will be safe.[41]

When two alpha males fight, this is usually over territory or breeding rights. Evolutionary biologists, however, translate this swashbuckling individual male drama into a more collective theater, as if it is not exactly two males competing, but *two sets of genes* warring against one another. In other words, gene *pools* may be in competition with each other.

Individuals who are akin and share similar genes tend to coalesce, form genetic coalitions, and ally themselves with like-minded (or like-gened) creatures. This is referred to as kin selection and inclusive fitness in the world of animal behavior and evolutionary biology. Since this is a possible new insight into those *us-versus-them* battles humankind obsessively engages in, it is necessary to look more closely at our animal cousins to see how this plays out.

Inclusive Fitness

W. D. Hamilton in 1964 proposed a unique idea that from the perspective of the gene, evolutionary success is determined by how many copies of itself it can leave in the population. Until that time, it was generally assumed replication occurred only on an individual level, by the single alpha male spreading his genes.

However, Hamilton argued that because other members of the population *share* similar genes, close genetic relatives have a natural tendency to form coalitions and maximize the spread of their genes through kinship. He developed a mathematical theorem for how these coalitions are formed known as Hamilton's rule, or the "coefficient of relatedness." "It is defined as the average proportion of alleles of individual A that are identical by descent to those in individual B."[42] In other words, genetic relatives aggregate together, care for one another, and confederate with genetically similar groups.

If one looks at Florida scrub jays, for example, not only do parents participate in rearing offspring, but other genetically related birds also tend to nesting sites to help assure the baby jay's survival.[43] The same phenomenon is found in social insects, prairie dogs, and squirrels. In shrimp, closely related adults protect juveniles, and in some species of monkeys grandmothers or older sisters help care for the young.[44] Closely related wasps aid female nest mates.

Studies of sun-tailed monkeys show kin related to mothers act favorably to help raise youngsters, while among more distant kinships (e.g., half-siblings) caregiving drops off significantly. Colonies of horseshoe bats are determined by matrilineal kinship. As kinship closeness *declines* so does kin-biased cooperation in foraging and roosting.[45]

Even at the cellular level, Hamilton's rule seems to hold: the sperm of a wood mouse seems to perform "kin-selective altruistic activity" due to genetic similarity with surrounding spermatozoa.[46] By helping close genetic relatives, altruistic acts increase one's own fitness: "The more of your genes that are in a relative, the more interest you have in helping them."[47]

The Cinderella Effect

It is well known that a dominant male who is victorious over another male often kills the offspring of his defeated opponent. Harvard professor Sarah Blaffer Hardy defines this kind of infanticide as a product of mammalian evolution. "By killing off babies of other fathers, a male improves his chances of having more of his own offspring."[48]

This phenomenon, translated into human populations, is called *The Cinderella Effect*. A stepparent, for example, is one hundred times more likely to kill a child than a natural parent. Battery, abuse, and neglect of children fall far more heavily on stepparents than natural biological parents. Stepparents show higher levels of abusive behavior and are less positive toward children than genetic parents.[49]

Evolutionary psychologists Martin Daly and Margo Wilson argue that the Cinderella effect is an outgrowth of inclusive fitness and kin selection. The same biases that favor spreading one's own genes predominate, whether in lions, gorillas, or man.[50] [51]

Us versus Them: Flags, Plumage, and Territoriality

Animals recognize kin ("Us") by various markers.[52] Birds have easily identifiable color patterns which allow them to sort out differences at great distance. Plumage is effectively a language in which members of a particular species can identify characteristics. White birds, for example, generally mate with white birds and dark birds with dark birds.[53]

Male territorial and competitive attacks also vary with differing plumages that act almost like flags or badges.[54] "The study of kin recognition is still relatively new, but the general thought today is that 'mechanisms' that permit individuals to recognize their kin can facilitate the evolution of social cooperation, and they may confer other selective advantages as well"[55]

Humans of similar kinship form a variety of like-minded groups. Chinese immigrants tend to move to Chinese neighborhoods. Italians gravitate to Little Italy. Hispanics mix in east Los Angeles. From Greektown to Chinatown to the barrio, kin aggregate in ethnic enclaves throughout the world.

Certainly many factors go into these coalitions: food preferences, language similarities, traditions, culture, sub-culture, and religion. However, what we do not seem to notice is Hamilton's rule, namely that those having a closer genetic relationship coefficient, or kinship, more strongly associate with, care for, and nurture one another. Just as the physical immune system recognizes *self-nonself*, human psychological behavior engages the same kinds of discriminations, all variants of *us versus them*.

Birds recognize kin by song or plumage, and humans recognize kin by a variety of signals too, not least of which is a flag. Flags are metaphorically like plumage, and national anthems like bird songs. Both define territory and both separate out proprietors (us) from intruders (them).[56]

The flag of the state of California, or the American flag, is associated with territory, but to psychohistorian, Lloyd deMause, it also signifies "blood kinship."[57] The most frequent color of all world flags is red, occurring 77 percent of the time, whereas brown appears less than 5 percent of the time.[58]

Not only does a flag reflect territoriality—and subliminally blood kinship—the kinship factor runs deeper and takes on the character of a revered and sacred icon. In Egypt, the Pharoah's placenta was often placed on a pole to show his origins. "The sanctity of the flag is due to the fact that originally it was supposed to be functionally active as the life-giving powers of the king, and the celestial source of all life represented by the king's placenta."[59]

Flags function like plumage and point to territoriality, kin recognition, and blood kinship. Terms like "patriotism," "patrilineal," "fatherland," "motherland" and "matrilineal" underscore the closeness of blood-genetic connections.

To defile the flag is psychologically synonymous with defiling one's mother, father, or ancestors. The venerated nature of the symbol cannot be underestimated, nor can the magnitude of reactions to its debasement. Flag desecration is a criminal act in most countries from China to Denmark, Australia to Algeria.[60] To burn a flag is generally regarded as an act of apostasy and blasphemy.[61] Robert Hinde teases out these implications further:

> On a broader canvas, the country may be seen as the Fatherland or Motherland, and other soldiers as brothers-in-arms . . . patriotism depends on an unconscious perception of fellow countrymen as kin, and it is therefore a biological propensity to help related individuals. Animal and human data support the view that familiarity does augment attraction to other individuals. It is also likely that natural selection has acted to promote group solidarity. Nationalism involves and is augmented by denigration of the enemy. Thus in propaganda, the enemy is portrayed in ways calculated to augment hostile feelings, most frequently as an aggressor blamed for the conflict who is to be feared and resisted. There is an implied association between the enemy and evil; he may be portrayed as the Devil or Anti-God, or a barbarian, or greedy invader trying to acquire what is not his. Racism is readily recruited to aid the denigration of the enemy.[62]

More on Self/Nonself: Xenophobia, Ethnic Cleansing, and Anti-Semitism

Deep inside the adaptive *physical* immune system, lymphocytes are constantly patrolling for intruders, seeking out and destroying nonself invaders and antigens. This physiological battleground reflects epiphenomenally in the adaptive *psychic* immune system, where the war of self-nonself—*us versus them*—invades the psyche in ways almost too numerous to count. From the Viet cong fighting off American intruders to the Chicago Bulls skirmishing with the Detroit Pistons, human *us versus them* competitions take on infinite forms and rituals.

Amidst this dizzying confusion, social psychology comes front and center with an intriguing discovery. A pregnant woman in her first trimester has a weakened physical immune system and is especially susceptible to diseases. Researchers asked if she is more vulnerable at this time, does her psyche change? Is she more *preoccupied* with disease in general? Is she afraid of pathogens, foreigners, intruders, or even more "ethnocentric?" Did her psychic system become hyper-vigilant in scanning for threats to herself and the unborn child's survival?

Actually, it is all of that and more. Measurements show a significant increase in ethnocentrism and preoccupation with disease in the first trimester. However, her susceptibility to physical disease *recedes* in the second and third trimester, along with her ethnocentrism.[63] Just as the physical immune system patrols for invaders and pathogens, the psychic immune system scans for signs of disease or threats too. When the physical immune system is weakened, the psychic immune system becomes even more vigilant in scanning for pathogens.

Evolutionary psychologists have taken this thought further. They suggest that disease-avoidant processes at the psychological level form the basis of xenophobia, prejudices against the disabled, and even anti-Semitism insofar as they fall into the outgroup, or them category, and are therefore perceived as more pathogenic.[64] This is a strange twist on our understanding of prejudice.

Jews, for example, have been historically seen as having a loyalty more to their own subgroup than to the nation in which they live. Thus, they were often viewed as disloyal and untrustworthy. In eighteenth-century France, Jews were considered "collectively disloyal."[65] In Czarist Russia, Jews were said to have no loyalty to the "motherland," and persecution and pogroms were rampant.[66] President Richard Nixon's recorded tapes revealed his anti-Semitism came from the perception that Jews were "disloyal."[67]

Curiously, a recently published global survey of fifty-three thousand adults in 102 countries concluded that 26 percent of the world's adults are anti-Semitic. Iraqi, Yemeni, and Algerian levels of anti-Semitism were highest and reach close to 90 percent of the population.[68] Jews, identified as the "outgroup," were traditionally subject to discrimination and persecution.[69] Evolutionary psychologist Kevin MacDonald explains how inclusive fitness and kin selection play a role in this perception:

> One type of evolutionary approach to anti-Semitism considers the possibility that humans have mechanisms that cause them to favor relatives or others who share genes. There is little doubt that kin recognition mechanisms exist among animals . . . and some evolutionists have proposed genetic mechanisms based on kin recognition as an explanation for xenophobia. Mechanisms based on kin recognition and phenotypic similarity may have some role in traditional anti-Semitism, since in traditional societies there would be much more phenotypic similar-

> ity among gentiles than between Jews and gentiles, due to differences in clothing, language, appearance (e.g., hair style), and quite often their physical features. Moreover, among Jews, there are anecdotal reports of very high levels of rapport and ability to recognize other Jews, which are consistent with the existence of some sort of kin recognition system among Jews.[70]

Creating a group evolutionary strategy results in the possibility of cultural group selection resulting from between-group competition in which the groups are defined by culturally produced in-group markings.

> Groups mark themselves off from other groups and thereby are able to remain reproductively isolated from other groups and adjust rapidly to new and variable environments. Judaism in traditional societies was indeed characterized by a highly elaborated set of in-group markings that effectively set Jews off from gentile society. The proposal here is that the process of creating in-group markings is central to understanding anti-Semitism."[71]

Therefore, as the adaptive *physical* immune system patrols against pathogens and intruders—obsessively identifying self from nonself—the adaptive *psychic* immune system refuses to be outdone. It also has developed an elaborate *us versus them* scanning process where kin with similar gene pools aggregate as coalitions of *us* banded in opposition to alien out-groups who need to be removed from close proximity.

This is certainly a novel interpretation on understanding xenophobia, anti-Semitism, and ethnic "cleansing."

Psychoanalyst Richard Koenigsberg, in *Hitler's Ideology*, showed how Hitler saw the Jew as a pathogen, an invader, and a poisonous infection or parasite in the body of the Germany state. The holocaust in this model becomes a form of pathogenic disease control, however delusional and psychotic it may have been. A sampling of Hitler's rhetoric makes this abundantly clear:

> the personification of the devil as the symbol of all evil assumes the living shape of the Jew. . . . The Jew is the parasite of humanity. He can be a parasite for an individual person, a social parasite for whole peoples, and the world parasite of humanity. The black-haired Jewish youth lies in wait for hours on end, satanically glaring at and spying on the unsuspicious girl whom he plans to seduce, adulterating her blood and removing her from the bosom of her own people. The Jew uses every possible means to undermine the racial foundations of a subjugated people.[72]

During the Rwanda genocide, the clarion call to majority Hutus was that the Tutsis were "cockroaches" and needed to be eradicated. From Rwanda radio: "You have to kill the Tutsis, they're cockroaches. We must all fight. We must all fight the Tutsis. We must finish with them, exterminate them, sweep them from the whole country. There must be no refuge for them. . . . They must be exterminated. There is no other way. Be proud of your Hutu blood."[73]

The image of the infectious, poisonous "other," which differs from genetically similar kin, is arguably the unconscious essence of xenophobia, prejudice, and anti-Semitism, and it certainly formed the nucleus of the collective hysteria that engulfed Rwanda's reign of slaughter and terror.

Disgust, Revulsion, and the Behavioral Immune System

Mark Shaller, a psychologist from the University of British Columbia describes a "behavioral immune system" that perpetually scans the environment to detect and protect from pathogenic situations and people. Here is a short review of his trenchant thesis:

> You know, that pesky little piece of your body that throws out fevers, sweating, swelling, et al. to deal with the stress you put your body through? Well, this system is actually very metabolically costly in its attempts to keep the body healthy. To mitigate the risk of these costs ever being incurred in the first place, human immune systems have also developed behavioral mechanisms that can prevent contact with foreign and harmful pathogens. . . . Any time that you feel the need to stay away from people with known illness, you're experiencing the most obvious results of this system.
>
> Other examples of this kind of proactive avoidant behavior can be seen in nature: Schaller lists tadpoles, mice, and chimpanzees as animals that are known to *actively avoid other members of their species that are noticeably ill.* The primary emotion that is associated with studies of this system is disgust. The Behavioral Immune System can be subdivided into two sorts of behaviors—detection and response. Detection primarily depends on smell and sight to find possible risks of infection around you. This includes both objects and behaviors of those . . . who may be a vector of disease. The objects that subjects experience revulsion towards seem obvious—fecal matter, vomit, etc. When it comes to how you react to those around you, however, that's where the research gets interesting. Test groups not only responded with avoidant behavior to those who were obviously sick or clearly unhygienic, but also to those who seemed visibly different from the cultural norm. The reasoning seems to be that those who are from outside of the local culture pose a threat not only because they may carry unusual pathogens, but also because they haven't been taught the local methods of hygiene. (emphasis added)

Shaller hypothesizes individuals are psychologically primed to detect and avoid pathogenic situations, which forms the basis for all sorts of prejudice. We avoid and subconsciously find ourselves physically or emotionally repulsed in the presence of unhealthy or unhygienic people, and this extends to obese, disabled, unattractive, and foreign individuals.

> We are prejudiced against all kinds of other people, based on superficial physical features: We react negatively to facial disfigurement; we avoid sitting next to people who are obese, or old, or in a wheelchair; we favor familiar folks over folks that are foreign. If I asked you why these prejudices exist and what one can do to eliminate them, your answer probably wouldn't involve the words "infectious disease." Perhaps it should. What does infectious disease have to do with these prejudices? The behavioral immune system is our brain's way of engaging in a kind of preventive medicine. This is a suite of psychological mechanisms designed to detect the presence of disease-causing parasites in our immediate environment.[74]

Shaller then reports on research by Paul Rozin and colleagues win which chocolate fudge was molded into the shape of "poop." Most people would not eat it even though they knew that it was fudge. He argues they are responding unconsciously (autonomically) and that these "disease-avoidant psychological processes contribute to prejudices against people who are disabled, obese or old. These same processes also contribute to ethnocentrism and xenophobia."[75]

Shaller's group also saw evidence for how autonomic and unconscious this process is. For example, the perceived threat of infection actually translates into psychophysiological changes. In one study the mere sight of another person's symptoms of sickness (sores, rashes, sneezes) led those who witnessed these events to actually increase their own white blood cell counts to "respond more aggressively to bacterial infection."[76]

These dramatic psycho-immune avoidant responses are quite evident in the animal kingdom too. Sheep avoid grass near their own fecal droppings. A female mouse can detect and differentiate the smell of a healthy male versus one infected with worms and will mate with the healthier specimen.[77]

Chimp and Human Prejudice

One of Jane Goodall's chimps named McGregor was often preened and fussed over by the other chimps in his early life. However, when he contracted polio and started dragging himself around by his arms after his legs became paralyzed, the other chimps systematically ignored him, "Before McGregor got sick, he enjoyed hours of grooming from other chimpanzees, who picked out fleas, mites, and other parasites from his fur. Goodall watched in amazement as the other chimpanzees stayed away from him once he became ill."[78]

Just like McGregor, human beings with disabilities similarly feel shunned.[79] More than 66 percent of them report experiencing aggression, hostility, or name-calling.[80] In a Rutgers experiment, identical applications for employment—one mentioning a disability the other not—showed a 26 percent reduced interest in the disabled applicant.[81]

Among obese people, more than 50 percent have experienced discrimination, and two-fifths felt shunned.[82] Of individuals with a non-contagious skin condition called rosacea, 63 percent have difficulty establishing relationships, 58 percent said they were the subject of "stares, misconceptions, rude comments, and jokes,"[83] and 37 percent felt socially isolated.[84] Fear of illness, the unhygienic, the obese, the disabled, the "other," the "outsider," the "foreigner" may therefore be the regrettable and unhappy expressions of how the adaptive psychic immune system works.

We decry its proclivity toward bias and prejudice, but we include this constituent of the adaptive psychic immune system, based in part on the nature of the physical immune system. Just as the physical immune system deploys armies of lymphocytes to scan and target nonself foreign pathogens for destruction, the psychic immune system behaves similarly when deploying its *us versus them* kin recognition process, often with regrettable results: "Scholars suggest that in evolutionary times we became hard-wired to make instantaneous judgments about whether someone is in our 'in- group' or not, because that could be lifesaving . . . its a feature of evolution, says Mahzarin Banaji, a Harvard psychology professor." [85]

Indeed, there is a question of whether this kinship factor might also be innate or heritable. Infants begin to show a fear of strangers at six months.[86] Babies also show a preference for their own race by three months.[87] Is this another side of the pathogen-avoidant *us versus them* mechanism of the psychic immune system—only this time it is innate or partially innate?

Without resolving that issue, one can at least note a built-in predisposition to look away when confronted by a person with a facial deformity, or sit further from someone who is obese, disabled, homeless, unhygienic, or who may be "colored." These primitive pathogen-avoidance mechanisms, most of them instinctive, are distinctly embarrassing. We don't believe in them, and often consciously confront these attitudes or behaviors in ourselves.

However, those efforts do not mean we are successful. Only 18 percent of whites believe racism is a "very serious" problem in the United States, while twice as many blacks feel that way.[88] Among whites, 52 percent feel that blacks and whites receive equal treatment under the law. Only 10 percent of blacks feel the same.[89] A black man under the age of twenty-five has a 28 percent chance of being stopped by a policeman while a white man's odds are less than 14 percent.[90] The victims of prejudice are not quite as convinced about the sanguinity of these matters as might be expected.

The role of color discrimination, by the way, is not merely an American issue. Darker skin people generally do not do as well on planet earth. In an international seminar on ethnic-racial statistics,

> it was evident that discrimination and racial discrimination is a current and worrisome problem in Latin America. The Seminar coincided with the release of the book, *Pigmentocracies.* In general terms, the study proves what many already knew intuitively: the darker the person's skin tone, the worse his quality of life in Latin America. For example, in Brazil, light skinned people finish nearly 9 years of education, while those with darker skin have 7.6 years of education. Similarly, in Peru, those with lighter skin obtain an average of 12 years of education, while those with darker skin finish an average of 10 years.[91]

Even though a number of India's gods have darker skin, the "colorism" phenomenon is prevalent in India too.[92]

A new psychological test has taken academic psychology by storm. The Implicit Association Test measures *unconscious bias.* Based on making rapid associations, what a person consciously believes (explicit) is often contradicted by how he implicitly perceives the world. More than four million people have taken this test and results are disquieting to say the least. In 1995 Anthony Greenwald and Mahzarin Banaji, two social psycholgists, proposed that

> social behavior may not always be under a person's conscious control. They argued that much of our behavior is driven by stereotypes that operate automatically and therefore, unconsciously. In 1997, they developed the Implicit Association Test (IAT), a computer-based test that measures people's unconscious attitudes. Since then over 200 studies have been published using the IAT. This data strongly suggests that many people hold implicit biases towards members of particular groups. For example, over 80 percent of people who completed an IAT on age bias demonstrated a negative implicit bias against the elderly. In addition, about 75 percent of Whites and Asians demonstrated an implicit bias in favor of Whites compared to Blacks.[93]

Whites, who scored well in polls regarding attitudes on racism, have taken this IAT test, which nonetheless showed about 70 percent hold unconscious biases against blacks.[94] Curiously, even a large number of blacks show an unconscious preference of white over black.[95] One can assume most of this is learned and a result of cultural conditioning, but it is possible the behavioral immune system's pathogen-avoidance mechanisms are operating at an autonomic level behind the scenes too.

The fact that this *us versus them* drama is more unconscious than we might wish to admit is underscored by a recent survey that sent thousands of resumes to employers with job openings. The resumes were identical except for the fact that they contained stereotyped names ("Jamal" for an African American, and "Brendan" for a white person.) The white-sounding name had a 50 percent higher probability of being selected for a callback.

The same phenomenon was replicated with university professors who rather pride themselves on their lack of bias. Despite their academic hubris on this issue, they responded to inquiries about their academic programs to white-sounding names significantly more often than to black-sounding names.[96]

The insidious nature of racist unconscious attitudes may be abhorred from the perspective of one's value system, but the adaptive psychic immune system's mechanisms of kin selection, inclusive fitness, and *us versus them* predilections bias us against those who appear different, strange, unhealthy, dark, foreign, or otherwise alien. Once identified, these individuals or groups are reflexively—read unconsciously—shunned, avoided, or kept at a distance.

Sounds awfully unrefined and primitive, but the data corroborate our disappointment. Even today, stay-with-your-own kin biases are alive and well. In 2008, the number of couples marrying outside their ethnicity was minimal. Only 9 percent of whites and 16 percent of blacks married outside their ethnic group.[97]

There is a strong centripetal pull toward kin-affinities. More than 75 percent of American whites have no minority friends whatsoever.[98] Similar results pertain to blacks: "Among black Americans, 83 percent of people in their social networks are composed of people who are also black, while eight percent are white and six percent are some other race."[99]

A study showed the situation is also problematic in Africa. Some 43.5 percent of South Africans rarely (or never) speak to someone of another race, and only 17.8 percent "often" socialize with people of other races in their homes. Indeed more than half (56 percent) rarely or "never socialize across racial lines."[100]

Religion and Us versus Them

Robert Hinde's *The Psychological Bases of War*, reflects on how religion also plays into this us *versus them* polarity:

> Surveying world religions, Thompson found that while virtually all have talked peace, religion has often supported an "*us versus them*" attitude. Many wars have been characterized as holy wars, and religious imagery is often recruited to justify the nationalistic cause. In the World Wars, the slogans "Gott mit uns," or "In God we trust" were used by both sides. . . . The Old Testament, concerned with what were effectively tribal conflicts, is full of bloody battles. In the Christian Church, the believer is portrayed as a soldier 'fighting the good fight,' and the Book of Revelations makes extensive use of the imagery of war and death.[101]

As Umberto Eco writes, "All the religious wars that have caused blood to be shed for centuries arise from passionate feelings and facile counter-positions, such as Us and Them, good and bad, white and black."[102]

Lymphocytes, Worker Bees, and the Media

Deep in the heart of the physical immune system are lymphocytes, the essential ingredient for the adaptive immune system. They occur in large numbers—there are 2×10^{12} lymphocytes in the human body—about *as big a mass* as the liver or brain. Their role in our immune system was not discovered until the late 1950s.[103] Lymphocytes constantly patrol the body for pathogens, intruders, infectious agents, tumors, and other invasive agents.[104] Let us explore some further implications of how the psychic immune system epiphenomenally mimics this physical disease sentry. First, another visit to the animal kingdom.

GUARD HONEYBEES

Just as lymphocytes patrol for intruders, honeybees show similar behavior. Worker bees differentiate from other bees in the hive, and patrol for danger and intruders. They can even chemically summon reinforcements when needed. The bees have special glands that help them perform certain functions. When worker bees are about twenty-one days old,

> the venom in the sting is at its maximum potency, so they serve the hive as guards for a few days. Guard bees stand at the hive entrance on their back four legs with their front legs raised. The guard bees inspect every bee entering the hive. Bees entering the hive allow the guard bees to examine them with their front legs and antennae. The guard bees can determine if a bee belongs to its colony by the bee's odor, as each hive has a distinct odor. Worker bees that belong to the colony are allowed to enter. The guard bees will sting and remove foreign intruders, such as bumblebees, wasps, and yellow jackets. They will also sting and attempt to drive away intruding skunks, raccoons, and beekeepers. The guard bees can extend their sting and release alarm pheromone to attract other guard bees if needed.[105]

What is curious is the guard honeybee dies once it stings the intruder, an altruistic act biologically engineered to protect the integrity of the group, the hive, the social unit, or, if you wish, the gene pool, but not the individual.[106] A guard honeybee will even attack another bee if it is not from the same colony.

THE MEDIA AND NEGATIVE HEADLINES

It might be asked, what does the media have to do with guard honeybees, or lymphocytes, or the psychic immune system for that matter? Isn't this getting too far out on the limb?

Actually, the discussion forms a rather interesting intellectual mosaic. First, note how researchers discovered that people react to negative news and headlines far more than to positive renderings. "Negative superlatives work 30 percent better at getting your attention than positive ones. The average click-through rate on headlines with negative superlatives was a staggering *63 percent higher than that of their positive counterparts.*" (emphasis added)[107]

This bias is corroborated by neuroscience showing the brain region that processes emotional stimuli, the amygdala, is more quickly activated from fearful and dangerous stimuli than more pleasant or positive types.[108] [109] In other words, our consciousness (attention) is drawn more toward negative news than positive, and the corporate media is quite aware of this neurological trait.

> Media studies show that bad news far outweighs good news by as much as seventeen negative news reports for every one good news report. Why? The answer may lie in the work of evolutionary psychologists and neuroscientists. Humans seek out news of dramatic, negative events. . . . Many studies have shown that we *care more about the threat of bad things than we do about the prospect of good things*. Our negative brain tripwires are far more sensitive than our positive triggers. We tend to get more fearful than happy. And each time we experience fear we turn on our stress hormones. (emphasis added)[110]

In other words, the media—and to some extent collective consciousness—behaves very much as an epiphenomenon of our physical adaptive immune system.

Perhaps this idea can be conveyed better with slightly more detail. As the adaptive *physical* immune system is ever on patrol for danger, dispatching lymphocytes at the slightest threat, up in the epiphenomenal world of collective consciousness, the media acts as if it were the perceptual apparatus of the adaptive psychic immune system. It alerts us to threats, tornadoes, hurricanes, smuggled nuclear material, civil unrest, rebellions, insurrections, airplane crashes, murders, rapes, fires, and burglaries, all far more prominent—in fact seventeen times more prominent—than any appealing or pleasant news.

The first news heard is negative, only later followed by more personal or positive stories. As media gurus say, "If it bleeds, it leads." The headline reporting "Worst tornado ever!" receives far more attention than the one saying "Best motorcycle ever built!"

Many opine against negative news, but just as the physical immune system is hyper-vigilant against pathogens, the media, an agency of the psychic immune system, is hyper-vigilant against threats and danger in the same way. As *Psychology Today* reported, "A recent study by the Pew Research Center for People and the Press synthesizes 165 separate national surveys and finds that . . . war and terrorism have consistently ranked at the top of the stack since 1986, where the study begins. So have bad weather, and natural or manmade disaster stories."[111]

At the end of 2014, a list of the major stories of the year appeared. Cited were a polar vortex freezing New Yorkers; the California drought; the revolution in the Ukraine; Russian annexation of the Crimea; the Ebola outbreak; school girls kidnapped in Africa; the sinking of a South Korean ferry; ISIS gaining ground in Iraq; the World Cup; Robin William's suicide; racial tension in Ferguson, Missouri; Hong Kong protests; Bill Cosby's rape scandal; the Rosetta satellite landing on a comet; Sony Corporation hacked by North Korea; and a black man, Eric Garner, strangled by police.[112] Of these sixteen mega news stories, 88 percent were negative and only two either neutral or positive. The media, in short, is obsessively scanning for danger and threat. It is the early warning system of the adaptive psychic immune system.

SUMMARY SO FAR

The journey undertaken in this chapter is like a river meandering into myriad rivulets, so perhaps it is time to bring it into focus by summarizing what has been discussed. The intent of this chapter was to explore the hypothesis that not only is there an innate psychic immune system, but an adaptive one as well. As the *physical* immune system adapts to the sudden appearance of a pathogen and uses "immunological memory" to develop antibodies, the question was asked whether the psychic immune system possesses a similar kind of adaptive, protective defense against danger.

The discussion started with Columbia psychology professor George Bonnano's work on resilience—the more experience you have with bereavement, the more resilient you are in facing the next one. Bonnano warned that the psychic immune system is specific, just like the physical immune system, and while experiencing the loss of a loved one may equip one to better handle a similar event in the future, it doesn't help deal more effectively with an assault, a bankruptcy, or a car accident. Just like a flu shot protects against one viral strain, it does not provide immunity from other types of influenza. The same is true for the adaptive psychic immune system's response to threat.

The next quest was to examine heritability of immunological memory—only this time, psychic immunological memory. As the physical immune system is able to transfer "inherited memories" of toxins and pathogens—at least in antibodies passed from mother to child[113]—we asked whether the psychic immune system had any natural or inherited memory of pathogenic situations. Here epigenetics appeared which dramatically shows how adaptations and memories may be psychologically inherited, though not necessarily in the old Lamarckian way.

Epigenetics asserts that experience and learning do not change DNA directly, but rather alter and influence gene expression. A mouse conditioned to associate pain with the smell of cherries can pass that memory trace on to its offspring. The pain-smell association is adaptive because it communicates to future generations environmental stimuli to avoid.

While epigenetics research is only beginning, it supports the idea that human beings may have the ability to pass on learned survival strategies to subsequent generations—biologically. The science certainly adds another foundation stone in our developing knowledge of how the natural adaptive psychic immune system and immunological memory might work.

This journey then moved to a third constituent of the adaptive psychic immune system—territoriality, kin-selection, inclusive fitness, self and nonself.[114] With kin selection and territoriality, comparative biology teaches about the remarkable survival strategies that animals share. Not only do single alpha males compete for dominance and the ability to spread their genes, the whole drama operates at a group level as well. Animals from similar gene pools aggregate to protect, preen, and nurture one another as if the gene pool itself was engaged in a conspiracy to spread across the landscape of evolution. Following Hamilton's law, the closer the genetic similarity of a group, the greater the acts of reciprocity, cooperation, empathy, altruism, and mutual protection. The further apart genetic similarity is, the stronger the competition, territoriality, and rivalry.

Kin selection and inclusive fitness go hand in hand with the self-nonself process. At the cellular level, leukocytes and lymphocytes[115] separate self from nonself—us from them—and attack foreign invaders and antigens. That drama is epiphenomenally reenacted in the social behavior of animals and man where unfamiliar kin, or out-groups, are identified, and the great antagonism between self-nonself, us and them, proprietors and intruders, furiously wages up and down the evolutionary ladder.

Genetically, more distant kin are perceived as "nonself" and, once pinpointed, the world of fear, avoidance, discrimination, mistrust, prejudice, xenophobia, anti-Semitism, and ethnic cleansing revs up full steam. How adaptive these strategies are is certainly up for debate. Many of our more embarrassing prejudices can be laid at the feet of this process.

Sometimes the system is correct in assuming that strangers who are non-kin, or distant, may be more dangerous, less trustworthy, and more of a threat. Fear of the unknown, of strangers, of non-kin can be, at its best, a manifestation of risk-aversion and a response to uncertainty. In that sense, it can be argued the system is adaptive in dealing with danger.

However, this very same system often fails to identify *genuine* threats and leaves behind a legacy of ancestral, maladaptive prejudice instead. We turn on other human beings, casting them as nonself aliens or intruders and behave despicably toward them even when they present no threat at all. We do not "catch" obesity from sitting next to an obese person, or contract rosacea from someone in our discussion group who we unconsciously avoid.

We may look at these expressions of human behavior—and our own deportment—with disdain and disappointment, but these attitudes are, *or were,* based on primitive survival strategies regardless of how atavistic they appear today. Psychologist Robert Leahy puts it in context with an evolutionary spin: "The fear worked 50,000 years ago. It's simply out of date. You're using outdated software in your brain."[116]

To cast it in a different light, the adaptive psychic immune system can be maladaptive, make mistakes, or improperly identify a threat where none exists. An overactive psychic immune system may indeed be the origin of our biases, prejudices, scapegoating, and witch burning.

More than five hundred witches were burned in Africa in 2014 because they were thought to create spells that bring disease,[117] including the outbreak of Ebola: "The persistent belief in witchcraft is putting a serious dent in efforts to stop Ebola in its tracks. Some refuse to get medical help because they believe witches and sorcerers are cursing people and causing them to die."[118]

These mechanisms are primitive pathogen-avoidant strategies. When our fellow man or woman is mistakenly accused of being dangerous because of nonself, alien, or foreign status, they become shunned, hurt, discriminated against—or burned at the stake.

But the physical immune system makes mistakes as well. It becomes hyper-vigilant and misidentifies self as nonself, too, and sometimes attacks *us* as if it were *them.* Such reactions are known as autoimmune disorders. "An autoimmune disease develops when your immune system, which defends your body against disease, decides your healthy cells are foreign."[119]

The result is rheumatoid arthritis, lupus, multiple sclerosis, Addison's disease, psoriasis, and eighty different syndromes in which one's own cells are treated as foreign. Just as lupus is an autoimmune disorder of a hyper-vigilant physical immune system—mistaking us for them—a hyper-vigilant psychic immune system misidentifies us—our fellow man or woman kin—as them and attacks inappropriately.

However, when things are working properly, the adaptive psychic immune system acts to separate safety from danger, self from nonself by using functions predicated on genetic similarity, kinship, and Hamilton's Law. The operational rule of thumb is that we have an affinity to blood kin who wave the correct flags signaling that they belong to the same gene pool, share the same home territory, and have the same anticipated patriotism and fealty. Blood kinship seems a critical key to who can be trusted and whom to avoid.

The final leg in the exploration of the adaptive psychic immune system took a closer look at the media. As lymphocytes are scanning for pathogens, danger, and threats at the physical level, the media deploys its parallel mission epiphenomenally in the psychic sphere. The amygdala is a major brain receptor for danger and threat. Humans react to negative stimuli more than for positive, and much more consciousness is devoted to negative signal detection. The media feeds this neurological bias by providing substantially more negative than positive stories. It scans the immediate environment (the local news) and macro environment (world news) for risk, hazard, or any situation that threatens collective safety. The hallmark of the psychic immune system is, after all, safety, security, and threat avoidance, and the media operates as its eyes and ears alerting individuals to daily dangers and future fears.

As the media draws attention to menacing events, people become more prepared to adapt to stresses and meet new challenges. We send armies off to annihilate invaders who would threaten our children, avoid neighborhoods with high crime rates, prepare for impending hurricanes, and support revising safety standards for bridges, airbags, airplanes, handguns, or child car seats. In other words, we act to insure the danger and threats we became conscious of through the media can now be faced, defused, and remedied. This inevitably leads to rational, deliberate, and conscious interventions for more aggressively securing our protection and safety.

And that pivot becomes the critical segue into the next chapter.

NOTES

1. Larissa Long, "Older Adults Less Sensitive to the Effects of Stress," Whole Health, 2011, http://www.wholehealthinsider.com/newsletter/older-adults-less-sensitive-effects-stress/.
2. QuickStats: "Prevalence of Current Depression Among Persons by Age Group and Sex," *Centers for Disease Control and Prevention,* January 6, 2012.
3. National health and nutrition examination survey, CDC, July 2015, http://www.cdc.gov/nchs/nhanes.htm .
4. Erica Edwards, "Resilience in Aging," Arizona Center on Aging, 2012, http://aging.arizona.edu/sites/default/files/resilience_in_aging_0.pdf.
5. APA "Mental and Behavioral Health of Older Americans," APA, 2015,http://www.apa.org/about/gr/issues/aging/mental-health.aspx.
6. J. Zhaobao, T Wenhua, et al., "Are the Elderly More Vulnerable to the Psychological Impact of Natural Disasters' BMC Public Health, 2010, http://www.biomedcentral.com/1471-2458/10/172.
7. Sabrina Tavernise, "Suicide Rates Hit a 30-year High in the United States," *New York Times*, April 21, 2016,
8. David Brooks, "Why Elders Smile, "*New York Times*, December 4, 2014.
9. Karen Schrock Simring, "Age Brings Happiness," *Scientific American*, April 11, 2013, http://www.scientificamerican.com/article/age-brings-happiness/.
10. Hammen, R. "Age and Gender as Determinants of Stress Exposure and Reactions in Youngsters," *Child Development* 3 (1999).
11. P. Gooding, A. Hurst, J. Johnson, and N. Tarrier, "Psychological Resilience in Young and Older Adults." *Int Journal of Geriatric Psychiatry* 3 (2012).
12. "Widowers," Encyclopedia of death and dying, accessed 2015, http://www.deathreference.com/Vi-Z/Widowers.html#b.

13. Bonanno, G. "Loss, Trauma, and Human Resilience: Have We Underestimated the Human Capacity to Thrive After Extremely Aversive Events," *American Psychologist*, 59 (2004).

14. G. A. Bonnano "Resilience to Loss in Bereaved Spouses, Bereaved Parents, and Bereaved Gay Men." *Journal of Personality and Social Psychology*, 88 (2005).

15. Historically, researcher Daniel Gilbert, may be the first to have coined the term the "psychological immune system."

16. Personal Correspondence, George A. Bonnano, Dept. of Counseling & Clinical Psychology, Teacher's College, Columbia University, December 2013.

17. Personal Correspondence, George A. Bonnano, Dept. of Counseling & Clinical Psychology, Teacher's College, Columbia University, December 2013.

18. C. J. Jung, *The Collected Works* (New York: Routledge, 2015), 4434.

19. Ewen Callaway, "Fearful Memories Haunt Mouse Descendants," *Nature*, December 2013, http://www.nature.com/news/fearful-memories-haunt-mouse-descendants-1.14272 .

20. "Inherited Memory," The Connectome, July 25, 2011, http://theconnectome.wordpress.com/2011/07/25 .

21. Kud Larsin, G. Vazov, K. Krumov, and J. Schneider, *Advances in International Psychology* (Sofia: Kassel University Press, 2013), 142.

22. Tim Stephens, "Study Shows How Epigenetic Memory is Passed Across Generations," UC Santa Cruz Newscenter, September 18, 2014, http://news.ucsc.edu/2014/09/epigenetics.html.

23. Alex Hutchinson, "Epigenetics and Fitness," *Runner's World*, September 22, 2014, http://www.runnersworld.com/health/epigenetics-and-fitness.

24. Maurizio Melon and Guiseppe Testa, "Scrutinizing the Epigenetics Revolution," BioSocieties, 2014, http://www.palgrave-journals.com/biosoc/journal/v9/n4/full/biosoc201422a.html.

25. Ethan Waters, "DNA is not Destiny: The New Science of Epigenetics," Discover, November 2006, http://discovermagazine.com/2006/nov/cover.

26. Waters, "DNA is not Destiny."

27. Meeri Kim, "Study Finds That Fear Can Travel Quickly Through Generations," *Washington Post*, December 7, 2013, http://www.washingtonpost.com/national/health-science/study-finds-that-fear-can-travel-quickly-through-generations-of-mice-dna/2013/12/07/94dc97f2-5e8e-11e3-bc56-c6ca94801fac_story.html.

28. Kim, "Study Finds That Fear Can Travel Quickly Through Generations."

29. Kim, "Study Finds That Fear Can Travel Quickly Through Generations."

30. Kim, "Study Finds That Fear Can Travel Quickly Through Generations."

31. Dan Hurley, "Grandma's Experiences Leave a Mark on your Genes," Discover, June 25, 2015, http://discovermagazine.com/2013/may/13-grandmas-experiences-leave-epigenetic-mark-on-your-genes.

32. Katie McGhee and Alison Bell, "Paternal Care in a Fish: Epigenetics and Fitness Enhancing Effects on Offspring," Proceedings B, The Royal Society, September 17, 2014, DOI: 10.1098/rspb.2014.1146http://rspb.royalsocietypublishing.org/content/281/1794/20141146.

33. Jeffrey Craig, "The New Science of Epigenetics and the Possibilities for Resilience," ABC, 2015, http://www.abc.net.au/tv/life/stories/s2994579.htm.

34. Angela Miller, *Violence and Abuse in Society* (Santa Barbara, CA: ABC-Clio, 2010),445.

35. Carl Zimmer, "Parents May Pass Down More Than Just Genes, Study Suggests," *New York Times*, December 3, 2015.

36. "Languages of the World," One World, Nations Online, 1998, http://www.nationsonline.org/oneworld/languages.htm.

37. Norwegian Nobel Committee. Retrieved 4 October, 2012, www.nobelprize.org/nobel_prizes/peace/laureates/2012/.

38. Jerry Coyne, "Why Evolution is True," Blog at Wordpress, 2011, http://whyevolutionistrue.wordpress.com/2011/09/26/epigenetics-again-will-it-cause-a-revolution-in-evolution/.
39. Coyne, "Why Evolution is True."
40. Harman Kagan, *The Psychological Immune System* (Bloomington, IN: Author House, 2006), 197.
41. Kagan,*The Psychological Immune System*,198.
42. "Kin Selection and Inclusive Fitness," Arizona.edu, accessed 2015, http://www.public.iastate.edu/~nvalenzu/EEOB514/Lectures/6-KinSelection.pdf.
43. Kara Rogers, "Inclusive Fitness," Encyclopedia Britanica, accessed 2015, http://www.britannica.com/EBchecked/topic/1710067/inclusive-fitness.
44. Marie Charpentier, Delphine Deubel and Patricia Peignot, "Relatedness and Social Behaviors in Cercopithecus Solatus,"*International Journal of Primatology* 29 (2008): 487–95.
45. S. Rossiter, G. Jones, R. Ransome, E. Barratt, "Relatedness Structure and Kin-biased Foraging in the Greater Horseshoe Bat," *Behavioral Ecology and Sociobiology* 51 (2002).
46. Harry Moore, et al. "Exceptional Sperm Cooperation in the Wood Mouse," *Nature* 418 (2002): 174–77.
47. Kin selection course materials, http://eebweb.arizona.edu/faculty/dornhaus/courses/materials/7%20evolution%20of%20cooperation%20bw.pdf.
48. Carl Zimmer, "Unraveling Why Some Mammals Kill Off Infants," *New York Times*, November 13, 2014.
49. "We Are at a Crossroads for How We Deal With People who Abuse Children," NPCC, July 2015, http://news.npcc.police.uk/releases/we-are-at-crossroads-in-how-we-deal-with-child-abuse.
50. M. Daly and M. Wilson, "Child Abuse and Other Risks of not Living with Both Parents," *Ethology and Sociobiology* 6 (1985): 197.
51. "Kin selection course materials, http://eebweb.arizona.edu/faculty/dornhaus/courses/materials/7%20evolution%20of%20cooperation%20bw.pdf.
52. Philip Edwards, "Plumage Variation, Territoriality and Breeding Displays of the Golden Plover Pluvialis Apricaria in Southwest Scotland, *International Journal of Avian Science*, April 2008, http://onlinelibrary.wiley.com/doi/10.1111/j.1474-919X.1982.tb03747.x/abstract.
53. Philip Whitfield, "Plumage Variability and Territoriality," *Animal Behavior* 34 (October 1986): 1471–82.
54. Laszlo Zsolt, Balaz Rosivall, et. al. "Determinants of Male Territorial Behavior in a Hungarian Flycatcher Population," *Behavioral Ecology Sociobiology* 60 (2006): 663–71.
55. Bruce Walden, "The Ecology of Kin Recognition," *Annual Review of Ecology and Systematics* 19 (1988): 543–71.
56. Tab Numlock, "Flags are the Equivalent of Bird Plummage," Flags Forum, January 2010, http://www.flagsforum.com/viewtopic.php?f=20&t=1005.
57. Lloyd deMause, *Foundations of Psychohistory*, 1982, accessed 2015, http://www.geocities.ws/kidhistory/found/p271x290.htm.
58. "Color Matters," 1995, accessed 2015, http://www.colormatters.com/color-and-marketing/59-color-symbolism/the-meanings-of-colors.
59. deMause, *Foundations of Psychohistory*.
60. "History and Debate on Flag Burning," Debate.org, accessed 2015, http://www.debate.org/flag-burning/.
61. Evan Charney and Roger Chapman, eds., *Culture Wars: An Encyclopedia of Issues, Voices, and Viewpoints* (Armonk, NY: M.E. Sharpe, 2009);"History and Debate on Flag Burning," Debate.org, accessed 2015.
62. Hinde, *The Psychological Causes of War*, http://www.unc.edu/depts/diplomat/AD_Issues/amdipl_7/hinde3.html.
63. Carlos Navarrete, Daniel Fessler, et al., "Elevated Ethnocentrism in the First Trimester of Pregnancy," *Evolution and Human Behavior*, 28 (2007): 60–65.

64. J. Faulkner, M. Schaller, et al., "Evolved Disease–Avoidance Mechanisms and Contemporary Xenophobic Attitudes," *Group Processes and Intergroup Relations* 7 (2004): 333–53.

65. David Aberbach, *The European Jews, Patriotism and the Liberal State, 1789–1939* (New York: Routledge, 2012).

66. Semion Goldin, "Antisemitism and Pogroms in the Military (Russian Empire)," in 1914-1918-online. International Encyclopedia of the First World War, ed. by Ute Daniel, Peter Gatrell, Oliver Janz, Heather Jennifer Keene Jones, Alan Kramer, and Bill Nasson, issued by Freie Universität Berlin, Berlin 2014-10-08. DOI: http://dx.doi.org/10.15463/ie1418.10283.

67. George Larner and Michael Dobbs, "New Tapes Reveal Depth of Nixon's Anti-Semitism," *Washington Post*, October 6, 1999, http://www.washingtonpost.com/wp-srv/politics/daily/oct99/nixon6.htm.

68. Rick Gladstone, "26 percent of World's Adults are Anti-Semitic, Survey Finds," *New York Times*, May 13, 2014.

69. Kevin MacDonald, "A Social Identity Theory of Anti-Semitism," accessed 2015, http://www.kevinmacdonald.net/chap1.pdf.

70. MacDonald, "A Social Identity Theory of Anti-Semitism."

71. MacDonald, "A Social Identity Theory of Anti-Semitism."

72. "Adolf Hitler about the Jews," Jewish Upps main page, accessed 2015, http://www.mosaisk.com/auschwitz/Adolf-Hitler-about-the-Jews.php.

73. "Rwanda, 1994," Genocide, Peace Pledge Union Information, accessed 2015, http://www.ppu.org.uk/genocide/g_rwanda4.html.

74. "Rwanda, 1994," Genocide, Peace Pledge Union Information.

75. "Rwanda, 1994," Genocide, Peace Pledge Union Information.

76. Mark Shaller, "The Behavioral Immune System: How Unconscious Fears of Infection Shape Many Aspects of our Psychology." *Scientific American* (November 20, 2014): 1–3.

77. Carl Zimmer, "Is Patriotism a Subconscious Way for Humans to Avoid Disease," *Discover*, March 2009, http//discovermagazine.com/2009/mar/17-is-patriotism-a-subconscious-way-for-humans-to-avoid-disease.

78. Zimmer, "Is Patriotism a Subconscious Way for Humans to Avoid Disease."

79. Debra Nussbaum Cohen, "Poll: American Jews with Disabilities Excluded from Community," *Haaretz*, July 31, 2015, http://www.haaretz.com/jewish-world/jewish-world-news/.premium-1.547310.

80. "Scope Tracer Survey of Disabled People," ComRes, 2011, http://comres.co.uk/polls/scope-tracker-survey-of-disabled-people/.

81. Noam Scheiber, "Fake Cover Letters Expose Bias Against Disabled," *New York Times*, November 2, 2015.

82. Amanda Gardner, "Many Obese Americans Struggle with Stigma," Health Day, August 2012, http://consumer.healthday.com/vitamins-and-nutritional-information-27/obesity-health-news-505/many-obese-americans-struggle-with-stigma-discrimination-poll-finds-667697.html.

83. "New Survey Highlights Significant Psychological Impact of Rosacea," *The Dermatologist,* accessed 2015, http://www.the-dermatologist.com/content/new-survey-highlights-significant-psychological-impact-rosacea.

84. "Survey Shows Facial Redness Takes Emotional Toll," National Rosacea Society, November 2013, http://www.rosacea.org/weblog/survey-shows-facial-redness-takes-emotional-toll.

85. Nicholas Kristof, "Our Biased Brains," *New York Times*, May 7, 2015.

86. Hinde, *Psychological Bases of War*.

87. John Blake, "The New Threat: Racism without Racists," CNN, November 27, 2014, http://www.cnn.com/2014/11/26/us/ferguson-racism-or-racial-bias/.

88. "Most Americans See Lingering Racism—In Others," CNN, December 12, 2006,http://www.cnn.com/2006/US/12/12/racism.poll/index.html?eref=yahoo.

89. "Race and Ethnicity," CBS/New York Times Poll, PollingReport.com, July 2015,http://www.pollingreport.com/race.htm.

90. Charles Epp and Steven Maynard-Moody, "Driving While Black," *Washington Monthly*, February 2014, http://www.washingtonmonthly.com/magazine/january_february_2014/ten_miles_square/driving_while_black048283.php?page=all.

91. Juan Andres Paez, "Racial Discrimination in Latin America: The 'Pigmentocracy' Approach," *Dejustica*, December 2014, http://dejusticiablog.com/2014/12/09/racial-discrimination-in-latin-america-the-pigmentocracy-approach/.

92. Nandini Chavan and Qutub Jehan Kidwai, *Personal Law Reforms and Gender Empowerment: A Debate on Uniform Civil Code* (India: Hope India Publications, 2006).

93. A. G. Greenwald, and M. R. Banaji, "Implicit Social Cognition: Attitudes, Self-esteem, and Stereotypes," *Psychological Review* 102 (1995): 4–27.

94. News staff, "Implicit Association Test: Are You Secretly Racist?" Scientific Blogging, August 2012, http://www.science20.com/news_articles/implicit_association_test_are_you_secretly_racist_hint_you_are-92783.

95. "FAQs" Project Implicit, accessed 2015, https://implicit.harvard.edu/implicit/demo/background/faqs.html#faq19.

96. Sendhil Mullainathan, "Racial Bias, Even When We Have Good Intentions," *New York Times*, January 3, 2015.

97. Mary Mederois Kent, "Most Americans Marry Within their Race," PRB, August 2010, http://www.prb.org/Publications/Articles/2010/usintermarriage.aspx.

98. "75 percent of White Americans don't Have a Close Minority Friend," *The Week*, August 27, 2014,http://theweek.com/speedreads/index/267130/speedreads-75-percent-of-white-americans-dont-have-a-close-minority-friend.

99. Britni Danielle, "75 percent of White People do not Have any Nonwhite Friends," Takepart, July 2015, http://www.takepart.com/article/2014/08/28/75-percent-white-people-have-no-nonwhite-friends.

100. David Smith, "South Africa Still a Chronically Racially Divided Nation, Finds Survey," Guardian Africa Network, December 2012, http://www.theguardian.com/world/2012/dec/06/south-africa-racially-divided-survey.

101. Hinde, *Psychological Bases of War*.

102. "The Religion for After," Religion quotes, accessed 2015, http://www.searchquotes.com/search/Religion_Causing_Wars/.

103. Bruce Alberts, Alexander Johnson, et al,"Lymphocytes and the Cellular Basis of Adaptive Immunity," *Molecular Biology of the Cell*, 4th ed. (New York: Garland Science, 2002), http://www.ncbi.nlm.nih.gov/books/NBK26921/.

104. "Innate Immunity," British Society for Immunology, accessed 2015, http://www.immunologyexplained.co.uk/HowItWorks.aspx.

105. Richard Underhill, "Guard Bees Protect the Hive," The Peace Bee Farmer Blog, August 21, 2009, http://peacebeefarm.blogspot.com/2009/08/guard-bees-protect-hive.html.

106. Ken Thomas, "Why do Honeybees Die After They Sting," EarthSky, June 2011, http://earthsky.org/earth/why-do-bees-die-after-they-sting-you.

107. Shawn Paul Wood, "Bad News: Negative Headlines Get Much More Attention," PRNewser, February 2014, http://www.mediabistro.com/prnewser/bad-news-negative-headlines-get-much-more-attention_b85912.

108. Joakim Norberg, "Fearful Attention" Stockholm University, 2012, http://www.diva-portal.org/smash/get/diva2:576589/FULLTEXT01.pdf.

109. R. Lane and L. Nadel, *Cognitive Neuroscience of Emotion* (New York: Oxford University Press, 1999).

110. Ray Williams, "Why We Love Bad News," *Psychology Today*, December 2010, http://www.psychologytoday.com/blog/wired-success/201012/why-we-love-bad-news.

111. Williams, "Why We Love Bad News."

112. "The Biggest News of 2014," Mashable, accessed 2015, http://mashable.com/2014/12/22/news-of-2014/.

113. "How Long do Babies Carry their Mother's Immunity?" NHS Choices, May 2015, http://www.nhs.uk/chq/Pages/939.aspx?CategoryID=54.

114. By the way, it is important to recognize the doctrine of inclusive fitness is controversial. To Professor Martin Nowak of Harvard, "Contrary to what is often claimed there exists no empirical test of inclusive fitness theory; nobody has ever performed an actual inclusive fitness calculation for a real population." http://www.ncbi.nlm.nih.gov/pubmed/12576125.

115. Lymphocytes are a type of white blood cells while leukocytes are equivalently termed in general as white blood cells. See http://www.differencebetween.net/science/difference-between-lymphocytes-and-leukocytes/.

116. Robert Leahy, "Are We Born to be Afraid," *Psychology Today*, May 2009, https://www.psychologytoday.com/blog/anxiety-files/200805/are-we-born-be-afraid.

117. "Tanzania Arrests 23 over Killing of Seven 'Witches,'" NEWS, October 2014, http://www.bbc.com/news/world-africa-29572974.

118. Estelle Thurtle, "10 Ridiculous Theories about Ebola Crisis," Listverse, October 2014, http://listverse.com/2014/10/10/10-disturbing-conspiracy-theories-about-the-ebola-crisis/.

119. "Autoimmune Disease," Healthline, July 2015, http://www.healthline.com/health/autoimmune-disorders#Overview1.

EIGHT

The *Artificial* Psychic Immune System

In earlier chapters, the *physical* immune system was described as having two primary subdivisions, innate and adaptive. In the case of human beings there is an additional adaptive immune system that does not seem to exist in our primate cousins—the *artificial* adaptive immune system.

The adaptive immune system divides into natural and artificial components. When we say natural, we might as easily say an instinctive or autonomic adaptation to our environment. Artificial, on the other hand, refers to consciously manipulating immunities through science, learning, and culture, in other words, augmenting our natural immunities. By deliberate devices like sanitation, quarantines, vaccination, medical care, or scientific discovery, we artificially boost the immune system's efficiency.

The results have been astonishing.

The best way of thinking about the artificial physical immune system is to wonder what life would be like without it. Vaccines impacted polio, whooping cough, diphtheria, Meningitis C, and smallpox. Smallpox once killed 30 percent of those infected; today it has all but vanished from the human disease pantheon.[1]

Routine vaccinations in the United States since 1994 saved an estimated 732,000 lives.[2] Worldwide, about 83 percent of infants are now vaccinated against diphtheria, tetanus, and pertussis, saving between two- and three million lives annually.[3]

In 1847, before the germ theory of disease became known, Ignaz Semmelweis suggested that doctors wash their hands in a chlorine solution when delivering babies. The result was a rapid decline in maternal death from puerperal fever.[4]

The artificial physical immune system—that is, our conscious, deliberate attempts to control disease—is enormously important to collective health. If one looks at life expectancy during the last century, it is easily seen how robust the results are. In developing countries life expectancy rose from twenty-five to sixty-one, and in industrialized countries it expanded from forty-five to seventy-three in a century.

If there was no artificial immune system and humanity was left only with the innate and adaptive immune systems that most other creatures have, humanity would be in a sorry state indeed.

Think about Ebola for a moment. The current mortality rate for this scourge is 40 percent. It is one of the most virulent infections mankind has encountered.[5] At this writing, only about thirty thousand people have been infected, but that is only because the artificial immune system is working overtime.

Flights from the region were screened. Anyone having contact with an Ebola patient was detained at U.S. airports. Large areas of Africa were under quarantine. New burial practices went into effect to minimize the spread of the disease.[6] Potential vaccines from Johnson & Johnson, Merck, and GlaxoSmithKline, plus Chinese, Russian, and Canadian products were fast-tracked for possible deployment.[7]

If humankind did not engage in these measures, if there was no World Health Organization (WHO), no Center For Disease Control (CDC), no ongoing research to develop vaccines—in other words *no artificial immune system*—humankind would be left with only its natural primate immune system. Ebola would spread to virtually every corner of the earth, and 40 percent of the human population would succumb to the disease, 2.8 billion people.[8]

One must extend kudos to consciousness, rationality, and those precious higher human powers. Indeed, by November of 2015, only one new case of Ebola was seen in Guinea, and many argued the Ebola epidemic was effectively over.[9]

THE ARTIFICIAL *PSYCHIC* IMMUNE SYSTEM

So let us turn our attention to the psychic immune system as an epiphenomenon of our physical immune system. How does the psychic artificial immune system work, and what is it made of? The term artificial immune system comes from immunology, but in the psychic sphere, one is talking about rationality, intention, and all purposive attempts to mitigate danger and protect against threat and injury.

When Jane Goodall was asked if human aggression, war and violence, were inevitable, she said "I would argue not because we have also evolved this amazingly sophisticated intellect, and we are capable of controlling our innate behavior a lot of the time."[10]

Humans have created myriad institutions dedicated to just that. School bus drivers, along with their buses, are certified as safe, secure, and trustworthy. Schools demand that children have all of their immunizations before they can attend. Volunteers fan out every morning helping children cross the street to get to school without danger. Inside, teachers educate children about crossing the street too—*stop, look, and listen*—or teach them about new varieties of addictive drugs or sexually transmitted diseases they might encounter.

Parents read books on how to raise a baby. Swaddling is abandoned or reclaimed based on new data gathered on sleeping behavior and calmness. California is currently considering a law prohibiting spanking a child with an implement.[11] Sweden, Austria, and German already have outlawed corporal punishment.[12] Policemen and fireman protect the community. The National Guard stands at the ready whenever there is a natural disaster or a major social upheaval. Armies, air forces, and navies are on patrol to protect the nation.

The human institutional focus on survival and protection is ubiquitous, and each component of our artificial psychic immune system is structured ever keeping in mind the survival of the individual, family, group, community, and nation. Trying to identify all of its elements is impossible. Let us tease out a few constituents where we can, however.

Nonviolence, the Golden Rule and Fratricide

Certainly one important ingredient of the artificial psychic immune system is religion. Virtually every denomination includes some variant of the golden rule, a Biblical edict to treat others as you would have them treat oneself.[13] This is at least a meager attempt to neutralize or transcend the dichotomy of *us versus them* and introduce a measure of altruism.

Religions provide behavioral prescriptions toward reciprocity, cooperation, and nonviolence, while issuing prohibitions against intraspecies killing. Clearly, these are devices or strategies for protection and security. Here is a short tour of humanity's religious prohibitions and admonitions to reduce violence and augment human security and safety:[14]

Brahamanism: This is the sum of duty: Do naught unto others which would cause you pain if done to you. (Mahabharata)

Buddhism: Hurt not others in ways that you yourself would find hurtful. Udana-Varga

Christianity: All things whatsoever ye would that men should do to you, do ye even so to them. (Matthew, 7:12)

Confucianism: Surely it is the maxim of loving-kindness: Do not unto others that you would not have them do unto you. (Analects)

Greeks: Do not do to others what angers you if done to you by others. [Socrates (469 BC–399 BC)]

Islam: No one of you is a believer until he desires for his brother that which he desires for himself. (Sunnah)

Judaism: What is hateful to you, do not to your fellowmen. That is the entire Law; all the rest is commentary. (Talmud, Shabbat, 31,a)

Indeed we know that religions have historically precipitated war and violence—so their record on this score is certainly blemished—yet virtually all make public prohibitions against killing and fratricide. The sixth commandment, thou shalt not kill, is not merely a Judeo-Christian invention. The prohibition dates to 2050 BC and is found in Sumerian chronicles.[15]

OTHER MECHANISMS PROMOTING COOPERATION, ALTRUISM, AND NONVIOLENCE

The innate and adaptive psychic immune system confers not only an instinctive aversion to intraspecies killing, but also toward a cooperative, altruistic, and nonviolent predisposition. However, the *artificial* psychic immune system brings to the table a host of additional devices that work toward the same goal.

There are hundreds of organizations devoted to peace, conflict resolution, and nonviolence, ranging from *Peace Now* to the *Catholic Worker Movement,* the *Plowshares Fund* to *Doctors Without Borders,* and the *Palestinian Center for the Study of Nonviolence* to *Jewish Voices for Peace.* These institutional efforts promote nonviolence and cooperative collective behavior. In addition, every government has a phalanx of diplomatic embassies whose missions encompass dialogue, communication, negotiation, and conflict resolution.

The human race expends a great deal of energy in developing conscious strategies promoting peace, safety, and security—factors that are constituents of the psychic artificial immune system.

TERRITORIALITY, DOMINANCE, WAR, AND THE PSYCHIC ARTIFICIAL IMMUNE SYSTEM

Unfortunately, there is a darker side to the psychic immune system: territoriality, dominance, and aggression. It would be foolish to deny this psychological process also has an abiding influence over collective protection, survival, safety, and defense.

When discussing the conscious, rather than instinctive side of the psychic immune system, attention is drawn to all conscious and—allegedly—rational human organizations that are prepared to fight on behalf of humankind, not just the nonviolent peace groups we have identified.

Here it is incumbent to mention entities involved in military activity, defense spending, and myriad other efforts undertaken to defend our own kind.

China currently fields 3.9 million soldiers; North Korea 7.6 million, India 4.7 million, the United States 2.3 million.[16] The human race spends $1.8 trillion annually—that is, the total defense expenditures for all countries on earth—*to protect itself from its fellow kin.*[17]

The United States, with 6 percent of the earth's population, possesses the world's largest economy, equal to 19 percent of all goods and services produced by the human race.[18] The United States is the leading global superpower and accounts for 39 percent of all military expenditures.[19] It maintains one thousand overseas military bases and projects its power to every continent on earth.[20]

In terms of waging war or waging peace, humankind gives much higher priority to prepare for the former. The UN budget for peace is less than 0.005 percent the amount allocated for military defense and war. Despite these discrepancies, expenditures for war and for peace actually have resulted in an overall diminution of deaths due to military conflict.

Surprisingly, and despite the barbarities of the World Wars, Korea, Vietnam, Pol Pot, Iraq, and the slaughter in the Congo, the total number of deaths from military conflicts has declined since 1947. In effect the world is getting safer. A report from the Human Security Report Project says,

> Deaths from war—either between state powers or by a government against its people—have been generally in decline since the end of World War II. . . . During 2012—the most recent year for which there are data—the number of conflicts being waged around the world dropped sharply, from 37 to 32. High intensity conflicts have declined by more than half since the end of the Cold War, while terrorism, genocide and homicide numbers are also down. The report . . . "counts wars and war deaths (international and civil), murders, and other violence (including political coups), and compares the numbers historically." It shows, for example, that the number of international wars has fallen hard since the 1950s (from more than six a year, to less than one a year now). Likewise, the number of war deaths has also plummeted. In the 1950s, there were almost 250 deaths caused by war per million people. Now there are less than 10 per million. There have been some pretty extraordinary changes and they haven't been recognized. Military leaders, for example, say we live in the most dangerous time ever. And yet, in statistical terms at least, this isn't remotely true.[21]

If one places pro-peace and anti-military biases to the side, they would discover that whatever the human race is doing to protect itself from its own kin and the penchant for territoriality, aggression, dominance, and war actually seems to be working.

Certainly, one might wish that nonviolent, peaceful, reconciliation would replace military bombast. However, to be square with the empirical data, it needs to be recognized that the artificial psychic immune system is hard at work, either by peace-making or military muscle-flexing, to robustly deter violence and aggression.

This argument may seem controversial, but Harvard Psychologist Steven Pinker corroborates the sentiment: in charting the decline of violence over the last two millennia, he argues that it may seem illogical, especially as we read today's headlines, but, in fact,

> "Violence has been in decline for thousands of years," he says. "We may be living in the most peaceful era in our species' existence." . . . Pinker, who is a psychological scientist from Harvard University, collected his research on the subject in a new book called *The Better Angels of Our Nature*. . . . To reach his conclusions, Pinker says he estimated the frequency of violence and violent deaths relative to the human population from prehistory up to the present day. His estimates are supported by ethnographies, archeological research, law enforcement records, victimization surveys, and statistics recording casualties in armed conflicts. From these records, Pinker determined that up to 15 percent of prehistoric deaths were violent. In contrast, only 0.3 percent of human deaths in 2005 were violent.[22]

This comes as a rather pleasant surprise.

Therefore, if we are to confer any medals on the *physical* artificial immune system—all those vaccines, antibiotics, and scientific advancements in medicine—we can credit it with almost doubling human life expectancy in a century. In fact, *global* life expectancy increased by six years just since 1990.[23] Medals, please!

But the psychic artificial immune system deserves a few medals too. All of the conscious and rationally crafted peace treaties, sanctions, threats of war, UN Security Council resolutions, peace-keeping operations, military shows of force, convoluted nuclear deterrence strategies—all of it lumped together—also managed to protect and defend human beings, and to do so rather remarkably:

> Yes, thousands of people have died in bloody unrest from Africa to Pakistan, while terrorists plot bombings and kidnappings. Wars drag on in Iraq and Afghanistan. In peaceful Norway, a man massacred 69 youths in July. In Mexico, headless bodies turn up, victims of drug cartels. . . . Yet, historically, we've never had it this peaceful. . . . Statistics reveal dramatic reductions in war deaths, family violence, racism, rape, murder and all sorts of mayhem. . . . In his book, (Steven) Pinker writes: "The decline of violence may be the most significant and least appreciated development in the history of our species. . . . And it runs counter to what the mass media is reporting. . . . The number of people killed in battle—calculated per 100,000 population—has dropped by 1,000-fold over the centuries as civilizations evolved. Before there were

> organized countries, battles killed on average more than 500 out of every 100,000 people. In 19th century France, it was 70. In the 20th century with two world wars and a few genocides, it was 60. Now battlefield deaths are down to three-tenths of a person per 100,000. The rate of genocide deaths per world population was 1,400 times higher in 1942 than in 2008."[24]

In an article, "The World is not Falling Apart," *Slate* magazine searched behind the negative headlines to find quantitative measures that show worldwide violence declining, not accelerating. There is less child victimization, fewer battle deaths, lower homicide rates worldwide, decreased rates of rape/assault rates and a decline in mass killings.[25]

If one defines the adaptive psychic artificial immune system as a system of conscious, judicious, and deliberate strategies to protect and insure human survival, it is obviously learning from prior mistakes and doing more than a decent job. Medals, please.

THE ARTIFICIAL PSYCHIC IMMUNE SYSTEM AND OUR DARKER PREDISPOSITIONS

The prior discussion of the innate and adaptive psychic immune systems leaves one ambivalent. On one hand, the human race has an innate aversion to killing its own kind. That is reassuring. Children also think their loving parents smell worse than strangers, an incest avoidance mechanism that seems more hard-wired than Freudian. That is rather agreeable as well.

At the same time, though, our species possesses an innate territorial fight response that will autonomically engage, releasing huge spurts of cortisol and adrenaline into our system if someone parks their car in our driveway, enters our apartment uninvited, blasts sub-woofer hip-hop directly into our ears, or acts inappropriately with our wife or children. In other words, a volcanic emotional reaction can be triggered when someone violates personal space, territory, or possessions.

When these stimuli occur, there is an urgent need to calm down and remove oneself from the rage reaction that reflexively imposes itself. The hostility rising from territory violations is similar to the besieged ancestral proprietor who swells up and releases a huge dose of Robert Ardrey's "inspired lunacy." If we don't control our emotions, we wind up in the same predicament as myriad others who act out dark, inherited sets of territorial impulses passed down to us over the millennia.

Ellie Nesler was in court for the trial of Daniel Driver, a church camp counselor accused of molesting her son. Driver, who had previous convictions for child molestation, looked at Mrs. Nesler from the docket *and smirked.* Driver's smirk of defiance unraveled Mrs. Nesler's rational demeanor. She pulled out a small handgun and shot him in the back of the head right in the middle of the courtroom.

> Witnesses said she appeared calm as she was led from the courtroom in handcuffs. "You might think that somebody who did something like that would be shriveled up, but she was proud," said Rick Shackley. . . . "She wouldn't have done it if he didn't have that cocky look in the beginning," she said. . . . Ms. Adams did not fault her sister for the shooting. "What's a mother going to do?" she asked.[26]

Human beings have whole sets of blind, inherited tendencies that accompany them. Whether good or bad, adaptive or atavistic, prosocial or antisocial, they are the trailings of our innate and adaptive psychic immune system. When these protective traits become aroused, all hell can break loose.

Let's not forget these emotional packages are—*or were*—programmed for survival and self-preservation. In the modern world, however, they need to be nuanced, made rational, and the Neanderthal colorings blended into accepted civil behavior. This is one of the jobs of artificial psychic immune system.

Territoriality and Civil Law

We are quick to respond to violations of our sense of territory. Our natural reaction to a territorial intrusion is similar to Mrs. Nesler's in the courtroom—take the law into our own hands. The choice is fight or flight, either seek retribution in a fit of rage through confrontation, or turn and briskly flee from impending danger, leaving others to fend for themselves. Fortunately, the artificial psychic immune system *tempers* these autonomic and reflexive territorial responses.

It is what prompts a 911 call, or a reliance upon external social institutions that are interpolated between ourselves and our instincts. The appropriate behavior in these critical moments is to call the police and let the authorities handle the problem; not carry out redress and revenge like Mrs. Nesler did by shooting the perpetrator.

Territorial incursions may psychologically involve assaults on our person or our children. They may also go by another name, property crimes. In the civil justice system these include auto theft, shoplifting, burglary, larceny, vandalism, trade infringement, and even identity theft. In the United States, which boasts the highest crime rate in the world—more than eleven million crimes committed annually—property crime is the largest category. Eight million illegal "territorial" incursions related to private property crimes occur each year.[27] In the United States, about 12 percent of households have experienced some kind of property crime. Worldwide, close to $128 billion is lost from shoplifting, $42 billion in the

United States alone.[28] Identity theft plunders $5 billion per year from people.

Despite problems in prosecuting property crimes,[29] the social order continuously tries to protect and defend individuals, families, and communities. These are the people one calls for safety. These are the agencies in which to place one's trust.

Polls show 78 percent of Americans believe police will perform adequately on their behalf when a property crime occurs. In Switzerland, 98 percent feel this way, while in Mexico a victim's confidence in getting help from authorities drops to 45 percent.[30] When faith in the external social order declines, as in Mexico, there is a corresponding desire to take the law into one's own hands, an atavistic regression to vigilantism. This is a phenomenon currently witnessed in Mexico.[31]

In places where people have confidence in the social order, a greater sense of security also exists. The social order, in this context, is an oblique reference to the artificial psychic immune system, or the conscious, deliberate, and institutionalized way to assure security, self-preservation, and survival. From police to the courts, militias to civil defense forces, the *system* is there for collective safety and as a buffer against instinctive territoriality and the great evolutionary fracas between proprietors and intruders.

By the way, property crime, what we are calling territorial intrusion, is not always to be blamed on the intruder while the proprietor is held harmless. Have we forgotten Jean Valjean and *Les Miserables*? The proprietor may be a high-level contributor to territorial property crime by hoarding resources. Scholars long ago correlated property crime with income and wealth inequality.[32] The fewer eating at the table, the more are on the outside demanding a fair share of the pie. In the United States, wealth and income inequality gaps are farther apart than ever. "The wealthiest 160,000 families own as much wealth as the poorest 145 million families, and that wealth is about 10 times as unequal as income."[33] One way of equalizing these imbalances is through property crime.

Surely we will not solve the problem of worldwide crime or its etiology in this chapter, but we can underscore the role of our immune system to keep us safe. Specifically, we can trust our artificial psychic immune system to give us a layer of protection that is conscious, rational, and deliberative.

The safety net interpolates temperance, civility, the rule of law, and the social order between individuals and their instinctual tendencies that lead to danger. Civil behavior steers people away from the territorial lunacy of Mrs. Nesler's gun-toting courtroom drama. It prevents people from emulating Walter Stephens, who, if you recall, killed and then incinerated his neighbor over a few feet of land in a property dispute.

Generally, the artificial psychic immune system kicks in and successfully interjects the "law" between ourselves and territorial instincts. Prosecution of property crimes, civil litigation, bankruptcy filings, adjudication of real property, tenancy, trust, and common law disputes are resolved politely and with civility outside the theater of instinctual skirmishing, banditry, vigilantism, and courtroom shootings.[34]

Collective Hysteria

Earlier, the discussion centered on fight-flight behavior and found that some collective flight responses are genuinely rational. More than fifty million refugees streamed out of Syria, Somalia, Congo, and Afghanistan in 2014 in order to avoid conflict and seek a safe haven.[35] Makes sense.

Flight responses can also be irrational, however. Consider panic and hysteria, especially of the collective variety when everyone decides to stampede out the door at the same time. The instinctive reflex occurs in outdoor gatherings, but it also happens in our minds. In China, a man fainted on a subway train. Fearing danger, passengers started to panic to get out of the train. Everyone assumed some unknown event occurred that put them at risk. Many of the commuters had no idea why they were running. They were driven by fear that something was terribly wrong, and they headed for the nearest exit.[36] Humans are reflexively prone toward fight and flight. The role of the artificial psychic immune system again is to interpose rationality, logic, and restraint to counteract the release of these reflexive, autonomic response patterns.

Schools and businesses have fire drills or post evacuation plans to instruct students and adults how to behave in the event of a fire, earthquake, or other natural disaster. The National Fire Association requires these drills.[37] Such rehearsals are consciously mediated strategies to prevent panic stampedes—irrational collective flight responses—in a real emergency. An example of collective hysteria affecting mental states is when stock market panics lead to serious financial losses based on little more than a rumor. These events have precipitated contagion with everyone running and shouting at the same time. A few examples:

- "The stock market panic of 1907 or the Bankers Panic began with a failed attempt by two men to corner the copper market and then runs on the Knickerbocker Trust Company. That night the president of Knickerbocker committed suicide and the next day there were runs on all of the banks."[38]
- "The stock market panic of 1987 was a panic that had everyone trying to sell their stocks and no buyers. The stock market had gone up 41 percent during the past two years and some worried the market had gone up too fast. By Mid October 1987, the S&P 500 lost 10 percent in three days. At the opening bell of Monday October 19, 1987, the DJIA dropped and didn't stop dropping. By the end of the

> day the DJIA lost 508 points or 22.6 percent for *the largest single day percentage drop in the history of the average.* There doesn't seem to be a major reason for this panic. One reason given was program trading, too many computerized sell orders. The market steadily climbed back to a pre-crash level 15 months later."[39]

These collective panic attacks are not adaptive and more likely irrational events. To prevent collective hysteria and contagion—the errant glitches of the innate psychic immune system—rational antidotes are needed to mollify and temper flight-fight reflexes.

On Wall Street, trading curbs and circuit breakers were introduced into markets to deal with selling frenzies. Trading is halted twenty-five minutes or longer if flash crashes are 7 percent or higher in a single day. If panic-selling is larger, markets are shuttered.[40] These are rational mechanisms which attempt to soothe and anneal reflexes, instincts, and urges. After all, hysteria is a flight response. The first one out of the burning subway survives. Everyone for himself. At its most banal level, flight response is a survival reflex. True, but when everyone is engaged, it metastasizes into collective mob rule, mass hysteria, and herd behavior that is outright dangerous for everyone.

This is how the artificial psychic immune system works, with its toolbox of conscious, purposeful strategies, to pull victims out of the instinctual abyss into which they repeatedly fall. Whether fire drills, circuit breakers, or 911 calls, one can be thankful for the intervention of the artificial psychic immune system to maintain protection, order, safety, and sanity.

Tolerance and Us versus Them

Earlier it was noted that children begin to show a fear of strangers at about six months of age. They show preferences for their own ethnic group (kin) within the first three months of life. It is likely these fears and preferences have innate or epigenetic dimensions.

When we discussed the adaptive psychic immune system, the us for them drama appeared as an epiphenomenon of how the physical immune system is always on patrol for intruders and antigens. The psychic immune system behaves in parallel scanning the external world for danger and operating with a built-in mind-set that strangers, aliens, and those not one's own kin are more dangerous than their particular and familiar in-group. The Nazis enshrined anti-miscegenation laws forbidding marriage or extramarital relations outside of German bloodlines. This included not only Jews but "gypsies, negroes, or their bastard offspring."[41]

Nazis, however, didn't corner this market. Anti-miscegenation laws were also prevalent in the United States. Oklahoma banned marriages between whites and any person of African descent, as did Louisiana, Maryland, and Alabama. The Supreme Court declared such laws unconstitutional only in 1967.[42]

So kin-selection, inclusive fitness, and all of these darker *us versus them* derivatives form the basis for egregious human tendencies toward intolerance, xenophobia, prejudice, and intraspecies conflict. Some of these tendencies may have been adaptive in the ancestral past, but they are often inappropriate in the modern world. The artificial psychic immune system has before it, therefore, an educational task to temper and mitigate racist and prejudicial stirrings.

Psychiatric studies of racism show that associating outgroups with infection, filth, dirt, and disease is part of the unconscious content of prejudicial inclinations, or what Mark Shaller calls the pathogen-avoidant behavioral immune system.[43]

The artificial psychic immune system is given a pedagogical role: to eradicate irrational beliefs and bring them into congruence with reality. The fundamental polemic that is found in our classrooms—and our media—occurs at a very basic level. Blacks are not dirty or infectious. The elderly and disabled are not contagious. Foreigners or immigrants are not threats to our safety that we have to avoid.

Despite all these efforts, within the international media particularly, one can still see the *us versus them* battle being waged between tolerance versus intolerance, prodigiously, and on a daily basis. A short trip to YouTube will reveal a Saudi journalist interviewing individuals on the street and asking "Would you, as a human being, be willing to shake hands with a Jew?" On Sesame Street, on the other hand, one can regularly see programs on tolerance and acceptance.[44]

Consider AIDS as an example. When the disease was running rampant, there were calls to quarantine all HIV positive people. In 1986, an organization called PANIC (Prevent AIDS Now Initiative Committee) put Proposition 64 on the California ballot and sought to quarantine all AIDS patients. Education and science—to wit, the artificial psychic immune system—stepped in to show that HIV was not communicable except through specific exchanges of bodily fluids. Science, education, and the media took down Proposition 64; the measure did not pass, and no state adopted a quarantine.

However, since AIDS was closely connected to gay issues, there was a spillover toward anti-gay prejudice, which was countered by a media initiative. The television show, *Will and Grace*, elevated American consciousness on gay issues, and the level of popular support for gay rights grew accordingly. In 1997, only 27 percent of Americans supported gay marriage; today a majority does.[45] Currently, same-sex marriages are permitted in more than thirty-six states and *Will and Grace* is seen in at least sixty countries.[46]

A similar example of how the artificial psychic immune system counters *us versus them* prejudice is found with anti-immigrant feelings. Just as lymphocytes and macrophages seek out intruders and destroy them in the physical immune system, so does the psychic immune system irresistibly and reflexively surveils invaders, intruders, and aliens—or illegal aliens—and tries to do the same.

The debate is whipped up by rhetoric such as appears in this immigrants-are-diseased screed:

> Ebola. Chikungunya. Dengue. Norovirus. Hantavirus. Swine flu. Varicella. Variola. The names sound like something out of a Sci-Fi movie. Yet, threats to Americans are real, and escalating by the week. The Department of Homeland Security (DHS) reported on August 1 that serious diseases are spreading at detention centers for illegal border crossers. Health care workers and Border Patrol agents, plus their children, have tested positive for tuberculosis (TB), swine flu, chicken pox, lice and scabies. Instead of being quarantined, illegal border crossers are being dispersed rapidly across the U.S., with those of school age being registered in public schools opening soon for all.
>
> They are bringing diseases not common to, or eradicated from, the U.S. . . . Illegals from those countries have been identified coming across our southern borders. . . . Mexico has serious outbreaks of dengue fever, which can produce debilitating physical and neurological effects, and also has more severe and deadly hemorrhagic forms. . . . Deadly Ebola hemorrhagic fever is raging out of control in multiple countries in West Africa. Border Patrol agents confirmed that West Africans have been apprehended coming via Mexico into the Rio Grande Valley in Texas, with a number of seriously ill individuals whisked away to undisclosed locations for treatment of undisclosed illnesses.[47]

This kind of article arouses panic in readers already alert to diseases that could impact them or their children. A more dispassionate analysis, however, shows that diseases like Swine flu outbreaks in Mexico were well under control all the way back to 2009.[48] There have been no cases of Ebola identified in the United States that came from illegal immigration,[49] and Cikungunya and Dengue fever are only contracted from mosquitos. To quote one health source: "Dengue is a non-contagious disease, i.e., it never transmits from one person to another."[50] Furthermore, vaccination rates in Central America are almost identical to U.S. vaccination rates, about 93 percent of all children.[51]

The panic-inducing, anti-immigrant article makes none of these important distinctions and instead plays upon predispositions to be suspicious of foreigners, invaders, and infectious agents, the quintessential ingredients of xenophobia and prejudice. The task of the artificial psychic immune system, then, is to temper these inclinations assuaging tendencies toward fight-flight (panic), and clarifying what is a rational versus an irrational threat in the modern world.

Whether the focus is on fire drills, trading curbs, *Will and Grace*, or factual presentations about AIDS, Ebola, or Dengue fever, the role of the artificial psychic immune system is to rationally protect and defend safety and security. And when ancestral impulses are aroused and these unconscious passions enflamed, its function is to quell the fight-flight emotion with intelligence, dispassion, and expanded consciousness.

MORE CONSTITUENTS OF THE PSYCHIC ARTIFICIAL IMMUNE SYSTEM: ALTRUISM AND MEDALS OF HONOR

If the artificial psychic immune system pursues conscious and willful strategies to assure protection and security, then it has a vested interest in promoting nonviolence, cooperation, tolerance, mutuality, altruism, and heroism. Virtually every society on earth celebrates and pays tribute to heroic deeds.

If Jung is correct that there is a hero archetype or imprint in every living human being, then the role of the artificial psychic immune system is to praise it, reinforce it, and encourage it whenever possible. In the United States, a soldier who sacrifices himself or is wounded while serving with his fellow comrades, is awarded a Medal of Honor. Close to 3,700 recipients have been given this honor since the Civil War.[52] In the days of the USSR, one of the highest medals given was "Hero of the Soviet Union"; over thirteen thousand were awarded. China has a "Hero's medal" and Australia its "Pride of Australia" awards. Egypt bestows the "Order of the Nile" on its heroes.

Every society, from ancient Rome to the present, sings hosannas for its heroes, the essence of the honor being to place the good of the other, the group, the nation, family, or country above self-interest. Awards of this sort are not merely for military heroism. Societies celebrate philanthropy and generosity, from canonized saints in the Catholic Church to the Carnegie medal for Philanthropy. Gentiles who saved or protected Jews during the Holocaust are awarded the designation, Righteous Among the Nations.

Heroism and altruism are prized by the artificial psychic immune system as well because such behavior promotes phylogenetic safety, security, and protection. Like the prairie dog thumping warnings, the guard honey bee prowling for intruders, or the brave flycatcher risking detection by screeching of approaching danger, the human community values, honors, memorializes and promotes similar heroic and altruistic behavior with uncanny ubiquity.

CONCLUSION

The adaptive artificial psychic immune system is certainly a mouthful, and exactly what it is and how far it reaches boggles the mind. It is, in fact, the name given for all conscious, rational, and deliberate strategies dedicated to human security, protection, and safety. This includes more behavior-oriented institutions, agencies, policies, and politics than we could possibly describe in a single text.

Admittedly, there are many government entities that promise protection and security but all too often are merely foils for suppression and control in the service of wealth, power, and privilege. Granted.

But at the same time, some human agencies on this planet actually exist for protection and security, and as such they belong to the artificial psychic immune system. From Russia's Federal Guard Service, to China's Ministry of Public Security, all the way to American agencies that seek to safeguard us from traffic accidents (National Traffic Safety Institute), criminals (FBI), terrorists (TSA), aircraft accidents (FAA), poisoning (FDA), communicable diseases (CDC), occupational hazards (OSHA), homelessness (HUD), weather emergencies (FEMA), boating accidents (Coast Guard), suicides (NIMH), or sex abuse (Child Protective Services), human beings are surrounded by collective security blankets of every color. Add into the mix charitable organizations worldwide that rescue and protect (UNICEF, International Red Cross, Red Crescent, HOPE, United Way), and then calculate the actual size of the artificial psychic immune system; it is inestimable.The ancestral, autonomic, and evolutionary security systems found in the animal kingdom—and in our innate and natural adaptive psychic immune system—have descended into present time. But all of that is *augmented* by the artificial psychic immune system.

The social order and the myriad institutions that belong to it make up a large part of that system, and its reach extends far beyond anything found amongst our primate cousins or the animal kingdom generally. As Trotsky observed, "The historic ascent of humanity, taken as a whole, may be summarized as a succession of victories of consciousness over blind forces in nature, in society, in man himself."[53]

Surely, the main function of the artificial psychic immune system is to use conscious strategies to provide safety, security, and protection from threats in a world that is constantly in flux.[54] But, it has a critical secondary function too which we cannot skim over.

When physicist Stephen Hawking was asked what he felt the greatest danger facing mankind was, he replied: "Human aggression. It may have had survival advantage in caveman days, to get more food, territory or partner with whom to reproduce, but now it threatens to destroy us all. . . . A major nuclear war could be the end of civilization and possibly the human race."[55]

Hawking's antidote for this existential condition is empathy, understanding, and greater consciousness. This second function of the artificial psychic immune system, then, is to interpolate consciousness, thought, and restraint between these baser, ancient survival instincts and actions.

It is critical that the human race increase the width and breadth of consciousness. The immediacy of this task is without question. The role of the artificial psychic immune system is to reduce both innate territoriality impulses and *us versus them* survival reflexes. We need to increasingly see ourselves as one species—humankind, brothers and sisters—rather than competing kinship groups that project, scapegoat, vilify and demonize one another. Virchand Gandhi perhaps best summarizes the need to overcome these *us versus them* ancestral predispositions: "This is my country, that is your country; these are the conceptions of narrow souls . . . the whole world is a family."[56]

NOTES

1. CDC, cited in Liz Szabo, "CDC: Vaccines Save Hundreds of Thousands of Lives," *USA Today*, April 24, 2014.
2. Behar Gholipour, "Vaccination has Saved 732,000 Children's Lives Since 1994," Livescience, April 24, 2014, http://www.livescience.com/45111-national-vaccination-effects.html.
3. "Immunization Facts and Figures," UNICEF, April 2013, http://www.unicef.org/immunization/files/UNICEF_Key_facts_and_figures_on_Immunization_April_2013(1).pdf .
4. O. Hanninen, M. Farago, and E. Monos, "Ignaz Philipp Semmelweis, The Prophet of Bacteriology," *Infection Control* 4, no. 5 (September/October 1983): 367–70.
5. Kevin Sack, Sheri Fink, et al., "How Ebola Roared Back," *New York Times*, December 29, 2014.
6. Jonathan Paye-Layley, "Ebola Outbreak: Quarantine Camps in West Africa at Breaking Point," *The Independent*, August 1, 2015.
7. Bahar Gholipour, "Here's a Look at the 3 Front Runners," *Live Science*, January 12, 2015, http://news.yahoo.com/ebola-vaccines-heres-look-3-front-runners-070326797.html.
8. WHO data cited in Julia Belluz, "America has Stopped Paying Attention but Ebola is still Ravaging Sierra Leone," Vox Health Care, December 2, 2014, http://www.vox.com/2014/12/2/7318913/ebola-virus-outbreak.
9. "Ebola Situation Reports," World Health Organization, November 18, 2015.
10. Hannah Osborne, "Happy 80th Birthday Jane Goodall: Inspirational Quotes from the Lady of the Apes," *Business Times*, April 3, 2014.
11. "California Anti-spanking Bill Passes First Hurdle," Campaign for Children and Families, *Christian News Wire*, April 15, 2015, http://www.christiannewswire.com/news/552126278.html.
12. Global initiative to end all corporal punishment of children, accessed 2015, http://www.endcorporalpunishment.org/.
13. Frank Kardasz, "Common Ground, World Religions," Ethics training for Law Enforcement, accessed 2015, http://kardasz.org/Ethics_CommonReligiousBeliefs.html.
14. "Ben Franklin quotes," The Golden Rule Organization, 2002, http://www.thegoldenrule.net/quotes.htm.
15. Miguel Civil. "The Law Collection of Ur-Namma." *Cuneiform Royal Inscriptions and Related Texts in the Schøyen Collection*, 221–86, edited by A. R. George, 2011.

16. "List of Countries by Number of Military and Paramilitary Personnel," accessed 2015, http://en.wikipedia.org/wiki/List_of_countries_by_number_of_military_and_paramilitary_personnel.

17. Anup Shah, "World Military Spending," *Global Issues,* June 30, 2013, http://www.globalissues.org/article/75/world-military-spending.

18. "GDP as Share of World GDP at PPP by Country," Quandl, accessed 2015, https://www.quandl.com/c/economics/gdp-as-share-of-world-gdp-at-ppp-by-country.

19. Shah, Anup, "World Military Spending," June 30, 2013, *Global Issues,* http://www.globalissues.org/article/75/world-military-spending.

20. David Vine, "The United States Probably has More Foreign Military Bases than any Other People, Nation or Empire in History," *The Nation,* September 14, 2015.

21. Colin Shultz "Globally, Deaths from War and Murder are in Decline," *Smithsonianmag.com,* March 21 2014, http://www.smithsonianmag.com/smart-news/globally-deaths-war-and-murder-are-decline-180950237/#wutvjswK1pGr4bvS.99.

22. "Is Violence Declining? APS fellow Steven Pinker says 'Yes,'" Association for Psychological Science, accessed 2015, http://www.psychologicalscience.org/index.php/video/is-violence-declining-aps-fellow-stephen-pinker-says-yes.html.

23. David McNamee, "Global Life Expectancy has Increased by 6 Years Since 1990," *Medical News Today,* December 2014.

24. Seth Bornstein, "World Becoming Less Violent," *Huffington Post,* December 22, 2011. http://www.huffingtonpost.com/2011/10/22/world-less-violent-stats_n_1026723.html.

25. "Statistical Risk Assessment" Early Warning Project, accessed 2015, http://www.earlywarningproject.com/risk_assessments.

26. "Accused Molester is Killed in Court," *New York Times,* April 4, 1993, http://www.nytimes.com/1993/04/04/us/accused-molester-is-killed-in-court.html.

27. "Crime in the United States," FBI, 2012, http://www.fbi.gov/about-us/cjis/ucr/crime-in-the-u.s/2012/crime-in-the-u.s.-2012/tables/1tabledatadecoverviewpdf/table_1_crime_in_the_united_states_by_volume_and_rate_per_100000_inhabitants_1993-2012.xls.

28. "Global Retail Theft Barometer Study," *Market Watch,* November 6, 2014,http://www.marketwatch.com/story/global-retail-theft-barometer-study-finds-shrink-cost-retailers-128-billion-worldwide-averaging-129-percent-of-sales-2014-11-06.

29. Lawrence Mower, "Most Burglaries Go Unsolved," *Las Vegas Review Journal,* February 10, 2008, http://www.reviewjournal.com/news/most-burglaries-go-unsolved.

30. Steve Crabtree, "U.S. Confidence in Police about Average for Wealthy Countries," Gallup, July 29, 2015, http://www.gallup.com/poll/180227/confidence-police-average-wealthy-countries.aspx.

31. Patricio Asfura-Heim and Ralph Espach, "The Rise of Mexico's Self-defense Forces," *Foreign Affairs,* July/August 2013, http://www.foreignaffairs.com/articles/139462/patricio-asfura-heim-and-ralph-h-espach/the-rise-of-mexicos-self-defense-forces.

32. Pablo Fajnzylber, Daniel Lederman, and Norman Loayza, "Inequality and Violent Crime," *Journal of Law and Economics* XLV (April, 2002), http://siteresources.worldbank.org/DEC/Resources/Crime%26Inequality.pdf.

33. Chris Matthews, "Wealth Inequality in America: It's Worse than You Yhink," *Fortune,* October 31, 2014, http://fortune.com/2014/10/31/inequality-wealth-income-us.

34. Edwin Fruehwald, "A Biological Basis of Rights," *Southern California Interdisciplinary Law Journal* 195 (2010).

35. Harriet Sherwood, "Global Refugee Figure Passes 50m for First Time Since Second World War," *The Guardian* June 2014.

36. To view a video of this event, see http://www.mirror.co.uk/news/weird-news/watch-crowd-stampede-chinese-subway-4090742.

37. Jerry Ball, "Employee Fire and Life Safety," National Fire Protection Association, 2001, http://www.nfpa.org/~/media/Files/Safety%20information/For%20consumers/Occupancies/Evacuation.pdf.

38. Robert Bruner and Sean Carr, *The Panic of 1907: Lessons Learned from the Market's Perfect Storm*, (Hoboken, NJ: John Wiley & Sons, 2007).
39. Sam Montana, "The History of Stock Market Panics," Knoji, 2010, https://stocks.knoji.com/the-history-of-stock-market-panics/.
40. "Circuit Breakers and other Market Volatility Procedures," U.S. Securities and Exchange Commission, July 2012.
41. S. H. Milton. "'Gypsies' as Social Outsiders in Nazi Germany," in Robert Gellately and Nathan Stoltzfus, *Social Outsiders in Nazi Germany* (Princeton, NJ: Princeton University Press, 2001), 216, 231.
42. Charles Lawing, "Loving v. Virginia and the Hegemony of 'Race'" (PDF), 2000, http://www.charlielawing.com/modhist_lovingv.virginia.pdf.
43. Note, racism is not just socialised; there are deep subconscious psychological reasons for it. "Dirt in the form of excrement is externalized to the outside world and projected onto dark-skinned people," cited in Ron Hall, "The psychogenesis of color based racism," Julian Samora Institute, September 1997, http://www.jsri.msu.edu/upload/research-reports/rr21.pdf.
44. For a video of a Saudi journalist asking passers by "Would you, as a human being shake hands with a Jew" see https://www.youtube.com/watch?v=_fiMO4VNvxY&spfreload=10] To view a program on tolerance appearing on Sesame St. see https://www.youtube.com/watch?v=QS-rJcm7jyQ.
45. "For First Time, Majority of Americans Favor Legal Gay Marriage," Gallup.com, May 20, 2011.
46. "Will and Grace," accessed 2015, http://en.wikipedia.org/wiki/Will_%26_Grace .
47. Elizabeth Vlet, "Illegal Immigrants Bring Risk of Ebola and Global Array of Viral Illnesses" CP Opinion, August 2014, http://www.christianpost.com/news/illegal-immigrants-bring-risk-of-ebola-and-global-array-of-viral-illnesses-124329/.
48. "Swine Flu, WHO Praises Mexico's Response to the Virus," *The Telegraph*, May 2009, http://www.telegraph.co.uk/health/swine-flu/5281924/Swine-flu-WHO-praises-Mexicos-response-to-virus.html.
49. "Cases of Ebola Diagnosed in the United States," CDC, December 16, 2014,http://www.cdc.gov/vhf/ebola/outbreaks/2014-west-africa/united-states-imported-case.html.
50. Vatsal Anand, "Can Dengue Transfer from Person to Person, " *OnlyMyHealth*, October 2012, http://www.onlymyhealth.com/is-dengue-fever-contagious-1301653693.
51. Racheal Pearson, "Disease Threat from Immigrant Children Wildly Overstated," Observer, July 10, 2014, http://www.texasobserver.org/disease-threat-immigrant-children-wildly-overstated/.
52. "Medal of Honor Recipients," Congressional Medal of Honor Society, 2015, http://www.history.army.mil/moh/mohstats.html.
53. Leon Trotsky, *The History of the Russian Revolution*, 1932, cited at https://www.marxists.org/archive/trotsky/1930/hrr/ch48.htm.
54. One curious coda to this discussion is that cutting edge computer security systems are increasingly modeling themselves after the human immune system. The name given for this new field is called The Artificial Immune System or AIS."The field of Artificial Immune System (AIS) is concerned with abstracting the structure and function of the immune system to computational systems . . . a sub-field of biologically inspired computing . . . currently new ideas along AIS lines, such as danger theory and algorithms inspired by the innate immune system are also being explored . . . the common techniques are inspired by specific immunological theories that explain the function and behavior of the mammalian adaptive immune system. . . ." In trying to examine biological or chemical terrorist threats, the DOD is financing computer based modeling of the artificial immune system awarding a $7.9 million grant to the Scripps Research Institute to build "what is, in essence, an artificial immune system, comprising vast 'libraries' of different types of molecules from which will emerge individual compounds to detect or neutralize an array of biological and chemical threats." The 7th, 8th, and 9th International Conference on the Artificial Immune System specialized

in reviewing intrusion detection systems based on mimicking the human artificial immune system. "Threat recognition," "danger theory," and "threat assessment networks,"are all strategies modeled on the human immune system, are part of cutting edge computer science today. See "Artificial immune system," World Public Library, accessed 2015, http://www.netlibrary.net/article/whebn0001589987/artificial%20 immune%20system.

55. "Stephen Hawking: Human Aggression Threatens to Destroy Us All," *Science*, February 24, 2015.

56. *Speeches and Writings of Virchand Ghandi*, Vallabh Smarak Nidhi, Bombay, 1970, cited at http://www.goodreads.com/quotes/640498-this-is-my-country-that-is-your-country-these-are.

NINE

The *Invisible* Psychic Immune System

In the prior pages the constituents of the psychic immune system in its innate, adaptive, and artificial incarnations were outlined. But we still have no idea how it works. How does it operate in bringing wars to an end or in preventing nuclear holocausts and misjudgments? How does it dampen impulsive, irrational human behavior that could unleash a worldwide cataclysm?

When Khrushchev brought the "thaw" to Soviet communism and emptied Stalin's gulags, was that positive outcome somehow connected to the operation of the human psychic immune system? When Pol Pot's barbarity was cut short by the Vietnamese, and the grotesque slaughter of the killing fields brought to an end, was the psychic immune system involved in this process—or are we imagining things? When those Russian submarine officers were engaged in their debate in 1962, which just happened to save the northern hemisphere from a nuclear winter, was the protective and positive force of the psychic immune system at play?

We have no idea. The psychic immune system we have been describing, if it exists at all, is, for all intents and purposes, palpably invisible. As Delo McKown rather sarcastically observed, "Sometimes the invisible and the nonexistent look very much alike."[1]

Humanity has gathered about 130 years of knowledge about the physical immune system. In that span of time, the role of white blood cells, killer T cells, and lymphocytes have been delineated, and we have a much stronger idea of how the physical immune system works in rejecting transplants, healing our wounds, and attacking antigens. It can be hobbled by HIV, or gain strength from engineered T cells, monoclonal antibodies, and stem-cell transplants.[2] [3]

With respect to the psychic immune system, our knowledge is still in the prenatal stage. Few psychologists are working in this elusive area.

There are no subdivisions in the American Psychological Association (APA) specializing in the psychic immune system. It is not at all possible to show how psychic antibodies operate. More importantly, we have no idea when the psychic immune system is functioning.

This entire discussion is based on inference, on observing some remarkable qualities about the human condition—especially that it hasn't yet blown itself up. Something seems to be operating to quash humanity's worst atrocities, murderous rampages (Genghis Khan) and stygian genocides (Adoph Hitler), after an average thirty-seven-year reign of terror.

We don't know why the dark side of the human condition doesn't thrive for centuries once it gains power, but who can deny the joy that comes when these barbarities come to an end? Nonetheless, one is simply at a loss to explain the innate survival mechanisms that are switched on to repel the ascendancy of these periodic evil empires.

What is known is that it isn't luck, but that's about as far one gets. The rest is inference. Something seems to have humanity's back. Some system or entity, which lies outside of awareness, appears to be functioning on humanity's behalf. That is the nub of this journey.

Higgs, Dark Matter, and Psychology

Physics has had much more experience with the invisible than psychology, and it has visited inscrutable terrain before. There is something for psychology to learn from this history. "Rutherford predicted the neutron . . . in 1920, 12 years before it was discovered. Dirac predicted anti-matter 27 years before *it* was first detected. Pauli predicted the existence of neutrinos in 1930, 26 years before they were discovered."[4]

More than seventy years ago, Peter Higgs predicted the existence of a new particle, the Higgs boson. Theoretically, there was an "invisible field of energy" that existed throughout the entire universe. The field, in turn, was accompanied by a particle, the Higgs boson.

How did the physics handle Higgs's work on this invisible field and unknown particle?

When particles of energy pass through this invisible field, they are "endowed with the property of mass," Higgs conjectured. If an object travels through a dense liquid like molasses, it becomes heavier. Similarly, when a particle with zero mass speeds through the Higgs field, it *acquires* mass. This explains how matter was created, and why the Higgs boson was affectionately called by journalists, "The God Particle."

When first proposing the theory, Higgs was considered little short of a crackpot. There was no proof for his conjectures, and no evidence of any Higgs field. The particle could not be verified, only inferred. There were no machines big enough to find it. When the European Organization for Nuclear Research decided to spend $10 billion to build the Large Hadron

Collider (LHC) there were deep questions posed about whether there was any true justification for such an investment. The machine shoots particles in opposite directions around a twenty-seven kilometer circle colliding at a rate which is just three meters per second slower than the speed of light.

> One of the primary missions of the LHC since its completion in 2008 has been to discover the existence of the Higgs boson. It is thought to hold the key to understanding the fundamental workings of the universe. . . . Nicknamed the "God particle" the Higgs would explain a rudimentary universal question yet to be answered: Where does mass come from? Or simply, why do things have mass?
>
> Researchers at the LHC facility announced that they'd detected a particle about 125 times the mass of a proton, which they firmly believe is the Higgs boson. "This is indeed a new particle. We know it must be a boson and it's the heaviest boson ever found. The Higgs is so rare that about one in every trillion collisions inside the LHC is likely to produce it. This is not a needle in a haystack—it's much worse," said Joe Lykken, a theoretical physicist.[5]

The 2012 acceleration test proving the Higgs boson particle's existence was ranked by *Science* magazine as the scientific discovery of the year. The final observation of the Higgs boson, "completes the standard model, perhaps the most elaborate and precise theory in all of science. . . . The discovery's announcement in Geneva was met by loud cheers usually only heard at football matches or rock concerts. The feat marks an intellectual, technological and organizational triumph."[6] Higgs triumphed indeed, but endured a fusillade of negative feedback all along the way. Stephen Hawking bet against the Higgs field and felt it was not a useful construct. Hawking admitted he lost the bet. Lawrence Krauss was also a critic of the Higgs field "It seemed too easy. It seemed to me that introducing an invisible field to explain stuff is more like religion than science. . . . Great, I invented invisible hobgoblins to make things right."[7]

When Higgs first submitted his paper to a prominent physics journal, it was rejected out of hand for having *"no obvious relevance to physics."*[8]

There are important lessons psychology can learn from this history. In this text, a theory has been proposed that attempts to explain certain human phenomena, like why grotesquely inhumane wars and barbarities always seem to come to an end or why the human race had twenty close calls with nuclear annihilation, but never crossed the threshold of unleashing a nuclear winter.

It has proposed an invisible system operating in the margins of human behavior that protects humanity from its own irrationality, impulsivity, folly, and stupidity. The psychic immune system, as it was proposed, was as an epiphenomenon of the physical immune system. Just like the physical immune system is perpetually on guard for danger and invasive agents, so is the psychic immune system ready at the quick to defuse and suppress threats to individuals, groups, societies, and the human race itself.

But like the Higgs boson and the Higgs field, we can't see it, and we know very little about it. It is illusive and, perhaps to some, a preposterous supposition where we have proposed nothing more than an invisible hobgoblin to explain just plain good luck.

What keeps it together? What keeps us together?

Physics seems almost addicted to proposing invisible entities to explain something it cannot comprehend. Take a closer look at dark matter. Dave Goldberg explains that he has written often about dark matter and always seems to get accusatory reactions which accuse physicists of being lazy or stubborn in adhering to dark matter as an absurd "fudge" to fix all of humankind's ignorance about the universe. He replies to that criticism as follows:

> Let's go back a bit. In the 1920s, the astronomer Fritz Zwicky found that galaxies were moving around in clusters so quickly that unless there was a lot of matter that wasn't in the form of stars or gas, the clusters should fly apart in no time. . . . The reason that some people are so dismissive of dark matter is that they're focusing on 90-year-old arguments. They are judgy because a) We've never detected a dark matter particle, and b) We're not even really sure what it is. But there are LOTS of reasons to believe in dark matter, besides the obvious (and damn compelling, if you ask me) fact that galaxies would fly apart without it. . . . If you're put off by the fact that we've never seen a dark matter particle, don't be. . . . We have a very good track record for figuring out what's out there long before we see it . . . I'll put my money on dark matter and general relativity any day.[9]

NASA's Charlie Plain speaks of it in a similar tone when he underscores that the way galaxies rotate, dark matter *must exist.*

> For the stars in a galaxy to remain in orbit around the galaxy's center, some force must be acting on them, and the only possible candidate, at such distances, is gravity. But the gravity attributable to the stuff we can see is way too feeble to "glue" galaxies together. It's dark matter—or more exactly, *the gravity it exerts*—that must supply the force holding galaxies together, and lots of dark matter is needed to do the job. The numbers seem to change each month, but roughly 80 percent of all matter in the universe is that unseeable flavor.[10]

Even though dark matter particles have never been identified, we infer its existence based on its effects. But like the Higgs boson, dark matter also has its critics. Physicist Paul Steinhardt who said the concept didn't explain anything: "I am disappointed with what most theorists are willing to accept."[11] Dragon Slavkov didn't think dark matter existed either;[12] another said it was an "unnecessary construct." Ditto for Prof. David Shiga in the *New Scientist* who said it was an "illusion." But Bob Nichol from the University of Portsmouth says, "we're more confident than ever that this exotic component of the universe is real—even if we still have no idea what it consists of."[13] However ever confident some physicists are, in 2014 *Scientific American* wrote that clear evidence for dark matter has eluded detection despite all efforts to capture it.[14]

Psychology is very much in the same place with the invisible positive psychic immune system. And certainly the critics of this thesis could easily argue we are barking up a nonexistent tree, chasing after ghosts, and making up invisible hobgoblins to explain things we cannot understand.

Admittedly, there is little to directly measure, only inferences, shadows, silhouettes, and, at best, correlations. As physics stared into the vacuum of space and postulated a field filled with unmeasured dark matter, we are similarly staring into a vacuum and postulating a field or force of undetectable positive energy enveloping human collective psychology which acts to prevent, temper, or subdue threats to human survivability and preservation.

To clarify the mystery we are chasing down: this text has not proposed some salubrious bromide that there will be no more genocides, tyrants, flash-crashes, race riots, social implosions, or nuclear accidents. These things will certainly appear again just as a flu or cold will happen in due course in a person's life.

But what wriggles its way on to the table for a fuller discussion is that an uncanny force, field, or entity exists in the theater of psychology that acts like an immune system and has a protective, self-preservative function for individuals, groups, nations, and the human race itself. As the physical immune system suppresses eruptions of disease, the psychological immune system suppresses negative eruptions with its own mysterious sets of antibodies, all of them effectively invisible to us. As physics infers the existence of dark matter to explain things—even though they have never seen nor measured it—we journey down an identical path.

Let us see in a contemporary example if we can parse out a few more tracings or footprints left by the invisible psychic immune system.

IRAQ

Iraq possesses one of the more ancient human capitals, Baghdad, commissioned in 762 AD, making it just over 1,200 years old. Contrary to what Westerners might think, Iraq never had any period of sustained parliamentary democracy in its history.

It was occupied and fought over by the Ottoman Empire for four hundred years beginning in 1533, then became part of the British colonial empire in 1917. That was followed by a monarchy in 1941, and then it evolved under a sequence of coups and military regimes until Saddam

Hussein grabbed the reins of power in 1979. Any notion that Iraq had a thriving democratic tradition is folly.[15]

Most Americans are aware the United States attacked Iraq in its campaign of "shock and awe" in March 2003. The reasons given for the invasion were two-fold—namely that Iraq was developing weapons of mass destruction and that it had some relationship to Al Qaeda and the attacks of 9/11.

President Bush said, "We're taking the fight to those that attacked us." Vice President Cheney was also quite explicit in arguing that Iraq had connections to 9/11.[16] Subsequent inquiries, however, showed that Iraq had no systematic program for WMDs,[17] nor did it have a role in the 9/11 attacks in New York and Washington. President Bush admitted as much in a news conference blunder many years later.[18]

The U.S. occupation forces oversaw the preparation of the new Iraqi constitution, wrote most of it,[19] and supervised the country's first elections. Nouri al-Maliki was ultimately installed as prime minister in 2006 and rapidly began excluding rather than including competing groups in Iraq's power circles. The majority Shiites retained coveted government posts while Sunnis and Kurds were given scraps from the table. As *Foreign Policy* opines:

> The 2010 government formation process turned out to be yet another opportunity for politicians of all stripes to grant themselves senior positions which they could use to plunder the state. . . . The failures of Iraq's governing class—and the U.S. occupation forces—to create even a single stable national institution will haunt the country for years to come.[20]

The unfortunate result is that Iraq is now a parliamentary democracy in name only and fractured into three regions: Shiites in the south, the Kurds in the North, and Sunnis in the central areas. Moreover, Sunni areas are rapidly being subsumed—or consumed—under the barbaric rule of ISIS, ISIL, or IS, "Islamic State."

Iraq has almost ceased being an organic country at all. Sunni Muslims refuse to salute Iraq's new flag.[21] The Kurds have their own national anthem and flag, which is not the Iraqi version, and ISIS militants fly their own colors. One Iraqi pointed out this barrier: "Geographically, we practically have to cross another country to get to Baghdad. We have to cross through territory that is governed and secured by forces that are not loyal to the federal government in Baghdad."[22]

Iraqi poet Ehah al-Aliki, tried to contribute his talents to a project that would create a deeper sense of unity consciousness on what it means to be Iraqi:

> His goal, he said, was to use his poems to promote national unity and the convergence of views, and to call for peaceful coexistence and nonviolence between communities. For this he has received numerous

death threats. One, in a text message read "you are a Shiite dog, a bastard, and we swear to God we will cut your belly out and give it to the dogs. You don't deserve life and we will hunt you down."[23]

The Enemy of My Enemy Is My Friend

The absurdity of Iraq politics grows daily. The fractious state is a swirling mass of contradiction. In 2015, the United States engaged in bombing ISIS in both Iraq and Syria, but America's latest adversary, Iran, is also fighting ISIS.[24] This puts Iran as a defacto ally of the United States in a campaign to stop the march of ISIS toward Baghdad.[25]

Note that ISIS is also at war with Bashar Assad's brutal dictatorship in Syria. America, too. The United States supplies weapons and support to rebel forces and mercenary groups trying to topple Assad's regime, which ironically then makes it a de facto ally of ISIS.[26] In other words, America is fighting ISIS at the same time Iran is battling the militant group. Meanwhile, ISIS is fighting Assad in Syria, and the United States is supplying arms to other rebels opposed to Assad. The United States thus appears to be fighting *for* the interests of ISIS (the removal of Assad) and *against* the interests of ISIS (the establishment of the ISIS caliphate in Iraq) and doing all this in consort with Iran, a powerful adversary.

After examining the perplexities in the war torn region, one may legitimately ask what any of this has to do with the psychic immune system? Certainly one might think no progress has been made in the Iraq conflict, and that contradiction, violence, competing interests, terrorism, corrupt governance, and killing are the dominant forces of this particular reality.

However, looking at a graph of violent deaths in Iraq—prepares one for a shock. It looks very similar to those old bell-shaped physical epidemic curves with a sharp crest and then a retreat into remission.[27] Mortality rises in 2003, reaches a peak in 2006, and then trails off in 2010 to virtually where it started in 2003.[28]

Despite the failures, broken democracy, rebellions, insurrections, and beheadings, the early rise in mortality rates suddenly retreats and falls like a stone.

This may seem a peculiar question—and an entirely unconventional way of looking at modern day Iraq—but let us explore a few more of the implications of how the psychic immune system might be involved in this contemporary venue.

Territoriality

In the prior charting of psychic epidemics, there was a repeated encounter with quasi-bell-shaped curves which rise with territoriality—that is, dominance, aggression, and the pernicious male chromosome that always seems ready for a fight. However, the path of that crisis chart curves and falls as a cooperative, nonviolent phase restores the system to its normal baseline and homeostasis.

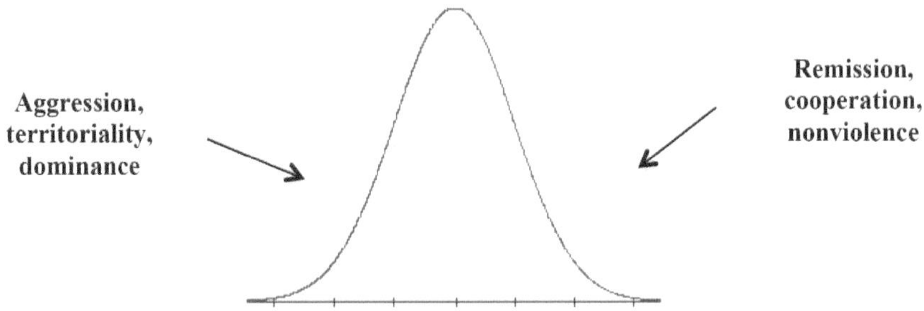

Figure 9.1 Remission Curve for Psychic Epidemics

If one adopts this model for understanding the Iraq conflict, the first question to ask is "where was the 'territoriality' issue?" It is not immediately apparent. If the United States attacked Iraq for territorial reasons, why did it leave? What was the prize? Where was the pot of gold at the end of the rainbow?

At this writing it is known that the real reason the United States invaded was not because of Hussein's plans to develop a nuclear weapon, nor was it his support of 9/11 terrorists. That has pretty much been agreed.

But why, then, did the United State lose 4,493 Americans, bring home 32,000 wounded veterans,[29] oversee the slaughter of between 100,000 and 400,000 Iraqis,[30] and spend close to $1.7 trillion doing it?[31]

If the war was territorial, what resources (territory) was it after, and why did it spend all this national treasure only to withdraw without taking any of the hard-won goodies home?

Some pundits assert the real reason we invaded was to remove Israel's major nemesis, Saddam Hussein. The quiet but aggressive inside lobbying of Paul Wolfowitz, Richard Pearle, and the Israeli lobby is often cited by academics or[32] wonks like Pat Buchanan[33] as the disguised causative agent for the war. According to conservative columnist Robert Novak: "This is really about change of regime in Iraq and change of the political outlines in the Middle East more to Israel's benefit. That's what this has all been about."[34] Marc Weber's "Iraq, a war for Israel,"[35] further underscores there are quite a few talking heads who espouse this idea.

But if the United States invaded Iraq for Israel's benefit, this does not lead one easily to the issue of territoriality at all.

A second real reason, may be closer to the truth, namely that the United States invaded Iraq over the issue of oil. The comments of former federal reserve chairman Alan Greenspan point to that direction in his memoirs: "I'm saddened that it is politically inconvenient to acknowledge what everyone knows. . . . The Iraq war is largely about oil."[36]

If oil supply was the true motive, it fits neatly into the discussion of territoriality and the ancestral, acquisitive fight for resources. American ground troops may have left Iraq, but oil companies did not. Indeed some of the largest oil companies like ExxonMobil, BP, and Shell stayed.

> On November 27 . . . Royal Dutch Shell announced its pursuit of a massive gas deal in southern Iraq. . . . Three days later, the US-based energy firm Emerson submitted a bid for a contract to operate at Iraq's giant Zubair oil field, which reportedly holds some eight million barrels of oil. . . . Iraq's supergiant Rumaila oil field is already being developed by BP, and the . . . Majnoon oil field, is being developed by Royal Dutch Shell. Both fields are in southern Iraq. . . . According to the US Energy Information Administration (EIA), Iraq's oil reserves of 112 billion barrels ranks second in the world, only behind Saudi Arabia. The EIA also estimates that up to 90 percent of the country remains unexplored.[37]

In 2015, Iraq oil production reached its highest level in thirty years.[38] A territorial war over oil becomes a more likely explanation, especially when one remembers that the United States attacked Iraq once before over the issue of oil too, in the Gulf War in 1990–1991.

Revanchism and Operation Desert Storm

Here is a brief summary of events for those unfamiliar with the Gulf Oil dispute:

- Saddam Hussein invaded and occupied Kuwait in 1990.
- U.S. president George H. W. Bush, responded with a call for liberation of Kuwait, calling Hussein the "butcher of Baghdad."
- Close to a million allied troops led by General Norman Schwarzkoff were deployed in the first Gulf War that lasted six months.
- The war ended with a death toll of 148 Americans[39] and at least 12,000 Iraqis, although some reports say 50,000 to 150,000 Iraqis may have been killed.[40] [41]

At the time, George H. W. Bush told Americans this was a war about freedom and against tyranny, and most people remained in the dark about the true motive, control of the oil supply. Kuwait sits on actual, not estimated, oil reserves second highest only to Saudi Arabia.[42]

The purpose of the war according to Paul Aarts, Michael Renner, Michael Lind, and other military analysts,[43] was to repatriate our oil from the acquisitive clutches of Hussein. The rallying cry of protestors at the time was, "No blood for oil." Obviously *some* Americans were not naive about the true nature of the conflict.

The mainstream media, however, continued to feed Americans a story line about fighting for freedom and democracy—and most people swallowed it. It didn't matter that Kuwait was never a democracy. It was ruled by an all-male monarchy led by the fourteenth richest man on earth, Jaber Al-Ahmad Al-Sabah. During the Gulf War, he was absent from almost all press coverage, and most never heard of him. When hostilities ended, Hussein's troops left Kuwait in a mass exodus, while the Emir quietly returned to his villas to redecorate.

It is painful to realize that fifteen American women gave their lives to restore an undemocratic, all-male monarchy to power.[44] Women were not allowed to participate in any significant part of the Kuwaiti government before the Gulf War, and after Kuwait was "liberated," the situation remained the same. Women were denied any practical rights to vote for another fifteen years in his highness' lavishly appointed sheikdom.[45]

Despite these sad details, if the Gulf War of 1990 was about our oil, perhaps the invasion of Iraq in 2003 was also about oil as Fed chief Greenspan averred. To commentator Dennis Berstein: "Oil has always been part of U.S. decision-making on Iraq, a key motive for the 2003 invasion and the bloody occupation that followed."[46]

If true, it certainly qualifies as a territorial conflict, and thus is eminently relevant to our discussion of the psychic immune system. Recall, if you will, a prior reference to Kalevi Holsti's study that found 79 percent of wars from 1648 to 1989 involved territoriality.

Kin Selection, Inclusive Fitness and Us versus Them

Beyond territoriality, there is another dimension of the Iraq conflict that relates to the concept of the psychic immune system. It is the tradition of "staying with your own kind." Shiite militias remain wary of Sunnis, and both have issues with Kurds. There is a great deal of *us versus them* sloshing about inside the borders of Iraq. About 78 percent of Iraq's population is made up of Arabs while Kurds are about 16 percent.

> In terms of religious sect, Iraqi Arabs are somewhat split: the survey found that most said they were Shi'a Muslims (62 percent), but about three in ten identified themselves as Sunnis (30 percent).[47]
>
> Of its 32 million citizens, 80 percent speak Arabic, 13 percent Kurdish, 4 percent Turkic, and 1 percent Persian.[48] The fractured nature of Iraq, in part, comes from being artificially carved out by colonial powers after the fall of the Ottoman Empire.
>
> For more than 500 years, the region was not homogeneous; it was divided into three separate and distinct areas, the Mosul region, populated by Kurds, the Baghdad region populated by Sunnis, and the Basra area populated by Shiites.
>
> The Ottoman empire was able to survive for more than 600 years and cover much of the world partly by respecting the natural political divisions of the territories it conquered such as those between Kurds, Sunnis and Shia. The split between Sunni and Shia dates from Caliph Ali's murder in 661 and there has been generations of cross sectarian grievance between the two groups ever since.[49]

In fact, Iraq today seems to be morphing into the same three geographic-ethnic regions that existed during the centuries of Ottoman rule. To some extent, the United States has naively attempted to forge—or even force—a multi-ethnic parliamentary democracy on Iraq, a colonial approach from the British that was tried and failed in the past.

One might think these ethnic-religious-linguistic differences are primarily theological, cultural, or historical, but there are also genetic differences between these populations. Sunni and Shiite, for example, have distinct gene differences,[50] and even Kurds in Iraq have a closer genetic affinity with the Yazidis than with other Iraqis.[51]

The *us versus them* battle, therefore, is sitting on very firm ground, and the natural tendency to prefer one's own kin is a formidable obstacle in creating any kind of homogenous country one could call modern day Iraq.

The Invisible Psychic Immune System and Iraq

Speculations about territoriality, remission, kin selection, and *us versus them* are interesting, but we simply do not know enough about the psychic immune system to tease out clear explanations for what is actually happening on the ground in this region of the human landscape.

We do not know the role of epigenes in this drama, and likely will not have any basis for drawing out implications for decades until research graduates from rat pups to human beings. We do not know precisely how kin selection and inclusive fitness help us understand the current conflicts between ISIS, the Kurds, the remaining Sunnis, and Shia populations. We are, in fact, speculating, but hopefully not wildly.

At least we can observe one important phenomenon—or epiphenomenon—that this text has proposed. There is an uncanny similarity in the charted curves of physical versus psychological epidemics. They rise precipitously, and then fall just as quickly, and sometimes they appear to do so for no apparent reason at all.

Iraq is as unstable today as it ever has been, but the level of mortality is down. That is a mystery. With all the divisiveness, the artificiality of the country, the multiplicity of languages, sectarian divides, and even genetic differences in populations, one is in awe at the decline in mortality almost *back to baseline and homeostasis.* Whatever is keeping this mortality curve down and in remission is uncanny. And to recall the physical pandemic of the Spanish flu, one is similarly reminded of the familiar decline into remission.

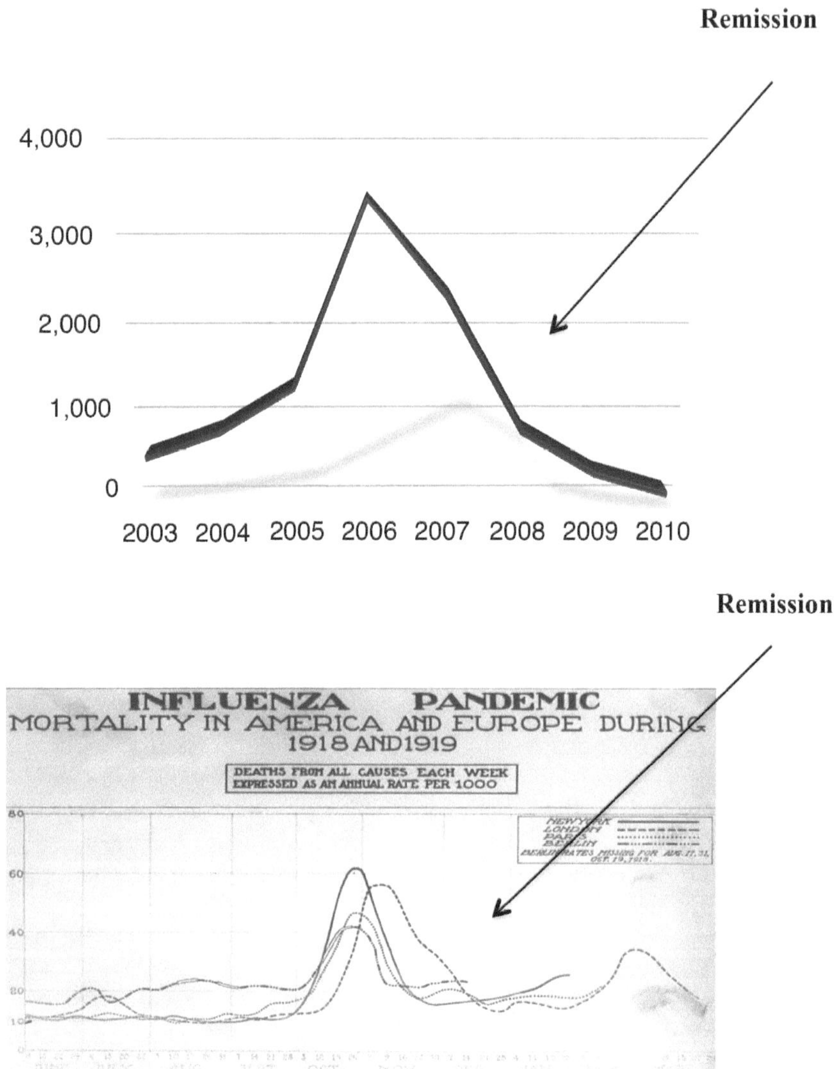

Figure 9.2 Remission Curves for Psychic Epidemics (Iraq) and Physical Epidemics (Spanish Flu)
Data used to create Iraq graphic from "Iraq Casualties: How Many Iraqis Died," Frontline, 1995, accessed 2015, http://www.pbs.org/wgbh/pages/frontline/gulf/appendix/death.html. Spanish flu graphic courtesy of the National Museum of Health and Medicine.

Remission and What It Means

For psychic and physical epidemics mortality curves rise and then decline. This is not universally true, but it is often true of both kinds of outbreaks. While territoriality is situational and cultural, it is also instinctive and a likely culprit driving these curves upward. But what is driving the curves down? We know that physical immunities are driving down the Spanish flu. Are psychic immunities driving down Iraqi mortality figures?

Is it possible that equally instinctive tendencies toward nonviolence, cooperation, altruism, and aversion to killing may be at play? Based on prior chapters, these processes are just as autonomic and hard-wired as territoriality and acquisitiveness. So while the *us versus them* dramas boil over into sectarian violence, could there be opposing affiliative, nonviolent tendencies quietly operating in the margins as well? For example, out of Iraq's six million marriages, two million are mixed marriages between Sunnis and Shiites. One such couple opines.

> We've been married for six years and our sectarian differences have never affected us. . . . For many years, we Iraqis viewed mixed marriages not as a problem but as an asset for uniting our country. . . . In the beginning, my family was worried about our marriage . . . But in the end, we convinced them that religious differences were not important enough to prevent a family from being built. . . . Mixed marriages between Arab Sunnis and Shi'ites—and also between the predominantly Sunni Kurds and Arabs of both sects—have been common, even in the days of former president Saddam Hussein.[52]

Strangely, there was a period during Iraq's downward pull (remission), that things seemed delightfully sanguine. An article in *Foreign Policy* speaks about sunnier times.

> By 2008, al Qaeda-affiliated militias and death squads no longer swarmed the country from Samarra to Mosul as they had just two years before. . . . Although unemployment, corruption, and failing public services were still major problems, ordinary Iraqis in the areas that had been dominated by al Qaeda still breathed a collective sigh of relief. They could go back to work, resume their studies, and relax outdoors without the constant ring of gunfire in the background. Families took their children to the river, where they swam and picnicked, while young men made regular trips to Kirkuk or Baghdad to stock up on local Iraqi beer.[53]

Despite strong sectarian differences, differences in language, traditions, genetic heterogeneities, plus ever-brewing *us versus them* dogfights, the movement toward nonviolence, affiliative reciprocity, cooperation, mutuality, empathy, and maybe even altruism—common in so many primate species—may be observed here as well. People not only have a tendency to fight, but they have rather miraculous capacities to get along.

The Unconscious and Invisible Nature of This Process

Still, newspapers are filled everyday with violence and atrocities. ISIS is beheading Christian Yazidis and apostates of every hue.[54] Shiite militias are revving up martyrs to defend Baghdad; Iran, the United States, Jordan, France, and even Russia are joining to bomb ISIS, and Kurds are battling to keep their villages from falling.

That is the state of affairs in mid-2016, and, at least from the press, the situation looks anything but pacific. But it is still possible to be baffled when reviewing curves of violent deaths in Iraq in the twenty-first century. They rise and then they fall, just as we saw with World War I and World War II, Pol Pot, Leopold, Genghis Khan, Mao, An Lushan, Stalin, Timur, and the three pashas of the Ottoman Empire.

Note that just like the Spanish flu, these curves may show occasional signs of relapse; currently in Iraq some nineteen thousand civilian deaths have been recorded in the prior twenty-two months, but these relapses do not generally exceed the high point previously reach, and they too begin to return to their downward trek and recede back to baseline.[55]

The process of remission and retreat from war is no less significant than the horrific beginnings of war, genocide, and barbarity of every flavor. When one is confused, flummoxed, and sees no reason why these curves should be declining, we are reminded of an important observation: a very large share of the psychic immune system is autonomic and unconscious. Just as the physical immune system operates outside of conscious awareness, the psychic immune system may do so as well.

To look at this controversial hypothesis in different colors: there is a safety net beside and beyond those conscious and deliberate strategies to end war and bring peace. Beyond peace treaties, troop withdrawals, or poets who opine about what it is to be Iraqi—all the admirable efforts of the artificial psychic immune system—there is something else that is at work.

There is another, remarkable process functioning inside the human condition that promotes safety, security, peace, and nonviolence, and, indeed, strong empirical reason to believe this is just as instinctive and autonomic as humankind's darker impulses toward dominance, war, aggression, and territoriality.

With the new and emerging collapse of Syria, we are seeing the curves once again rise as over 470,000 Syrians have died including twenty-thousand children and millions fled the country as a new psychic pandemic takes hold. But we can legitimately, albeit tentatively predict, that this curve will also reverse and retreat into remission in due course as all others have.[56] [57]

CORRELATIONS AND CAUSATION

When the physical immune system revs up, it has its own rhythm. It takes a few days to learn its targets, ramp up production of antibodies, attack, and this is followed by a decline which points to a return to health, remission of the disease, and a fall back to homeostasis.[58]

With psychic epidemics there are similar rhythms. In the American Civil War, the graph of battle deaths for Confederate soldiers takes on a shape that rises and then falls into, in this case, victory for the Union armies and the formal end of slavery.[59] In the Vietnam War, a war most feel the United States lost, the curve of casualties looks the same. Mortality rises and then falls into retreat.[60]

More recently, in the Congo, close to 4.5 million people have perished due to an unusual conglomeration of warlords, malefactors, rapists, gangs, marauding militias, child soldiers, disease, and starvation all *combining together* with a failed state to produce nightmarish outcomes.

This conflict is the second deadliest since World War II. Unlike both Vietnam and the Civil War, in this case there does not appear to be any clear winner. The actual situation on the ground today (2016) is disorganized. There is the M23 rebellion, Mutanga's Mai Mai, the Iruri conflict, the Lord's Resistance Army,[61] Boko Haram and a continuing problem of raping marauding militias.[62]

Like so many others, this war appears to have a territoriality dimension to it as well—mineral rights. But even as the humanitarian crisis continues,[63] especially with famine and disease,[64] the mortality rates for battle deaths in sub-Saharan Africa, strangely enough, show the same familiar rise and decline (see figure 9.3).[65] [66]

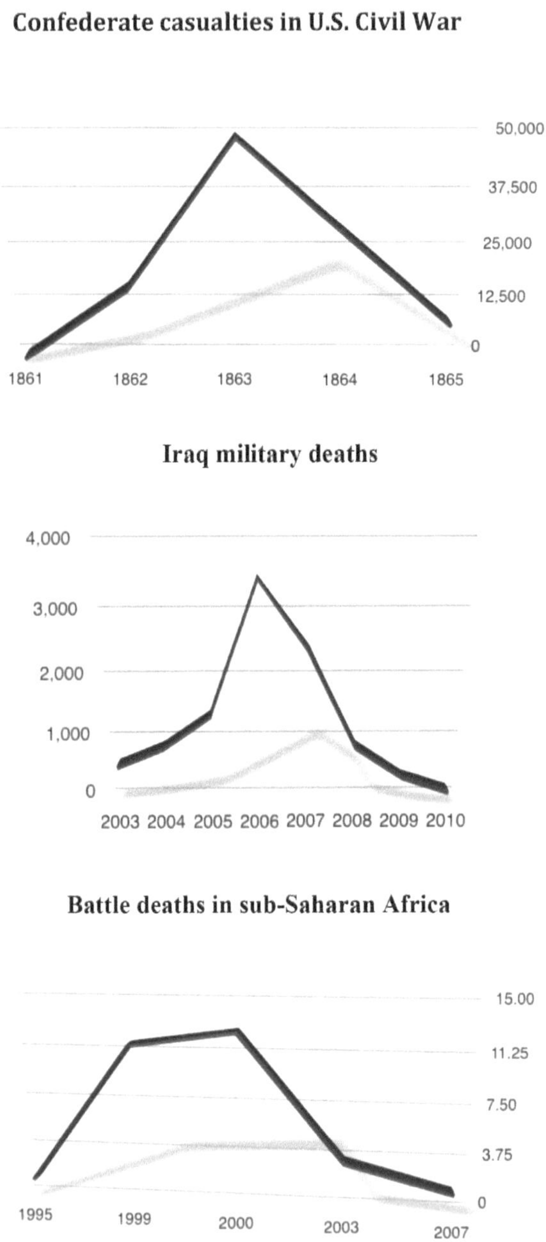

Figure 9.3 Contemporary Psychic Epidemic Mortality Curves
Charts developed from the following sources: Iraq casualties: http://musingsoniraq.blogspot.com/2011/01/2010-ends-with-slight-drop-in-iraqi.html. Confederate casualties: http://www.brcweb.com/alplm/BRC_Counting_Casualties.pdf, appendix VIII. Sub-Saharan Africa: "Mortality in the Democratic Republic of Congo, 2007"; deaths are expressed as per-thousand per month, http://www.rescue.org/sites/default/files/migrated/resources/2007/2006-7_congomortalitysurvey.pdf.

This war is not over. There is no winner, no loser. Maybe battle deaths will again ascend to an even greater level, but, for the present, we draw upon the same increasingly redundant observation that the mortality curve of battle deaths even in the unresolved war in the Congo, falls into remission.

There is an uncanny parallel and correlation between the progression of physical epidemics and psychic ones. They rise at the outset and then fall. With physical epidemics, the immune system works overtime deploying armies of antibodies to bring the disease into remission—or in the case of pertussis (whopping cough), a vaccine was introduced in 1949 and the decline again in evidence. Incidence of pertussis today is about one twenty-third what it was in the 1940s.[67] With psychic epidemics and wars similar remissions occur.

These multiple symmetries between physical disease charts and psychic epidemics cause one to sing the same familiar refrain: the psychic immune system behaves toward psychic epidemics, war, and barbarities just as the physical immune system behaves toward infectious diseases and pandemics.

Generally we tend to be very conscious-centric in such matters. We think that when the Civil War ended, it was the Battle of Appomattox and General Ulysses S. Grant who defeated General Robert E. Lee. But was something else at play? Was there another process—an invisible press or force—working to bring this episodic intraspecies killing spree to a conclusion? Whether the war is won, lost, or undecided, as is the case in the Congo, the curves rise to a peak and then relapse to baseline, as if an invisible force drives them back into homeostasis.

Of fourteen major conflicts America participated in since World War II, their average duration was 4.2 years.[68] Was this the time needed for our generals to defeat their adversaries, or was this the time needed for the human psychic immune system to do the work necessary to bring back balance and health to the system? *Or do both processes occur simultaneously and in tandem?*

We are consummately wedded to a conscious-centric, historic bias whenever discussing wars and how they end. One side surrenders, and the other pins medals on itself with a victory parade. "General X surrendered at the battle of XYZ." That is the conventional, formulaic means by which we understand events of war and peace.

We do not think of these interludes in human psychology as manifestations of our darker side—aggression, territoriality, dominance, violence, murder, genocide—which is then counterbalanced by nonviolence, cooperation, reciprocity, mutuality, nurturance, and an instinctive human aversion to killing.

The theory of the psychic immune system proposes that these are real forces and trends swirling within the volcanic magma of the human condition. One erupts, and the other quells the disturbance to neutralize it.

Curves rise and then they fall.[69] Both forces are intimately related to human survival. Both have innate and adaptive aspects. Both are biologically rooted with instinctive elements. Both have conscious as well as autonomic and unconscious dimensions.

We do not know exactly how this system works. And, most importantly, we do not know when it works. It is effectively invisible. As Felix Palma writes, "I'm convinced the true history of our time isn't what we read in newspapers or books. . . . True history is almost invisible. It flows like an underground spring. It takes place in the shadows, and in silence."[70] Dark matter has never been seen or verified either, but certain phenomena in galaxies—like why they just don't fly apart—are explained by the hypothetical "invisible hobgoblin" called dark matter.

The same question is being asked in this psychology text: why don't things just fly apart? What glue is holding us together? Today, there are 7.3 billion earthlings whose average age is twenty-four, who have less than seven years of schooling, while 16 percent are functionally illiterate.[71] [72]

What is keeping this young, uneducated, impulsive, unstable, ravenous, volatile, capricious, prone-to-the-irrational and superstitious human race steady, forward moving, healthy, growing, progressing, living longer, and not blowing itself up with stupidity, misjudgment, barbarity, fanaticism, bigotry, passion, and miscalculation?

There is no clear answer to that, but we can at least take note of our good fortune. Like Higgs, we notice strange effects, tracings, and shapes, and a theory has been proposed to explain them. It is, after all, only a theory, a theory based on a few correlations of curves which rise and curves which fall.

A theory is only good insofar as it can be tested. Is there a way to test the theory of this invisible psychic immune system? Is there any laboratory on earth where one could see how the theory might take a step beyond correlations and symmetries and look more closely at cause and effect—or at least be able to predict a future outcome?

In the next chapter, we will see how close we can come to just that.

NOTES

1. Delow McKown, cited in http://www.goodreads.com/quotes/17434-the-invisible-and-the-non-existent-look-very-much-alike
2. "About Engineered T Cells," Adoptive engineered T-cell targeting to activate cancer killing, accessed 2015, http://www.attack-cancer.org/AboutengineeredTcells/.
3. Denise Grady, "T-cell Therapy Puts Leukemia Patients in Extended Remission," *New York Times*, October 15, 2014.
4. Dave Goldberg, "Ask a Physicist: Why Believe in Dark Matter" *io9*, May 2010, http://io9.com/5528758/ask-a-physicist-why-believe-in-dark-matter.

5. Theunis Janen van Rensberg, "Large Hadron Collider Detects Higgs Boson Particle," BWTH Blog, July 4, 2012, http://www.bandwidthblog.com/2012/07/04/large-hadron-collider-detects-higgs-boson-particle/.
6. Robert Booth, "Discovery of Higgs Boson Rated Year's Top Scientific Achievement by Science," AAAS, December 2012, http://www.guardian.co.uk/science/2012/dec/20/top-scientific-discoveries-higgs-boson.
7. Robert Wright, "Why Some Physicists Bet Against the Higgs Boson" *The Atlantic*, July 17, 2012.
8. Brian Greene, "How the Higgs Boson was Found," *Smithsonian Magazine* (August 2013), 27.
9. Dave Goldberg, "Ask a Physicist."
10. Interview with Richard Muschotzky, Wilton Sanders, and Kimberley Weaver, *Xray Vision*, 1999, http://whyfiles.org/092x_ray/4.html.
11. Jenny Hogan,"Unseen Universe: Welcome to the Dark Side," *Nature* 448, no. 7151 (2007): 240–45.
12. Lisa Zyga, "Dark Matter May Be an Illusion Caused by a Quantum Vacuum," Phys.org, August 11, 2011, http://phys.org/news/2011-08-dark-illusion-quantum-vacuum.html.
13. Space.com staff, "Elusive Dark Energy is Real, Study Says," Space.com, September 12, 2012, http://www.space.com/17549-dark-energy-real-universe-expansion.html.
14. Clara Moskowitz, "Dark Matter Still Hiding: Latest Experimental Sweep Comes up Empty," *Scientific American*, October 30, 2013.
15. "Timeline of Iraq's History and Culture," Cultural property training resource, U.S. Dept. of Defense, accessed 2015, http://www.cemml.colostate.edu/cultural/09476/iraq02-01enl.html.
16. J. Kroth, *Duped: Delusion, Denial, and the End of the American Dream* (Cupertino, CA: Genotype, 2013) 11.
17. Michael Norton-Taylor and Ewen MacAskillk "A Litany of Failure, but No One to Blame" *The Guardian*, July 14, 2004.
18. "George Bush Admits Iraq had Nothing to do with 9/11," https://www.youtube.com/watch?v=6U66ab4cMCE.
19. "Bremer: US will help Iraq Write Constitution," Fox News, November 16, 2003, http://www.foxnews.com/story/2003/11/16/bremer-us-will-help-iraq-write-constitution/.
20. Zaid Al-Ali, "How Maliki Ruined Iraq," *Foreign Policy*, June 19, 2014.
21. Leila Fadel and Hussein Kadhim, "Some Sunni Muslims won't Salute New Flag," McClatchy DC, January 25, 2008, http://www.mcclatchydc.com/2008/01/25/25471/some-sunni-muslims-wont-salute.html.
22. Wilson Arya, "Iraq: West's Failed Democracy Project," *International Policy Digest*, June 16, 2014.
23. Tim Arango, "In Struggle for National Identity, Iraqis Rally Around Many Flags," *New York Times*, December 22, 2014.
24. Ian Black, "Iranian Air Force Bombs ISIS Targets in Iraq, Says Pentagon," *The Guardian*, December 3, 2014.
25. Helene Cooper, "U.S. Strategy in Iraq Increasingly Relies on Iran," *New York Times*, March 5, 2015.
26. Ed Payne, "Pentagon: US to Begin to Train and Equip Moderate Syria Rebels," CNN, January 16, 2015.
27. Chart developed from data from the following source: http://musingsoniraq.blogspot.com/2011/01/2010-ends-with-slight-drop-in-iraqi.html.
28. Iraq Body count, accessed May, 2016, http: https://www.iraqbodycount.org/.
29. Margaret Griffis, "Casualties in Iraq," Antiwar.com, May 2015, http://antiwar.com/casualties/.
30. Dan Vergano, "Half-million Iraqis Died in War, Study Says," *National Geographic*, October 16, 2013.

31. Daniel Trotta, "Iraq War Costs U.S. More than $2 trillion: Study," Reuters, March 14, 2013, http://www.reuters.com/article/2013/03/14/us-iraq-war-anniversary-idUSBRE92D0PG20130314.
32. John Mearsheimer and Stephen Walt, *The Israeli Lobby and U.S. Foreign Policy* (New York: Farrar, Straus and Giroux, 2007).
33. Mark Weber, "Iraq, a War for Israel," Institute for Historical Review, accessed 2015, http://www.ihr.org/leaflets/iraqwar.shtml.
34. Carl Estabrook, "Israel and the US War on Iraq, Counterpunch, February 26, 2003, http://www.counterpunch.org/2003/02/26/israel-and-the-us-war-on-iraq/.
35. Ibid.
36. "Greenspan's Book Asserts 'Iraq war is largely about oil,'" *The Nation*, September 17, 2007.
37. Dahr Jamail, "Western Oil Firms Remain as U.S. Exits Iraq," Al Jazerra, January 2012, http://www.aljazeera.com/indepth/features/2011/12/2011122813134071641.html.
38. Sarah Kent, "Iraq's Oil Output Surges to Highest Level in over 30 Years," *Wall Street Journal*, March 14, 2014, http://www.wsj.com/articles/SB10001424052702304914904579438860227481506.
39. Doug Rokke, "Gulf War Casualties," Trapock Peace Center, Rense.com, September 30, 2002, http://www.rense.com/general29/gulf.htm.
40. "How Many Iraqis Died," Frontline, 1995, accessed 2015, http://www.pbs.org/wgbh/pages/frontline/gulf/appendix/death.html.
41. Caryle Murphy, "Lingering Gulf War Mystery: How Many Iraqis Really Died?" *Washington Post*, June 30, 1991.
42. Aarti Nagraj, "Top 10 Countries with the World's Biggest Oil Reserves," *Gulf Business*, April 14, 2013.
43. Michel Lind, "The Wars that Really are about the Oil," *The Spectator,*, August 30, 2014.
44. "Killed in Operation Desert Shield/Desert Storm," Desert Storm, accessed 2015, http://www.nooniefortin.com/desertstorm.htm.
45. "Kuwaiti Women Win Right to Vote," BBC, May 17, 2005, http://news.bbc.co.uk/2/hi/middle_east/4552749.stm.
46. Dennis J. Bernstein, "Iraq and the Oil Wars," Consortiumnews, August 17, 2014, https://consortiumnews.com/2014/08/17/iraq-and-the-oil-wars/.
47. Besheer Mohamed, "Who are the Kurds?" The Christian Century, September 4, 2014, http://www.christiancentury.org/article/2014-09/who-are-iraqi-kurds.
48. "Languages," Looklex encyclopaedia, accessed 2015, http://looklex.com/e.o/iraq.languages.htm.
49. Mike Rosenberg, "Time to Partition Iraq?" Doing Business on the Earth Blog, June 23, 2014, http://blog.iese.edu/doing-business/2014/06/23/time-to-partition-iraq/#sthash.cyfAHIfM.Ql2kpmAP.dpuf.
50. M. Eaaswarkhanth, B. Dubey, et al., "Micorsatellite Diversity Delineates Genetic Relationships of Shia and Sunni Populations," Hum Biol 81, no. 4 (August 2009): 427-45. doi: 10.3378/027.081.0403.
51. Levon Yepiskoposian, Ashto Margarian, et al, "Genetic Affinity Between the Armenian Yezidis and the Iraqi Kurds," *Iran and the Caucases* 14 (2010): 37-42.
52. "Iraq: Mixed Marriages Confront Sectarian Violence," *Irin*, April 6, 2006, http://www.irinnews.org/report/26268/iraq-mixed-marriages-confront-sectarian-violence.
53. Zaid Al-Ali, "How Maliki Ruined Iraq," July 8, 2014, *The Week*, http://theweek.com/articles/445631/maliki-ruined-iraq.
54. Ted Thornhill, "Raped, Tortured, Forced to Watch Beheadings, then Beaten when They Tried to Kill Themselves: Yazidi Girls Reveal the Hell They Endured During ISIS Captivity," Daily Mail, October1, 2014, http://www.dailymail.co.uk/news/article-2776268/Raped-tortured-forced-watch-beheadings-beaten-tried-kill-Yazidi-girls-reveal-hell-endured-witnessed-ISIS-captivity.html.
55. Nick Cumming-Bruce "UN Reports Nearly 19,000 Iraqi Civilian Deaths in 22 Months," *New York Times*, January 19, 2016.

56. "I am Syria," accessed 2015, http://www.iamsyria.org/daily-death-toll.html.
57. Anne Barnard, "Death Toll from War in Syria now 470,000, Group Finds," *New York Times*, February 11, 2016.
58. Chart developed from the following source: http://www.bbc.co.uk/bitesize/ks3/science/organisms_behaviour_health/disease/revision/6/.
59. Chart developed from the following source: http://www.brcweb.com/alplm/BRC_Counting_Casualties.pdf, appendix VIII.
60. Accessed 2015, http://www.lies.com/images/entire_war.gif.
61. Rick Gladstone, "Former Lord's Resistance Army Commander Appears at War Crimes Court," *New York Times*, January 26, 2015.
62. Christian Bennett, "Rape in a Lawless Land", *The Guardian*, March 27, 2010.
63. "Congo War-driven Crisis Kills 45,000 a Month-Study," *Reuters*, January 22, 2008.
64. Benjamin Coghlan, Pascal Ngoy, et al., "Morality in the Democratic Republic of Congo, An Ongoing Crisis," accessed 2015, http://www.rescue.org/sites/default/files/migrated/resources/2007/2006-7_congomortalitysurvey.pdf.
65. "Democratic Republic of Congo Country Profile," BBC, accessed 2015, http://www.bbc.com/news/world-africa-13283212.
66. "The Invisible War," Social Design Notes, February 2009, http://backspace.com/notes/2009/02/ also based on UCDP/HSRP dataset.
67. "Surveillance & Reporting," CDC, accessed 2015, http://www.cdc.gov/pertussis/surv-reporting.html.
68. U.S. Participation in major wars, accessed 2015, https://en.wikipedia.org/wiki/List_of_the_lengths_of_American_participation_in_major_wars.
69. Freudians have referred to this bipolar flux as a battle between the life instincts (Eros) and the death instinct (Thanatos). Jungians may see it more as a cosmic dance between animus and anima.
70. Felix Palma, *A Map of the Sky: A Novel* (New York: Simon & Schuster, 2011), 36.
71. UNESCO Institute for Statistics, accessed 2015, http://www.sheppardsoftware.com/worldgeographymainpage/worldstatistics8.htm.
72. Robert Barro and Jong-Wha Lee, "Educational Attainment in the World, 1950–2010," VOX, May 18, 2010, http://www.voxeu.org/article/educational-attainment-world-1950-2010.

Part III

An Experimental Test of the Theory

TEN

Hypothesis Testing

Where the Rubber Meets the Road

Nobel laureate, Richard Feynman, once remarked, "It doesn't matter how beautiful your theory is, it doesn't matter how smart you are. If it doesn't agree with experiment, it's wrong."[1] There actually may be a way to test this controversial theory, but the laboratory is rather large in size: planet earth.

Global warming represents an ideal litmus test. After all, this book is about a few serious dilemmas human beings created like nuclear weapons which managed not to explode, or mass murders, genocides, and wars which, instead of metastasizing into something worse, waned or washed out entirely very much to our collective favor.

The issue of global warming is another corner humanity painted itself into, another disease it contracted, and how it is cured—and *if* it is cured—will stand as the ultimate test of this theory.

If there is a psychic immune system, it should work tirelessly in getting humanity out of this mess. If we've been barking up the wrong tree—and there is no psychic immune system—then there is no safety net to catch us, no rescue coming, no internal force inside the human condition which will neutralize this threat for our own self-preservation and survival.

The test of the hypothesis is clear. Either there is such a system or there isn't. Either humanity triumphs over global warming and mitigates its effects, or it progressively succumbs to the conditions it created.

Before exploring the possibilities of this experiment, some homework on the global warming problem itself is required.

GLOBAL WARMING

A 2010 Gallup poll showed that almost half of the American population felt global warming was "greatly exaggerated."[2] The following year, republicans, in a Pew poll showed 75 percent of staunch conservatives, 63 percent of libertarians, and 55 percent of Main Street republicans said there was "no solid evidence of global warming."[3] In the year after that, 2012, 48 percent did not think the earth was warming at all,[4] and 69 percent of the American public were skeptical of global warming and believed scientists falsified research.[5]

Even among youth ages eighteen to twenty-nine, only 30 percent ranked it significant or important.[6] And as late as 2014, a poll showed 25 percent of Americans thought global warming was a downright lie.[7] An even more recent October 2015, study showed 40 percent of Americans were not worried about climate change.[8]

The major media talking heads disseminating these ideas are John Stossel, George Will, Michael Steele, Robert Samuelson, Steve Moore, Rick Santorum, Sean Hannity, Benny Peiser, Senator James Inhofe, Michael Crichton, William Kristol, Sarah Pailin,Tucker Carlson, Rush Limbaugh, Fox News, in general, and Glenn Beck in particular, who called it the "greatest scam in history."[9]

This is only a sliver of the rhetoricians repeating the canard that global warming is either not to be believed, a left-wing conspiracy, or a liberal hoax.[10]

Any cursory review of the evidence, however, is entirely contrary to this view and overwhelming in certifying the reality of global warming. A study in the journal *Nature* found that of 928 peer-reviewed articles on the subject, not one took issue with human-caused global warming.[11]

A Gallup poll of scientists showed only 10 percent had doubts in 2003.[12] Compare that to 40 percent of an entranced public who absorb John Stossel's spin or the scientific journalism of *Fox and Friends*.[13] Popular weatherman, John Coleman, can be seen on YouTube reassuring the public that global warming presents no threat.[14]

In the first decade of the twenty-first century, the hottest years on record occurred, and countless scientific bodies affirmed the seriousness of global warming. A short summary: the Polish Academy of Sciences, the National Research Council, the Royal Society of the United Kingdom, the American Chemical Society, the Union of Concerned Scientists, the American Institute of Physics, the U.S. National Academy of Sciences, the European Physical Society, the American Geophysical Union, the European Geosciences Union, and the European Federation of Geologists . . . the list is too long to enumerate.[15] [16]

A most recent poll of 1,372 scientists by the National Academy of Sciences in 2011 showed 97 percent of scientists believe global warming is real and man-made.[17] Only 3 percent harbored any lingering doubts, but, as late as 2012, 30 percent of Americans believed global warming was "not a serious" problem.[18] [19] [20] Corroborating that survey an independent review of twelve thousand scientific articles reported that 97.1 percent alleged climate change was real and human-caused.[21]

This is very much an American serving of delusion wrapped in a pastry shell of denial.[22] Unlike their American cousins, only 2 percent of Canadians entertain any doubts at all about global warming.[23] As Elizabeth Kolbert remarked in the *New Yorker,*

"As best as can be determined, the world is now warmer than it has been at any point in the last two millennia, and, if current trends continue, by the end of the century it will likely be hotter than at any point in the last two million years."[24]

The Problem in Brief

Global warming is the single gravest threat *Homo sapiens* faces, and "the greatest challenge of our time" says Thomas Stocker, co-chairman of the UN Intergovernmental Panel on Climate Change. [25] Eleven of the past twelve years have been the hottest since 1850. The hottest year on record—originally—was 2005, and the third hottest year ever recorded was 2010.[26] But 2012 then took top ranking in the contiguous United States.[27] Not to be outdone, *Scientific American* reported 2014 topped all prior years as the hottest ever recorded, not just in the United States, but globally.[28] And the first six months of 2015 another record was set.[29] Two months later NOAA announced the first eight months of 2015 smashed all global records for heat.[30] Not to be outdone, October 2015, set a new heat record as well.[31] Still NASA's Mark Serrez said that January 2016 "was a truly extraordinary month. Coming off the hottest year ever recorded (2015). . . . And it was, I would say, absurdly warm across the entire Arctic Ocean . . . more than 6 degrees Celsius above average for the month."[32]

A few summers ago, France experienced an unusual heat wave, and ten thousand seniors in retirement homes, which did not have air conditioning, perished in a month. Later, a "thermal invasion" from the Sahara desert created a scorching heat wave in southeast Europe with temperatures reaching as high as 111 degrees in Turkey, Bulgaria, Greece, Romania, and Italy.

In the far north, Inuit leader Sheila Watt-Cloutier said: "For the first time in history, my community has had to use air conditioners. Imagine that, air conditioners in the Arctic."[33]

A plague affecting over one thousand dolphins off the coast of Florida occurred recently. Ditto for a mass extinction of moose in North America; one area of Minnesota had its population of four thousand Moose drop to less than one hundred. Both die-offs were believed related to global warming.[34] Eight thousand dead murres were found in Whittier, Alaska, another twelve thousand discovered in Prince William Sound, and 120,000 saigas (antelope)—almost half the entire species—expired in Kazakhstan, all die-offs thought to be related to global warming.[35] [36] Between 1970 and 2008, there has been a whopping 52 percent decline in the world wildlife population.[37] A consortium of scientists recently warned that by 2050, 37 percent of species on earth would become extinct due to warming.[38] [39]

The percentage of Earth's surface regularly suffering drought has more than doubled since 1970.[40] Western snow packs in the United States now melt up to a month earlier than they did a half century ago, creating a burning season scorching 6.5 times more acreage than two decades ago.[41] The California snowpack in 2015 was the lowest in five hundred years, spawning gigantic forest fires covering hundreds of square miles.[42]

In August of 2010, three hundred to four hundred forest fires were starting every day in Russia due to the most intensive heat wave in 130 years of record-keeping.[43] And globally wildfire seasons have lengthened 25.3 percent since 1979.[44]

A similar 2010 heat wave caused temperatures to reach 128 degrees in Pakistan. The Indus river valley flooded with two million homes damaged, a fifth of the country under water, and twenty-million people impacted, due to unprecedented torrential rains.[45] As environmentalist Lester Brown says, "What happened to Russia and to Pakistan in the summer of 2010 are examples of what lies ahead for all of us if we continue with business as usual . . . more crop withering heat waves, more intense droughts, more severe floods, and more destructive storms."[46] Record highs are now twice as frequent as record lows on the planet.[47] As of February 2012, there were 324 consecutive months in which global temperatures exceeded their long-term averages.[48] That is twenty-seven years in a row, and that trend continues into 2016.

In Iran, in July 2015, the heat index soared to 163 degrees, as one meteorologist remarked, "This was one of the most incredible temperature observations I have ever seen, and it is one of the most extreme readings ever in the world."[49] In Australia an unprecedented heat wave scorched the country in 2013:

> A searing heat wave is baking central and northern Australia . . . topping 48 degrees Celsius in the central west. . . . In the remote town of Marree, 700 kms (435 miles) north of Adelaide in South Australia, one resident tested the folklore that you can fry an egg on the road during an outback heat wave. You hear stories of people frying an egg on a shovel, so we set up a shovel this morning . . . yep, we fried an egg on a shovel.[50]

In 1910, there were 150 glaciers in Montana compared to only 27 today.[51]

Glaciers are melting in the Andes, Rockies, Alps, the Himalayas, and the Tibetan Plateau. The giant Gangotri Glacier keeps the Ganges River flowing, but it is retreating, impacting 407 million people who live in the Gangetic basin.[52] Virtually the entire nine million strong population of Lima depends on the water from Peru's glaciers. Glacial ice in the Andes that took 1,600 years to form significantly melted in just the last twenty-five years.[53] Everest is expected to be ice free by the end of the century.[54]

Scientists believe the Arctic Ocean could be free of ice as early as the summer of 2020.[55] The last time that occurred is said to have been 125,000 years ago.[56] Surface temperatures in Greenland are four to six degrees above average, and the melting index 2.5 times the annual average, an all-time high.[57] The Greenland ice sheets are shedding two hundred cubic kilometers of ice per year, and as the earth's ice sheets melt, they stop reflecting sunlight back into the atmosphere. The poles turn darker as they absorb heat at unprecedented rates, and the albedo of the earth changes. Scientists from the University of California in San Diego analyzed Arctic satellite data over twenty-two years and found the average albedo levels decreased twice as much as prior models suggested.[58] All of this is happening so rapidly that in 2007 Arctic sea ice was at the lowest level ever recorded, "*twenty percent less than in 2005*."[59] That record was topped in 2012.[60]

From 1992 until 2011, the Greenland ice lost 2.7 trillion metric tons of ice, while the Antarctic ice sheet divested itself of 1.35 trillion metric tons.[61] By 2015 Greenland and Antarctica together lost 5 trillion tons of ice since 2002.[62] The temperature of the water in the Arctic is higher than at any time since 1870, and recently bluefin tuna were caught in waters off Greenland, a thoroughly unprecedented event.[63]

One of the implications is that the Gulf Stream may change as a result of this melting—it is now slower than it has been in 1,100 years—and this could ultimately convert the Northern European landscape into one far similar to Siberia, no longer warmed by these temperate ocean currents.[64] [65]

In Australia, the largest coral reef in the world slowed its growth due to the warmest water trend in four hundred years.[66] Rising ocean temperatures are causing a proliferation of the Bibrio genus of bacteria that cause food poisoning, gastroenteritis, septicemia, and cholera.[67]

Barbel Honisch, from Columbia University writes in *Science* that not only are oceans becoming warmer, but also more acidic, threatening coral reefs, oysters, salmon, and other species. The rate of acidification is greater than in the last fifty-six million years. "We are entering an unknown territory of marine ecosystem change," says Honish.[68] A follow-up 2013 study reported ocean acidification increasing at a faster pace than at any time in the last three hundred million years.[69] Douglas McCauley, an ecologist from the University of California, concurs and warns, "We may be sitting on a precipice of a major extinction event."[70]

HABITAT DESTRUCTION BEYOND WARMING

Humanity is destroying its environment in matters that go beyond global warming. Unregulated economic activity and burgeoning population are causing numerous other tipping points. In 2015, the population of the world will reach 7.3 billion, double the amount of a half-century ago. The planet is increasing its population by seventy-four million people, adding a new Iran or Turkey each year. The result is increasing population chasing dwindling resources.

For example, 80 percent of the ocean's biomass has been depleted due to industrialized fishing in the last fifteen years. For every pound of shrimp sold, twenty pounds of other sea creatures are caught in nets.[71] All seventeen of the world's oceanic fisheries have been harvested beyond capacity, and the oceans have lost more than 90 percent of predatory fish, tuna, swordfish, shark, and marlin.

Open ocean sharks have fallen to 1 percent of their 1950 level.[72] It is said only twenty-five thousand blue fin tuna remain on the planet.[73] The average weight of an Atlantic swordfish used to be one thousand pounds. Today it is ninety.

A marine biologist from the University in Halifax says, "People have fished for as long as we've dwelled on this planet. Within our lifetime, it's going to be over."[74] Fish stock depletion comes from commercial fishing and bottom trawling. Bottom trawling drags huge nets weighted down by various gear. The net is then connected to two large doors made of steel which can weigh up to five tons.

> These doors are designed to drag along the seafloor and keep the nets open. On average, a commercial trawling boat can catch an average of 15 tons of fish in a single haul. The sheer size and weight of trawls allow them to capture virtually everything in their path, from unwanted fish and mammals to sea turtles and deep-sea corals. Their gear and chains literally scrape the ocean floor and flatten anything in their path. The massive trawl doors create tracks on the ocean floor as the huge engines from the boats are able to take this operation further and further out to sea.[75] [76]

As the Marine Conservation Institute reports, "Bottom trawling is unselective and severely damaging to seafloor ecosystems. The net indiscriminately catches every life and object it encounters. . . . This collateral damage, called bycatch, can amount to 90 percent of a trawl's total catch."[77] Worldwide deep sea bottom trawling covers an area roughly half the area of the entire United States every year.[78]

Water Depletion

Another consequence of overpopulation is the depletion of water and fossil aquifers. Saudi Arabia tapped into its ancient aquifer and started harvesting wheat, but because of over pumping, its three-million ton wheat harvest ended abruptly, and the crop was entirely gone by 2012.

India's over-pumped aquifers are following Saudi Arabia's lead. Yemen's water tables have fallen so much that tap water is available in its capital only once every four days, and its grain harvest declined by 30 percent. The underground basin that supplies the capital city, Sanaa, may be entirely depleted in 2015.[79]

Close to half the world's population lives where water tables are falling, including China, India, and the United States.[80] A fifth of the U.S. grain harvest comes from irrigated land; for India it is three-fifths; for China, four-fifths. Underground water now meets 75 percent of Beijing's needs. The city currently drills down one thousand feet to reach water, five times deeper than twenty years ago.[81]

The Middle East, however, has the most serious water crisis, particularly Saudi Arabia, Yemen, Syria, Algeria, Libya, and Iraq.[82] It takes only fourteen tons of water to produce a ton of steel, but over a thousand tons of water to produce a ton of wheat.[83] As one might expect, the world's top nine wheat importers are in the Middle East.[84]

In 2015, a UN study predicted that within fifteen years there will be a 40 percent water shortfall. Humanity will have only 60 percent of the water that it requires.[85]

Deforestation

Another symptom of habitat destruction is the increasing level of deforestation. In 2015, scientists reported that the speed of deforestation is larger than previously supposed, increasing 62 percent faster than the prior decade. Today the planet is losing twenty-five thousand square miles of forest, "roughly the size of Sri Lanka" every year.[86] The UN Environmental Programme estimated that since the dawn of *Homo sapiens*, humans have reduced the number of trees on the planet by 50 percent.[87]

The Most Alarming Statistic

Most of these facts are known, and there is no need to recite even more. One piece of data, however, stands out and deserves repetition. It is the single most ominous statistic confronting the human race: "Researchers pulling up samples of Antarctic ice cores find air bubbles in the samples. They can determine the amount of carbon in the air as far back as 650,000 years. Their work reveals current CO2 levels in the atmosphere today are *27% higher than at any time in the last 650,000 years.*"[88] There were four ice ages during this period, and in each CO2 levels rose, but *none* as high as the levels experienced today. That ghastly statistic comes from the journal *Science* and is not likely embroidered. A subsequent study examined an ice core going back 800,000 years, and the conclusion was the same. In eight hundred millennia of accumulated CO_2 concentrations, there was simply "no analogue to the present time," said Dr. Eric Wolff of the British Antarctic Survey.[89] [90] [91] The tundra of Siberia contains frozen methane. If the tundra continues to thaw, there is a chance methane will be released, a greenhouse gas twenty-three times worse than CO_2.[92] [93]

Many lakes in Siberia have simply disappeared in a single day. As the tundra that supports the lake melts, the water seeps underground and the lake simply vanishes. Of almost eleven thousand Siberian lakes that shrank significantly, researchers "found 125 disappeared entirely and were refilled with vegetation."[94] As these lakes succumb to melting tundra, accelerating methane emissions will not be far behind, compounding an already foreboding problem of the atmosphere now containing the highest levels of CO_2 in eight hundred thousand years.

Consequences

If one is between eighteen and thirty years of age—and, luckily, one of the 30 percent of Americans who believe this problem is serious—by the time they reach retirement, the following planetary circumstances will likely greet them:

- Over a million species of plant and animal life will have gone extinct, more than one-fourth of all plant and vertebrate species.[95] There will likely no longer be tigers, pandas, rhinos, sturgeon, alligators, parrots, sharks, gorillas, tuna, elephants, blue whales, golden lions, red wolfs, snow leopards, trumpeter swans, northern hawk owls, polar bears, or gazelles.[96] [97]
- Half of America's bird species will have emigrated to other climates.[98]
- In the summer, there will be no ice sheet in the Arctic Ocean.
- Most coral reefs and the species they protect will be gone.
- One quarter of all land animals and plants will not have survived climate change and will have gone extinct.[99]
- Diseases formerly associated with equatorial climates will reach into Europe and North America: malaria, encephalitis, ticks, and sand flies, which carry visceral leishmaniasis, the Zika virus, Lyme disease, and Bluetongue, West Nile Virus, Chagas, Dengue, Chikungunya; these along with yellow fever are only some that are predicted.[100] [101] [102]
- Wildfires, heat waves, droughts, and extreme weather events like hurricanes and cyclones will be run-of-the-mill occurrences.[103] [104] [105]
- There will be large-scale food shortages and famines.

- The disappearance of glaciers in the Andes is expected along with a drop in agricultural production in South America of up to 50 percent, and a collapse of the Caribbean ecosystem.[106]
- The volume of fresh water in the Arctic Ocean from melting could convert the thermal landscape of Europe to one more resembling Siberia.[107]
- Ocean levels will rise to inundate and destroy many islands, archipelagos like Fiji, the Marshall Islands, Micronesia, the Cook Islands, portions of New Guinea, Tuvalu, the Maldives, Bangladesh, and over 150 million shoreline-dwelling humans will have been displaced inland.
- Most glaciers will have disappeared, affecting the down river communities that depend on runoff for their survival.
- The number of people who have lost their homes due to desertification, water pollution, and famine will reach a billion "climate refugees" by 2050.[108]

In her book, *The Sixth Extinction: An Unnatural History,* Elizabeth Kilbert says that warming today is occurring ten times faster than in the last ice age "one-third of all reef-building corals, a third of all freshwater mollusks, a third of sharks and rays, a quarter of all mammals, a fifth of all reptiles, and a sixth of all birds are headed for oblivion."[109]

Comments of the World Bank are timely:

> Around the world, the deep oceans are heating, the tundra is thawing, ice shelves are breaking up, sea levels are rising, fish, insects, birds, and ecosystems are migrating, violent weather is increasing, and the timing of the seasons has changed—all from a one degree Fahrenheit temperature increase. The scientific consensus is that temperatures will rise an additional two to 10 degrees by the end of this century. Two years ago, the biggest insurer in Great Britain, CGNU, said that unchecked climate change could bankrupt the global economy by 2065. Nature's message is remarkably simple: Cut carbon emissions quickly, globally, and dramatically, or prepare for a future of environmental and economic disintegration.[110]

Indeed, a recent peer-reviewed scientific report says that once CO2 concentrations reach a certain level—we are not quite there yet—the effects become irreversible for at least one thousand years, regardless of mitigation efforts.[111]

Despite all the evidence, however, the level of denial is pronounced, particularly in the United States. In 2015, a bill introduced by Senator Bernard Sanders contained an amendment that "climate change is real and is caused by humans." The bill was defeated fifty-six to forty-two.[112]

MAJOR CULPRITS: THE UNITED STATES AND CHINA

Currently, the United States and China are the world's largest emitters of CO2.[113] From 1990 to 2007, the United States and China, together, increased their carbon emissions by 60 percent. China now emits more CO2 than the United States and Canada.[114] Almost 75 percent of China's energy production and electricity comes from the burning of dirty coal in old-fashioned coal-fired facilities. In addition, an estimated eight hundred million of China's 1.2 billion people use coal in their homes. In many rural communities, the fuel is full of arsenic, lead, mercury, fluorine, and poisonous metals that can pose a serious health threat.[115] In 2013, the *New York Times* published a study showing that life expectancy in northern China—where coal and soot pollution are greatest—already declined 5.5 years due to cardio-respiratory diseases.[116]

China currently *burns more coal than the United States, Japan, and Europe combined,* and its coal burning is increasing every year. China and the United States together account for close to 40 percent of the world's carbon emissions. This was true in 2007,[117] in 2010, [118] and in 2014.[119] [120]

While China's emissions exceed the United States today, on a per capita basis the United States carbon footprint is twice that of China.[121] They may produce more CO2 than the United States does, but they have three times the population.

China has increased its carbon emissions three-fold in the last seventeen years. It is building two sooty, coal-fired power plants every week in an attempt to manufacture all the products the United States and Western Europe request.[122] The majority of what Americans buy at Walmart is made in China. Shop at Target, Longs, K-Mart, and the story is similar.

China also consumes half the world's cement, and its industrial machine is so heavily polluting its own country that 70 percent of China's major lakes and rivers are polluted.[123] The once pristine Yangtze River, said one author, is virtually devoid of birds and visible signs of life.[124]

In the city of Harbin in 2013, the air quality index reached one thousand micrograms per cubic meter. Any number above five hundred is considered "heavily polluted" and "hazardous."[125]

Chengdu and Chongqing dump billions of tons of mostly untreated human, animal, and industrial waste directly into the river. Today, most of the acid rain in Japan and South Korea is "Made in China."[126]

China is considered the most polluted country on the planet today.[127] More than 1.2 million premature deaths are attributed to air pollution alone.[128] A more recent 2015 paper increased that estimate to 1.6 million people. [129]

China has more than one hundred cities of more than a million people, and nearly everyone is shrouded in a toxic haze of sulfur dioxide and lung-piercing particulates. Of the twenty largest cities in the world with the absolutely worst air pollution, "sixteen of these gaseous metropolises are in China."[130] Of 360 Chinese cities sampled, 90 percent failed to meet national air quality standards.[131] In addition Greenpeace reported in 2015 that 16 percent of China's soil and 19 percent of its farmland was polluted from lead, nickel, cadmium and arsenic.[132]

As the United States transfers its manufacturing to China, the Chinese, in turn, build coal-fired power plants far faster than all the hybrids the American middle class might ever buy to mitigate this planetary damage. Coal is now the source of 30 percent of the world's energy, up from 25 percent in the 1990s.[133]

To most experts, it is necessary to retreat to CO2 levels that existed in the early 1990s if humanity is to make any impact on global warming. The target of 350 ppm which existed in 1990 is considered the threshold that must be reached to prevent a planetary disaster.[134] As James Hansen of NASA writes: "If humanity wishes to preserve a planet similar to that on which civilization developed and to which life on Earth is adapted, paleoclimate evidence and ongoing climate change suggest that CO2 will need to be reduced from its current 385 ppm to at most 350 ppm."[135]

Mr. Hansen wrote those words when earth measured a level of 385 ppm. Unfortunately, at the end of 2013, emissions went in the opposite direction and reached 400 ppm.[136] As of March, 2015, they reached 401 ppm.[137]

Thousands of foundries in China run on industrial-grade coke with no pollution control devices on their smokestacks, creating a plume of smoke that stretches across the Pacific.[138] As *Time* reported:

> The soot-blackened city of Linfen in China's inland Shanxi province makes Dickensian London look as pristine as a nature park. Shanxi is the heart of China's coal belt, and the hills around Linfen are dotted with mines, legal and illegal, and the air is filled with burning coal. Don't bother hanging your laundry, it'll turn black before it dries.[139]

The pollution is now easily visible from space. Satellite photos often show more than one thousand kilometers of pollution stretching over China. The "Asian Brown Cloud" is a haze of pollution about three km thick sometimes covering an area as big as Australia.[140]

As the cloud crosses the earth, soot darkens arctic snow. Soot is known as "black carbon" and new estimates of its heat trapping power are double that made by a UN panel in 2007. To Mark Jacobson, an atmospheric scientist at Stanford, "When black carbon settles on glaciers or arctic ice, it renders them darker, and they absorb more heat and melt at a faster rate."[141] The Arctic, thus, warms four times faster than the rest of the earth.[142] Largely because of this, the disappearance of summer ice cap in the Arctic is expected.

Recorded human civilization from ancient Sumeria to the present, from the Roman Empire to the Ottoman, never knew a planet without an ice-covered North Pole.

President Bush refused to sign the Kyoto protocols to reduce CO2 emissions, because he felt it would be bad for the U.S. economy and create a recession. He managed to create the Great Recession, even without Kyoto's help, but in the longer view, there were financial panics, stock market crashes, and depressions in 1819, 1836, 1857, 1873, 1921, 1929, 1987, and dozens more recessions and waves of unemployment, civil war, starvation, and world war. But there was always a polar ice cap.

Antarctica is not faring much better. Since 1958, it warmed by 4.4 degrees Fahrenheit, roughly twice as much scientists predicted and three times the overall rate of warming on earth.[143] On a Tuesday in 2015, a temperature of +63 degrees Fahrenheit was observed, the highest temperature ever recorded there in the last 150 years.[144]

Lester Brown

Lester Brown's *World on the Edge* represents one of the most gloomy assessments on global warming ever written while struggling to find a few slivers of optimism. On the drearier side, Brown frightens his reader with a litany of statistical evidence, similar to what has been reviewed here, and predicts that if the Western Antarctic Ice Sheet breaks off (portions already have) or the Greenland ice sheet disappears, "the word that comes to mind is chaos . . . *we probably cannot save civilization as we know it.*"[145]

Brown is president of the Earth Policy Institute and proposes the most draconian remedies:

> At the heart is a call to reduce global carbon dioxide emissions 80 percent by 2020—far more aggressive than anything you'll hear from political leaders or even most activists. It's an ambitious plan, one that is less concerned with political feasibility than the survivability of the planet. "This is not Plan A, business as usual," Brown writes. "This is Plan B—a wartime mobilization, an all-out response proportionate to the threat that global warming presents to our future."[146] [147]

He believes by acting decisively we could reverse global warming in the next eight years. We actually don't have much more time than that. Some say less. Richard Betts of the British Meteorological Office, for example, says if emissions continue climbing *beyond the next three years*, there will be long-term disastrous consequences.[148]

Brown's remedies involve *extremely* stoic measures that no politician would ever dream of endorsing. But Brown casts the problem in the most dramatic light:

> In World War II, the sale of new cars was banned. Residential construction was halted. Driving for pleasure was banned. People were recycling and planting victory gardens. Gasoline, fuel, and sugar were ra-

> tioned in 1942. The US wanted to produce 60,000 planes, and built 229,000.[149] A merry-go-round factory made gun mounts. A toy company made compasses. A corset manufacturer produced grenade belts. A pinball machine plant made armor piercing shells. The point is that it did not take decades to restructure the U.S. industrial economy. It did not take years. It was done in a matter of months. If we could restructure the U.S. industrial economy in months, then we can restructure the world energy economy during this decade.[150]

Unfortunately the United States is not anywhere close to Brown's hope for a new American resolve. There is virtually no support in Congress or the Senate for *any* of his ideas.

In sum, humanity is headed into one of the greatest crises it has ever faced and one that is entirely of its own making. "The best available evidence suggest that amount of the gas in the air has not been this high for at least three million years."[151] The Mauna Loa Observatory measured four hundred ppm in 2013 and 401.6 in 2015, and the last time the Earth's CO2 concentration was that high was in the Pliocene era when summers in the Arctic were eight degrees Celsius warmer than today.[152] That is two independent investigations bellowing the same incomprehensibly bad news. Unfortunately, in May 2016 the same observatory published new and astonishing findings that CO2 levels had reached 407.9 ppm.[153]

Furthermore, the situation is not improving despite all efforts at conservation. Joseph Alcamo of the UN Environmental Program said that in 2010 global greenhouse gas emissions reached the equivalent of 50.1 gigatons of carbon dioxide, and without significant action, that number will reach fifty-nine gigatons by 2020, an expected 16 percent increase of emissions in the next five years.[154]

There are millions of concerned youth attempting to live more minimalist lifestyles who are deeply concerned and committed to a greener planet, but unfortunately whatever conservation measures we think we may be making, they are not producing tangible planetary results. Thomas Friedman's remarks are of interest:

> For thousands of years up to the dawn of the industrial age 200 years ago, the Earth's atmosphere contained 280 parts per million of the heat-trapping greenhouse gas carbon dioxide. Today that number is nearly 400 ppm. . . . Melting the permafrost in Alaska, Canada, and Siberia, for example would release massive amounts of carbon that would further increase global warming. Permafrost is packed with CO2 and frozen methane which is 25 times more potent a greenhouse gas than CO2. If the tundra continues melting," says Hal Harvey, the chief executive of Energy Innovation, "we could basically release the equivalent of all the carbon that all humanity has emitted from the start of history to now."[155]

It will be curious how, and if, a way is found out of this predicament.

There are a few glimmers of good news. British carbon emissions dropped in 2014 by 8.4 percent.[156] U.S. carbon emissions decreased slightly, in part due to the recession, the conversion of coal power plants to natural gas, and conservation.[157] But some would call that mere chump change. U.S. emissions actually increased in 2013[158] and once again in 2014.[159] [160]

The situation worldwide is much more alarming. The World Meteorological Association reported that "the concentration of carbon dioxide in the atmosphere actually increased last year *at the fastest rate for nearly 30 years*."[161] Indeed, in the first two months of 2014, global emissions increased 7.45 percent.[162]

Moreover, a staggering assessment by British Petroleum predicts global emissions will increase 29 percent between 2012 and 2035, primarily from emerging economies.[163] The Intergovernmental Panel on Climate Change (IPCC) penned a similar prognosis.[164] This same group predicted current greenhouse gas emissions will *double* by the end of the century.[165]

So, with that litany of bad news, this sojourn into global warming concludes with a report sponsored by the Global Humanitarian Forum. It asserts that climate change is

> already responsible for 300,000 deaths a year . . . *making it the greatest humanitarian challenge the world faces*. . . . The world is at a crossroads. We can no longer afford to ignore the human impact of climate change. This is a call to the negotiators to come to the most ambitious agreement ever negotiated or to continue to accept mass starvation, mass sickness and mass migration on an ever-growing scale.[166]

NOTES

1. "Science and Technology Picture Quotes, Feynman," www.quotesoflife.info.
2. Frank Newport, "Americans' Global Warming Concerns Continue to Drop," Gallup, March 11, 2010, http://www.gallup.com/poll/126560/americans-global-warming-concerns-continue-drop.aspx.
3. "Where did Global Warming Go?" *New York Times*, October 16, 2011, p. 7.
4. University of Michigan and Muhlenberg College poll reported in *The News*, Mexico City, February 29, 2012.
5. "Fox's Huddy Falsely Claims Skeptic's Questionable Study 'Seems to Debunk' that Global Warming is Man-made," Media Matters, August 6, 2011, http://mediamatters.org/mmtv/201108060002.
6. "Fox's Huddy Falsely Claims Skeptic's Questionable Study 'Seems to Debunk' that Global Warming is Man-made."
7. Jeffrey Kluger, "Americans Flunk Science Again," *Time*, April 22, 2014.
8. "40% of Americans 'Not Too Worried' about Climate Change," *The Guardian*, November 3, 2015.
9. http://www.youtube.com/watch?v=Ft8LfE7AI2w.
10. Joseph Romm, "Experts Debunk Polls Claiming Fewer Americans Believe in Climate Change," Grist, November 16, 2011, http://www.grist.org/climate-change/2011-11-16-experts-debunk-polls-claiming-fewer-americans-believe-in-climate.

11. Naomi Oreskes, "The Scientific Consensus on Climate Change,"*Science* 3 (December 2004).
12. Peter Hart, "In Denial on Climate Change," FAIR, May 1, 2007, http://www.fair.org/index.php?page=3418.
13. Newport, "Americans' Global Warming Concerns Continue to Drop."
14. See https://www.youtube.com/watch?v=Lk8SSqc7ekM.
15. IPCC, Synthesis Report, Section 1.1: Observations of Climate Change, in IPCC AR4 SYR 2007. Also IPCC, Synthesis Report, Treatment of Uncertainty, in IPCC AR4 SYR 2007. IPCC, Synthesis Report, Section 2.4: Attribution of climate change, in IPCC AR4 SYR 2007.America's Climate Choices: Panel on Advancing the Science of Climate Change; National Research Council. Advancing the Science of Climate Change (Washington, DC: The National Academies Press, 2010).
16. Seth Boresnstein, "Science Academies Explain Global Warming Reality," *Associates Press*, February 26, 2014.
17. Doyle Rice, "Report: 97 percent of Scientists Say Man-made Climate Change is Real," *USA Today*, June 22, 2010.
18. "Energy Update," Rasmussen Reports, July 7, 2015, http://www.rasmussenreports.com/public_content/politics/current_events/environment_energy/energy_update.
19. Richard Horwitz, "American's Problems with Global Warming,"*American Studies* 45, no. 1 (Spring 2004): 5–37..
20. Alana Horowitz, "Global Warming Poll: Climate Change a 'Serious Problem' to 68% of Americans, *Huffington Post*, November 12, 2012, http://www.huffingtonpost.com/2012/11/09/global-warming-poll-climate-change_n_2105600.html. Original source: Rasmussen Reports, "Energy Update," July 7, 2015, http://www.rasmussenreports.com/public_content/politics/current_events/environment_energy/energy_update.
21. Anna North, "Why Misleading Americans about Climate Change is Dangerous," *New York Times*, August 11, 2015.
22. A 2013 study confirms that global warming is human induced. See Justin Gillis, "Climate Panel Cites Near Certainty on Warming,"*New York Times*, August 19, 2013.
23. Rebecca Leber, "Just Two Percent of Canadians Deny Climate Change," ClimateProgress, August 16, 2012, http://thinkprogress.org/climate/2012/08/16/697911/canada-climate-change/.
24. Elizabeth Kolbert Quotes, *The New Yorker*, April 25, 2005.
25. Justin Gillis, "UN Climate Panel Endorses Ceiling on Global Emissions," *New York Times*, September 27, 2013.
26. Arthur Max, AP, "2010 on Track to be of 3 Hottest Years on Record," *San Francisco Chronicle* December 31, 2010.
27. Justin Gillis, "Not Even Close: 2012 was the Hottest Ever in U.S.," *New York Times*, January 8, 2013.
28. Gayathri Vaidyanathan, "2014 to be Hottest Year Ever Measured," *Scientific American*, December 4, 2014.
29. "Another Month, Another Global Heat Record Broken by Far," *New York Times*, July 20, 2015.
30. "Earth's Record Streak of Record Heat Keeps on Sizzling," *New York Times*, September 17, 2015.
31. Seth Borenstein, "Absurdly Hot October as Earth Sets 8th Heat Record this Year," AP, November 19, 2015.
32. Chris Mooney, "Scientists are Floored by What's Happening in the Arctic Right Now," February 2016, *Washington Post*.
33. Sheila Watt- Cloutier, *Sierra Club Currents* 6, no. 54, March 2007.
34. "The Disappearing Moose," *New York Times*, October 16, 2013.
35. James Gorman, "Animals Die in Large Numbers, and Researchers Scratch their Heads," *New York Times*, January 18. 2016.

36. Carl Zimmer, "More than Half of Entire Species of Saigas Gone in Mysterious Die-off," *New York Times*, November 2, 2015.

37. John Heilprin, "Wildlife Populations Plummet for 3,000 Species," Associated Press, September 30, 2014.

38. James Gorman, "Scientists Predict Widespread Extinction by Global Warming,"*New York Times*, January 8, 2004.

39. Photo of ice shelf collapse courtesy of NASA's Terra satellite, supplied by Ted Scambos, National Snow and Ice Center, University of Colorado, Boulder.

40. Jeffrey Kluger, "The Turning Point," *Time*, April 3, 2006.

41. "The Long Burn," *Science News* (July 8, 2006):19.

42. Matt Ferner, "Snowpack in Sierra Nevada at 500 Year Low," Huffington Post, September 14, 2015. Original source: Soumaya Belmecheri, Flurin Babst, et al., "Multi-century Evaluation of Sierra Nevada Snowpack," *Nature Climate Change* doi:10.1038/nclimate2809.

43. Lester Brown, *World on the Edge*, (Colorado: Earth Policy Institute, 2011), location 30.

44. "Wildfire Seasons have Lengthened," *Science News*, August 22, 2015.

45. Lester Brown, *World on the Edge*, (Colorado: Earth Policy Institute, January 2011), location 34.

46. Brown, *World on the Edge*, location 37–40.0

47. Brown, *World on the Edge*, location 151.

48. "With Erratic Weather, Scientists Look to the Ice," *New York Times*, March 29, 2012.

49. Thomas Friedman, "The World's Hot Spot," *New York Times*, August 19, 2015.

50. Matt Siegel and Colin Packham, "Australia Swelters after Record Hot 2013," Reuters, January 3, 2014, http://ca.news.yahoo.com/australia-swelters-record-hot-2013-farmers-slaughter-cattle-044230636.html.

51. Brown, *World on the Edge*, (Colorado: Earth Policy Institute, January 2011), location 164.

52. Brown, *World on the Edge*, location 167

53. Justin Gills, "In Sign of Warming, 1600 Years of Ice in Andes Melted in 25 Years." *New York Times*, 2013.

54. "Everest Could Lose Most of Its Ice by the End of the Century," *Science News*, June 27, 2015.

55. Craig Medred, "Expert Predicts Ice-free Arctic by 2020 as UN Releases Climate Report," *Alaska Dispatch News*, November 2, 2014.

56. "Polar Caps and Global Warming," globalgreenhousewarming, 2015, http://www.global-greenhouse-warming.com/polar-caps.html.

57. "In 2007, Greenland Set a Melting Record." *Science News*, January 5, 2008.

58. Laura Poppick, "Warming From Arctic Sea Ice Melting More Dramatic than Thought," LiveScience, February 17, 2014, http://news.yahoo.com/warming-arctic-sea-ice-melting-more-dramatic-thought-202504784.html.

59. *USA Today*, September 13, 2007, p. 3.

60. Justin Gillis, "Ending its Summer Melt, Arctic Sea Ice Sets a New Low that Leads to Warnings," *New York Times*, September 19 2012.

61. Eric Wayman, "Polar Ice Sheets Shrinking Overall," *Science News*, March 9, 2013.

62. NASA data cited in Phil Plait, "5 Trillion Tons of Ice Lost Since 2002," *Slate* magazine, September 3, 2015.

63. "Bluefin Tuna are Showing Up in the Arctic, and That's not Good News," Takepart.com, September 15, 2014, http://news.yahoo.com/bluefin-tuna-showing-arctic-thats-not-good-news-203045736.html.

64. Chris Mooney, "Global Warming is now Slowing Circulation of the Oceans with Dire Consequences," *The Washington Post*, March 23, 2015.

65. A more recent study makes this conclusion even more foreboding. See http://www.washingtonpost.com/news/energy-environment/wp/2015/09/24/why-some-scientists-are-worried-about-a-surprisingly-cold-blob-in-the-north-atlantic-ocean/.

66. James Morgan, "Coral Reef Growth is Slowest Ever," BBC News, January 2, 2009, http://news.bbc.co.uk/2/hi/science/nature/7807943.stm.

67. "Warming Oceans," *San Francisco Chronicle*, September 14, 2011, p. A2.

68. Wynne Parry, "Oceans Turning Acidic Faster than Past 300 Million Years," Live Science, March 2, 2012, http://news.yahoo.com/oceans-turning-acidic-faster-past-300-million-years-164401538.html.

69. Brad Plumer, "Carbon-dioxide Levels in the Atmosphere Rose at a Record Pace in 2013," World Meteorological Association, accessed in 2015, http://www.vox.com/2014/9/9/6126245/carbon-dioxide-levels-in-the-atmosphere-rose-at-a-record-pace-in-2013.

70. Carl Zimmer, "Ocean Life Faces Mass Extinction," *New York Times*, January 15, 2015.

71. Russ Kick, ed., *Everything You Know is Wrong* (New York: The Disinformtion Company, 2007), location 4667.

72. Janet Raloff, "Empty Nets," *Science News*, June 4, 2005, 167.

73. Catch Zero, *Science News* 164 (July 26, 2003): 59.

74. "Worthless Waters: By Mid-century Seas Value May be Drained," *Science News*, November 4, 2006, 291.

75. Craig Voros, "Commercial Bottom Trawling and Deep Sea Corals," June 2006, http://jrscience.wcp.muohio.edu/fieldcourses06/PapersMarineEcologyArticles/CommercialBottomTrawlingaA.html.

76. The European Parliament recently voted against a ban on deep sea trawling, but it did agree to restrict some of the worst practices. David Jolly, "Europe Moves to Prohibit Some Deep-sea Trawling," *New York Times*, December 10, 2013.

77. Marine Conservation Institute, accessed 2015, https://www.marine-conservation.org/what-we-do/program-areas/how-we-fish/destructive-fishing/.

78. "Scraping the Seafloor Smooth," *New York Times* editorial, October 22, 2012.

79. Brown, *World on the Edge*, location 271.

80. Brown, *World on the Edge*, location 103

81. Brown, *World on the Edge*, location 95.

82. Thomas Friedman, "The Other Arab Spring," *New York Times*, April 2012.

83. Brown, *World on the Edge*, location 105.

84. Thomas Friedman, "The Scary Hidden Stressor," *New York Times*, March 2, 2013.

85. "UN: World Could Face 40 percent Water Shortfall by 2030," Al Jazerra, March 20, 2015, http://america.aljazeera.com/articles/2015/3/20/un-world-faces-40-percent-water-shortfall-by-2030.html.

86. Ariel Min, "World's Tropical Forests Vanishing More Rapidly than Previously Thought," PBS Newshour, March 2, 2015, http://www.pbs.org/newshour/rundown/worlds-tropical-forests-vanishing-rapidly-previously-thought/.

87. Elizabeth Howell, "Earth Lost Half its Trees to Humans," Live Science, September 3, 2015.

88. "Carbon Dioxide at Highest Level in 650,000 Years," Mongabay.com, November 24, 2005, http://news.mongabay.com/2005/1124-climate.html.

89. Jonathan Amos, "Deep Ice Tells Long Climate Story," BBS News, September 4, 2006, http://news.bbc.co.uk/2/hi/science/nature/5314592.stm.

90. Another study corroborates this data. See Justin Gillis, "Study of Ice Age Bolsters Carbon and Warming Link," *New York Times*, February 28, 2013.

91. Graphic provided by EPA:http://epa.gov/climatestudents/scientists/proof.html.

92. Brendan Koerner, "The Other Greenhouse Gases," The Green Lantern, November 27, 2007, http://www.slate.com/id/2178595/. Note that the Arctic not only stores methane, but the top meter of Arctic tundra contains 200 trillion kilograms of carbon, which, if released through warming, some have called "the big Arctic carbon bomb," *Science News*, July 5, 2008, 29.

93. A recent study contradicts this hypothesis and alleges that the methane may be more secure than previously thought. See" Warming may not release carbon in Arctic tundra," *Science News*, June 15, 2013.

94. "Siberian Lakes Disappearing," *Washington Post*, June 6, 2006.

95. Brian Handwerk "Global Warming Could Cause Mass Extinctions," *National Geographic News*, April 2006.

96. In 2012, for the first time in recorded history, the Monarch butterfly did not arrive in Mexico for its annual migration. Jim Robbins, "The Year the Monarch didn't Appear," *New York Times*, November 23, 2013.

97. Felicity Barringer, "Climate Change Will Disrupt Half of North America's Bird Species, Study Says," *New York Times*, September 8, 2014.

98. Barringer, "Climate Change Will Disrupt Half of North America's Bird Species, Study Says."

99. Nigel Morris, "Climate Change Could Force 1 billion from their Homes by 2050," *The Independent*, August 6, 2015, http://www.independent.co.uk/environment/climate-change/climate-change-could-force-1-billion-from-their-homes-by-2050-817223.html.

100. Margaret Gilmore, "Global Warming Disease Warning," BBC News, June 18, 1999, http://news.bbc.co.uk/1/hi/sci/tech/372219.stm.

101. Justin Gillis, "Zika Could be Omen of Global Warming Threat," *New York Times*, February 18, 2016.

102. Donald McNeil, "U.S. Becomes More Vulnerable to Tropical Diseases like Zika," *New York Times*, January 4, 2016.

103. Justin Gillis, "Study Indicates a Greater Threat of Extreme Weather," *New York Times*, April 27, 2012.

104. Kate Galbraith, "Wildfires and Climate Change," *New York Times*, September 4, 2013.

105. Christopher Schwalm, "Hundred-Year Forecast: Drought," *New York Times*, August 11, 2012.

106. See Andrew Whalen, "World Bank Warns of Danger in Andes," *Associated Press*, February 18, 2009.

107. "Arctic Water May Cool off Europe," report by University College London, Reuters, *The News*, January 23, 2012.

108. Stephen Messenger, "Climate Refugees Could Number 1 billion by 2050," Treehugger, December 8, 2009, http://www.treehugger.com/corporate-responsibility/climate-refugees-could-number-1-billion-by-2050.html.

109. Michiko Kaktuna, "Cataclysm has Arrived: Man's Inhumanity to Nature," *New York Times*, February 3, 2014.

110. Ross Gelbspan, "The Big Name Game," *Grist* magazine, July 31, 2002.

111. S. Solomon, Gian-Kasper Plattner, et al., "Irreversible Climate Change Due to Carbon Dioxide Emissions," Proc Natl Acad Sci USA 106, no. 6 (February 10, 2009): 1704–9.

112. Coral Davenport, "Senate Rejects Human Role in Climate Change," *New York Times*, January 22, 2015.

113. The United States accounts for nearly 90 percent of North American GDP about 68 percent of its population, also is responsible for 85 percent of North America's carbon emissions. Kroth, *Duped* ibid.

114. Simon Rogers and Lisa Evans, "World Carbon Dioxide Emissions Data by Country: China Speeds Ahead of the Rest," *The Guardian*, January 31, 2011, http://www.guardian.co.uk/news/datablog/2011/jan/31/world-carbon-dioxide-emissions-country-data-co2.

115. Peter Navarro and Greg Autrey, *Death by China* (New York: Pearson FT Press, 2011).

116. Leslie Hook, "China Smog Cuts 5.5 Years from Average Life Expectancy," CNBC, July 8, 2003, http://www.cnbc.com/id/100871380.

117. "World CO2 Emissions Rose by 3.1 percent Last Year," Sustainable development, 2007,http://www.elrst.com/2008/06/16/world-co2-emissions-rose-by-31-percent-last-year/.

118. CO2 Emissions from Fuel Combustion -2011 Highlights" International Energy Agency, 2011, http://www.iea.org/media/statistics/CO2highlights.pdf.
119. "The Largest Producers of CO2 Emissions Worldwide in 2014," Statistics Portal, 2015, http://www.statista.com/statistics/271748/the-largest-emitters-of-co2-in-the-world/http://www.statista.com/statistics/271748/the-largest-emitters-of-co2-in-the-world/.
120. The Global Carbon Project report "singled out China as the world's biggest carbon emitter, accounting for 27 percent of global fossil fuel emissions in 2012. The US ranked a distant second place at 14 percent, followed by the European Union countries with a combined 10 percent and India at 6 percent." James Foley, "Global Carbon Emissions Projected to Reach Record in 2013," Nature World News, November 19, 2013, http://www.natureworldnews.com/articles/4990/20131119/global-carbon-emissions-projected-reach-record-high-2013.htm.
121. Ben Wolford, "Global Carbon Emissions Keep Rising; Expected to Reach New Record in 2013," *International Science Times*, November 18, 2013, http://www.isciencetimes.com/articles/6342/20131118/global-carbon-emissions-keep-rising-expected-reach.htm.
122. Eric Larson, "China's Growing Coal Use is World's Greatest Problem" Climate Central, January 27, 2014, http://www.climatecentral.org/blogs/chinas-growing-coal-use-is-worlds-growing-problem-16999.
123. "China's Rivers: Frontlines for Chemical Wastes," Worldwatch Institute, 2013,http://www.worldwatch.org/chinas-rivers-frontlines-chemical-wastes.
124. Peter Navarro, ibid.
125. Mia Li "Chinese City's Pollution Goes off the Charts," *New York Times* October 20, 2013.
126. Peter Navarro, *Death by China* (New York: Prentice Hall, 2011) 366.
127. Navarro, ibid, location, 1017
128. Edward Wong, "Air pollution linked to 1.2 million premature deaths in China." *New York Times*, April 1, 2013.
129. Dan Levin, "Study links polluted air in China to 1.6 million deaths a year," *New York Times*, Aug 13, 2015
130. Navarro, ibid, location, 2689
131. Edward Wong, "Hundreds of Chinese Cities don't Meet Air Standards, Report Finds," *New York Times*, April 21, 2015.
132. Cherie Chan, "Soil Contamination Found Near Huge Mine in Western China," *New York Times*, June 12, 2015.
133. Deiter Helm, "To Slow Warming, Tax Carbon," *New York Times*, November 11, 2012.
134. James Hansen, 350.org, 2009, http://350.org/en/about/science.
135. Helm, "To Slow Warming, Tax Carbon."
136. "Earth's CO2 Home Page," July 2015, http://co2now.org/.
137. Robert Scribbler, "CO2, Earth's Global Thermostat Dials up to Record 401.6 ppm," Robertscribbler.com, http://robertscribbler.com/2014/03/14/co2-earths-global-thermostat-dials-up-to-record-401-6-ppm-daily-value-in-march/.
138. Ian Fletcher, *Free Trade that Doesn't Work*, Washington DC, US Business and Industry Council, 2010, location 199.
139. Navarro, ibid, loc. 2632
140. Viv Forbes, "Clearing the Smog of Beijing with 'Coal by Wire,'" Canada Free Press, August 4, 2008, http://www.canadafreepress.com/index.php/article/4274.
141. Elizabeth Rosenthal, "Burning Fuel Particles do more Damage to Climate than Thought, Study Says." *New York Times*, January 15, 2013.
142. "Arctic Warming Linked to Combination of Reduced Sea Ice and Global Atmospheric Warming," *Science News*, July 6, 2012.
143. Justin Gillis, "Scientists Report Faster Warming in Antarctica," *New York Times*, December 23, 2012.

144. "It hit 63 degrees in Antarctica on Tuesday," CNBC, http://finance.trendolizer.com/2015/03/it-hit-63-degrees-in-antarctica-on-tuesday.html.
145. Brown, *World on the Edge*, location 575.
146. Bryan Walsh, "Plan B- How to Stop Global Warming," *Time*, January 4, 2008.
147. Walsh, "Plan B- How to Stop Global Warming."
148. Janet Raioff, "Studies See 4 Degrees of Warming," *Science News*, December 18, 2010.
149. Brown, *World on the Edge*, location 586.
150. Brown, *World on the Edge*, location 58.
151. Justin Gills "Heat-trapping Gas Passes Milestone, Raising Fears," *New York Times*, 2013.
152. "Atmospheric CO2 hits milestone," *Science News*, June 1, 2013.
153. Earth System Research Laboratory, Global Monitoring Division, NOAA, June 3, 2016.
154. David Jolly, "United Nations Group Warns on Emissions," *New York Times*, November 5, 2013.
155. Thomas Friedman, "The Market and Mother Nature," *New York Times*, January 8, 2013.
156. "Britain's Greenhouse Gas Emissions Down 8.4 percent in 2014," *Reuters*, March 26, 2015,http://news.yahoo.com/britains-greenhouse-gas-emissions-down-8-4-percent-113927997--business.html.
157. The EPA recently attempted to set limits on coal fired power plant emissions, but the opposition is strong. Mitch McConnel, Senate Republican leader, said "It's a devastating blow to our state, and we're going to fight it in every way we can." Michael Shear, "Administration Presses Ahead with Limits on Emissions from Power Plants," *New York Times* September 19., 2013.
158. Brad Plumer, "After Years of Decline, U.S. Carbon Emissions Rose 2 percent in 2013,"*Washington Post*, January 13, 2014.
159. "Rising Coal Use Reverses Three Years of CO2 Declines," *Wall Street Journal*, January 13, 2014.
160. Wendy Koch, "U.S. Carbon Emission Rise Despite Obama Climate Plan," *USA Today*, September 26, 2014, http://www.usatoday.com/story/money/business/2014/09/26/us-carbon-emissions-rise-despite-obama-climate-plan/16276811/.
161. Matt McGrath, "Greenhouse Gas Levels Rising at Fastest Rate Since 1984," BBC, September 9, 2014, http://www.bbc.com/news/science-environment-29115845.
162. Kevin Schultz, "Carbon Dioxide Emissions Rise with Rebounding Economy," *Scientific American*, June 6, 2014, http://www.scientificamerican.com/article/carbon-dioxide-emissions-rise-with-rebounding-economy/.
163. "BP Energy Outlook, 2035 Shows Global Energy Demand Growth Slowing, Despite Emerging Economies," British Petroleum, January 15, 2014, http://www.bp.com/en/global/corporate/press/press-releases/energy-outlook-2035.html.
164. "Projected Climate Change and its Impacts," IPCC, 2007, https://www.ipcc.ch/publications_and_data/ar4/syr/en/spms3.html.
165. Robert Stavins, "Climate Realities, *New York Times*, September 20, 2014.
166. John Vidal, "Global Warming Causes 300,000 Deaths a Year, says Kofi Annan Thinktank," *The Guardian*, May 29, 2009, http://www.guardian.co.uk/environment/2009/may/29/1.

ELEVEN

How Global Warming Might Test the Theory of the Psychic Immune System

Very few species will destroy their own habitat. Termites eat up theirs, but then they move to another delicious conifer. Elephants may be one of the rare species evolution produced which destroys its habitat, but recent research argues even against this. Before the elephant population completely sullies its domain, its birth rate declines in proportion to what remains.[1] So, it may be that *Homo sapiens* is a unique evolutionary experiment and the only species—or at least one of the few—that Nature produced which puts at risk its own survival by destroying the habitat on which it depends.

Global warming is a man-made tragedy. It is the worst conundrum the species put itself in during its 160,000-year history. In contrast to some far distant hundred years war found in time-honored history books, the menace is here, now, in our lifetimes, staring us in the collective eye. It is a living laboratory to test the hypothesis developed in this text.

But in science there is the hypothesis and the null hypothesis. There are really two ideas to evaluate. The null suggests that there is no effect, no psychic immune system, no mysterious, invisible, or inscrutable entity that exists to protect and preserve mankind from its follies. The psychic immune system simply does not exist and is just a mirage in this perspective.

The hypothesis, on the other hand, by now we are quite familiar with, the notion of a psychic immune system, similar to a collective self-preservative instinct. It has an innate and adaptive side—much of which is instinctual and operates autonomically to protect individuals, groups, nations, and the species from threat and harm. And its adaptive dimension also has an artificial side, which develops conscious and deliberate strategies to defuse danger, threat, and enhance survival. The global warming crisis represents a clear litmus test—and the Earth the laboratory—where this hypothesis could be tested.

We will separate out these two antithetical "voices" in the next section, the first will take the position of the null, that there is no psychic immune system and will explore how the global warming crisis evolves without it.

The second will postulate that there is indeed a flourishing psychic immune system and a force in human collective psychology which acts as a safety net that is protective, programmed to insure human survival, and which will resolve this crisis as it has all other darker manifestations of human frailty, barbarity, misadventure and malfeasance. There will be some notable differences in these points of view, but the intent of this exposition is to clarify for the reader what the psychic immune system might look like in this experimental situation.

THE VOICE OF THE NULL HYPOTHESIS: THE PSYCHIC IMMUNE SYSTEM AS A MIRAGE

From this stance, the news is not going to make anyone feel any better. Here there is no psychic immune system to bail humanity out of trouble, no unusual force or field inside the human topography flashing emergency rescue messages, and no safety net to catch humanity from its precipitous fall.

That means that global warming is going to march forward. There is no exceptional, unusual, mysterious or "invisible" system protecting humankind from its idiocy, from war and aggression, or from nuclear close calls and miscalculations. The psychic immune system is a fictional construction, a chimerical false hope . . . a pipe dream.

With respect to global warming, the human race will continue to soil its habitat and threaten its viability with escalating greenhouse gas emissions. Virtually no progress can be seen in controlling, stopping, or even slowing CO2. Emissions continue on a full upward course and without letup. From 1990 to 2010 humanity tacked on a 30 percent increase.[2]

Any objective review of the data shows there has been no retreat from human-induced global emissions. Most recently CO2 jumped 3 percent in 2011, another 2.6 percent in 2012,[3] and in 2015 it reached 401 ppm. That's the first time the planet achieved this level in two million years. In 2016 it hit 407 ppm.

The "psychic immune system" theory tried to explain how deaths under Stalin, An Lushan, or Pol Pot declined in a parallel fashion to how physical epidemics retreated, as so-called "resistance," or immune responses developed. These declining numbers were compared to physical epidemics like measles or polio.

The question then becomes, where is the expected decline in this data? Quite obviously global warming has a psychological basis—and certainly humanity's failure to do anything substantive about it, as well as the incredible level of denial over it, argues it has a prodigious psychological dimension. So where is the psychic immune system? Where is the anticipated negative slope in these curves? One can see no such "resistances" developing anywhere.

CO2 emissions continue escalating without even a hint of any intervening immune system. No topping has occurred on this curve, and absolutely no downward movement in emissions is even remotely on the horizon.

Where, we might ask, is that beloved bell-shaped curve? It isn't here. No remission. No decline back to baseline. No homeostasis. Absolutely nothing.

Certainly one can understand the desire to be optimistic, but if one faces reality and stops grabbing for straws, there is a very unhappy conclusion: Despite green revolution idealism, and the millions of world citizens changing conserving, and recycling, total CO2 emissions accelerate and just keep going higher.

The Global Carbon Project reports the growth of C0O2 has been increasing roughly 3 percent a year on average. . . . "At the moment, it's very hard to see any evidence that we're going to peak any time soon," says Dr. Glen Peters for the Center for International Climate and Environmental Research.[4]

In addition, we have seriously underestimated our production of methane which is twenty-one times more toxic than CO2.[5] The Proceedings of the National Academy of Sciences reported that methane effusions were 2.7 times greater than prior conventional estimates.[6] It is estimated 3.6 trillion cubic feet of methane escaped worldwide in just one year.[7] Those who champion fracking fail to understand that fugitive gases like methane are a serious byproduct. An even more recent study from MIT concluded there is "50 percent more methane in the atmosphere than previously estimated . . . a signal that more methane is leaking from the natural gas production chain than previously thought."[8] In effect, anyone pretending things are getting better is doing just that, pretending.[9]

The Kyoto accords were signed in 1997 with promises to reduce emissions, and instead they only went up, up, and up in the ensuing eighteen years. CO2 emissions today are 65 percent above the fanciful Kyoto promises to reduce down to 1990 levels.[10]

If Kyoto represents the so-called conscious and deliberate artificial psychic immune system at work, with a rational well-conceived treaty, then we must reluctantly observe it hasn't happened and is not happening. The conclusion one would be forced to draw clearly is that there is no artificial psychic immune system, and therefore, very likely no psychic immune system either.

Unfortunately, the Arctic meltdown just means "we are open for business." The Arctic holds 25 percent of the world's undiscovered oil and natural gas, and world powers, particularly Russia, seem intent on doing nothing else but try to exploit it.[11] [12]

Global warming initiatives like Kyoto were entirely ineffective; humanity is headed into a climatological storm, which will permanently damage its habitat, and no sweet, palliative, rescuing psychic immune system exists to prevent it. As M. F. Moonzajer says "by the time we are convinced of the climate change impacts; there would be nothing we could do to help."[13]

President Obama hoped to lower greenhouse gas emissions by 17 percent by 2020.[14] The first observation is that is not enough,[15] second, it is not likely he will succeed, and finally, he has no genuine plan to stop China's emissions. His milquetoast policies[16] are merely feckless attempts to kick the can down the road.[17]

The recent two-hundred-country Convention on Climate Change held in Paris in 2015 failed to make any discernible commitments. As Justin Gillis for the *New York Times* opined,

> In effect, the countries are vowing to make changes that collectively still fall far short of the necessary goal, much like a patient who, upon hearing from his doctor that he must lose 50 pounds to avoid life-threatening health risks, takes pride in cutting out fries but not cake and ice cream.[18]

Gillis is not the only critic. Jim Hansen, former NASA scientist and advisor to Al Gore said the Paris accords were "a fraud . . . really a fake . . . just worthless words." Eleven other climate scientists signed a declaration with him saying the accord has "deadly flaws."[19] So, in effect, there is no plan currently to concretely address the issues and most particularly China's emissions.

In order to stop global warming, Chinese coal burning must be cut back by a huge amount, and the only thing that could do that would be a worldwide boycott of its products. If, short of war, Americans decided that to stop Chinese coal burning was to forbid trade, there would be an immediate decline in Chinese emissions, by at least 7 percent and perhaps greater.[20]

Walmart would be forced to close its 8,500 stores, and the six heirs to the Walmart fortune—whose net worth is greater than the combined net worth of forty-two million American families—would be more than bitterly disappointed.[21] They would be livid.[22]

For some background on why this paralysis exists in the United States, consider the following. At the end of 2013, close to nine in ten

Americans disapproved of Congress.[23] At the same time, 90 percent of incumbents who sought to be reelected were.[24] How is it possible that nine in ten disapprove of Congress, and yet nine in ten incumbents get reelected by the very people who disapprove of them?

The answer is that skillful gerrymandering has quietly taken place for more than a decade. Polls show that more Americans identify with the Democratic Party than the Republican,[25] and yet Republicans have a majority in Congress, very much the result of insidious realignments and redefinitions of districts, a process which was supported, funded, and applauded by special interests. As one opinion piece put it: "GOP Gerrymandering is a clear and present danger to America. It is destroying the fabric of the American society. . . . The party that has gerrymandered majority representation out of a minority has used race, class, and economic deception to achieve its goals."[26]

The usurpation of the American political system by wealth, where the voice of the people becomes less and less relevant, is what is behind the huge number of Americans who disapprove of Congress. They feel disenfranchised, because they actually are.

America has quietly become a corporate state and a plutocracy. This is not an original observation. The super-rich, 1 percent occupy most of the seats in the Senate, made a cat's paw out of Congress, have a majority on the Supreme Court, at least up until Justice Scalia's death, and they have captured most of the governorships.[27] With respect to the upcoming 2016 presidential campaign, four hundred of the nation's richest families "have supplied almost half of the money raised so far by presidential candidates of both parties."[28] The level of wealth concentration and the growth of the plutocracy is beyond egregious. Today one hundred of the richest families in the United States have more wealth than the entire black population of the United States.[29] The twenty richest people in the United States possess more wealth than half the population of the country.[30]

Not only is this venal concentration of wealth completely unrepresentative of the American people, it has huge relevance to the issue of global warming. The American political system is so infected with special interests that the Walmart heirs and their cohorts—who profit from trading with gross polluters like China—will not quietly sit by as their winnings disappear. The practice of hiring Chinese labor at $3.50 per hour and importing those products into the United States duty-free will not be halted, impeded, or inhibited by any green initiatives.[31]

Take as an example another 1-percenter, Mitch McConnell, the Republican majority leader who is a steadfast supporter of coal companies like Peabody Energy. He has been pugnacious in undercutting, if not eviscerating, any climate change legislation calling it "Mr. Obama's war on coal."[32] Obama's initiative to implement new climate change regulations were defeated fifty-two to forty-six in the senate, all heavily orchestrated by Senator McConnell.[33] But note that McConnell's personal net worth rose from $9 million to $22.8 million during his tenure in office, and he now ranks as the tenth richest senator in the United States.[34] McConnell is not alone. Of 278 Republicans in Congress only eight have made comments accepting the reality of global warming.[35] That is only 3 percent.

The Supreme Court is complicit as well, recently blocking Obama's effort to reduce carbon emissions from coal-fired power plants with a five to four decision in February, 2016.[36]

To be realistic, the fandango will march forward, and the propaganda that global warming is a hoax will continue to spew from the mouths of Republicans, and from media outlets like Fox News. Glenn Beck earns $90 million per year; Rush Limbaugh $66 million;[37] Bill O'Reilly $16 million.[38] There's a fortune to be made as a global warming denier.

Recently, one scientist who is routinely cited by anti-global warming activists as their favorite intellectual apologist was outed by the *New York Times* for having published eleven peer-reviewed articles while accepting over $1 million from fossil-fuel interests and the Koch brothers.[39] (The Koch brothers, have spent $67 million funding climate denying front groups.)[40]

The *Times* also reported that Exxon knew about the dangers of climate change as far back as the 1970s but concealed its research while strongly advocating that the United States not sign the Kyoto Protocol in the 1990s.[41]

The U.S. government is so paralyzed by this process, the chances that a global carbon tax, or any restriction on trade with gross polluters will pass is exiguous, regardless of how much people believe something like that should happen.

In sum, the United States, China, and the EU will continue playing Nero's fiddle for the foreseeable future, promising much and delivering little. In 2014, China accounted for 29 percent of all the world's CO2 emissions.[42] Last year China burned 3.6 billion tons on coal, and by 2020 it plans on burning 4.2 billion tons—a 15 percent increase in the next six years.[43]

In 2015 China approved 155 new coal-fired power plants which will have a capacity equal to 40 percent of all the coal power plants in the United States. And these are just the new ones it is planning.

Finally, a recent 2015 study shows that estimates of Chinese coal burning have been incorrect. They are burning 17 percent more coal a year than the government previously disclosed: "Even for a country of China's size, the scale of the correction is immense. The sharp upward revision in official figures means that China has released much more carbon dioxide, almost a billion more tons a year . . . than previously estimated."[44] In short, there will be no political resolve appearing any time soon with any teeth.

Daniel Gilbert, professor of psychology at Harvard, talks about our inability to do anything to deal with the crisis as the "dragons of inaction." Indeed, that is precisely how the United States and humanity at large are dealing with this unfolding disaster.[45]

Regrettably a realist can only agree with the recent British Petroleum study which predicts that a 29 percent increase in global emissions will greet humanity in the next fifteen years, and this bad news will not be mitigated by any "mysterious" and "invisible" forces outlined in this text. For those who have more optimistic sentiments, a realist can only offer condolences.

Arctic sea ice in the summer reached its lowest level in 150 millennia, and that was on a Sunday in 2012.[46] And it is important to remember that the "Arctic Methane Apocalypse" is also arriving. The melting of the tundra and the possibility of releasing methane is more than just an hypothesis. A number of suspicious holes appeared in Siberia in 2014, more in 2015, with huge concentrations of methane measured. It appears methane exploded upward to form these strange craters. The release of methane as a result of global warming is already happening.[47]

More immediately, "If you poke your head outside of the U.S., coal-fired plants are being built left and right."[48] China and India were building four such plants between them *every week* in 2014. Global demand for coal is expected to grow a billion tons in a couple of years.[49]

If humanity is to stay below a two degree Celsius increase in global temperature—read disaster if it doesn't—it cannot add more than thirty-two to thirty-three gigatons of CO2 by 2030. But China alone is expected to exceed fifteen gigatons by that time all by itself, while planning to build 363 new coal-fired power plants to accomplish that pornographic colossus.[50]

India also plans to double its coal burning by 2019 and its "coal rush could push the world past the brink of irreversible climate change."[51] In late 2015 it announced that it is expected to triple its current carbon emissions by 30 percent.[52]

So from the perspective of a realist, there is no applause for conservation. No medals to distribute. No rescue. No accolades given for the Kyoto Accord kabuki dance. No discernible progress globally. And, no psychic immune system which will save humanity either.

Beyond the psychic immune system "dream world," there are a few scenarios which might indeed reduce greenhouse gas emissions. None are very pleasant, and all entirely catastrophic. Here are three:

1. World War: Whenever burgeoning population is confronted with dwindling resources, war is the likely result. Wars tend to get out of hand. They start locally, like a Serbian peasant shooting an Austrian duke, but become global quickly. In the nuclear age, not only is humanity overdue for a serious incident, but population in-

creases and resource depletion are the fuses which ignite the explosion. A loss of half a billion people in a major world war would likely have a mitigating effect on CO2. That is one catastrophic scenario to consider.

2. Worldwide Depression: Robert Prechter, a financial pundit, predicts a worldwide depression in 2016.[53] Fourteen others make similar calls.[54] Since George Bush's Great Recession, the major governments of the world have been trying to print their way out of it and artificially prop up the world economy. There is no greater culprit than the United States which prefers to call its money printing "quantitative easing." The Federal Reserve is fundamentally unregulated. "It can print and lend any amount of money for any length of time to any person or entity."[55]

   No one precisely knows how much money has been printed, perhaps close to $4.6 trillion, and any efforts to audit the Fed have resulted in failure.[56] [57] In fact, what the Fed may be hiding is just how much it has committed to prop up foreign central banks. Rumors swirl the amount may exceed $16 trillion, more than "four times the budget of the United States."[58] History teaches that a debased currency, runaway credit, and money printing is a precursor to depression.[59] It was exactly that way in the roaring twenties leading up to the Great Depression, and it could prove to be true again.

   If one looks at a long term graph of CO2 emissions, a small uncharacteristic drop appears beginning in 2008.[60] That was the first global drop in CO2 in decades. It wasn't caused by the green revolution, by conservation, or by any psychic immune system.

   It was caused by the global recession, a sharp decrease in industrial production, and a drop in Chinese coal burning due to shrinking exports during this period.[61] A worldwide depression would accomplish the same only to a larger degree. So, if there is going to be a significant decline in greenhouse gases, it might result from this second kind of catastrophic event.

3. Epidemics: A third possible tragedy which might mitigate global warming is disease. Unsafe industrial grade agricultural practices, both in the United States and China, are very likely to produce a pandemic like Swine flu, SARS, MERS, the latest superbug, CRE,[62] the spread of MCR-1 a gene variant that appears resistant to all antibiotics,[63] or any other variety of viral attack which could function like the Black Death of the thirteenth century, culling the human population by a significant degree. The latest mortality rate for bird flu ranges from 30 to 70 percent of those infected.[64] [65] MERS (Middle East Respiratory Syndrome) has a mortality rate of about 45 percent.[66] Any such outbreak could spread, but this time with enhanced mobility through airline travel. The pandemic

could cross the globe rapidly, and we could see a severe reduction in the human population and a corresponding drop in CO_2 as a consequence.

So, absent horrific events like a depression, pandemic, or world war, global warming is not going away. It will march forward unabated.

- The arctic summer ice cap will disappear as predicted.[67]
- Increasingly severe droughts, hurricanes, tornadoes, and forest fires will happen as predicted.
- 25 percent of species will drop off this planet into extinction by 2050 as predicted.
- Agricultural implosions that depend on mountain runoffs from vanishing glaciers in India will occur as predicted.
- The Caribbean ecosystem will be eviscerated, and agricultural production in South America will be half of what it is today as predicted.
- The spread of warming induced diseases will occur as predicted.
- The 40 percent water shortfall will occur as predicted.
- The death of millions of people due to global warming will occur as predicted.
- The estimate of a billion climate refugees who have lost their homes and habitat by 2050 will happen as predicted.[68]

And from a new text by Naomi Oreskes, a historian from Harvard, comes a prediction that floods, droughts, and mass migrations will result in the end of humanity in Africa and Australia. [69]

In summary, there is no quixotic psychic immune system operating anywhere on the horizon. This is certainly a voice of a Cassandra, but it is also the voice of realism. The news is as bad as it gets, and probably worse.

THE VOICE OF HYPOTHESIS: THE PSYCHIC IMMUNE SYSTEM AS APPARITION

If the psychic immune system theory is true, however, we encounter a different scenario entirely. Our second attempt to parse this data operates on the idea that the psychic immune system is not an invisible hobgoblin, not a "pipe dream," and not a mirage, but something very much to look forward to with respect to global warming.

The only things that the former and allegedly "realistic" point of view share, unfortunately, are that the global warming threat may be the most formidable crisis ever encountered by our species, and that the threat is entirely man-made.

With that said, how one views the success in dealing with it is quite another matter. If the theory of the psychic immune system holds, then there may be stirrings already happening in the human psychological landscape.

Although the psychic immune system is currently as elusive and inscrutable as dark matter, it is likely scurrying about boosting consciousness here, there, and everywhere so that mankind, once again, might find a way out of the mess it created for itself. Let us tease out the systems' attributes in order to get an idea of what we might anticipate.

Territoriality

There are two opposing tendencies within the psychic immune system which account for the bell-shaped curves earlier discussed. Both of these forces are connected to human viability and survival. The first is aggression, dominance, and territoriality, which is then followed by a downdraft on that fight-flight curve in which cooperation, nonviolence, and for lack of a better term, altruistic reciprocity comes to prominence to return the system to homeostasis.

With respect to global warming, territorial conflicts are expected. With shrinking resources and increasing population, conflicts erupt more frequently. If over three-quarters of human wars in the last 150 years have been territorial, then a skein of ancient evolutionary battles over food, water, and raw materials is clearly to be anticipated.

The battle between proprietors and intruders—have and have nots—will happen with greater frequency counterpointed, of course, with myriad *us versus them* propaganda blitzkriegs. Territorial wars of this sort, however, will not have any appreciable impact on CO2 levels.

This expectation should not be confused with the suggestion that world war is one of the three catastrophic scenarios that might bring CO2 levels down. A conventional world war, similar to World War II, would "cull" the human population by only a few percent—2.5 percent in the case of World War II.

On the other hand, if a thermonuclear war is what is imagined, it would probably usher in a nuclear winter, and that scenario in no way could be considered a positive outcome. It is estimated that a nuclear winter could kill as much as the human race.[70]

The theory of the psychic immune system implies that wars and internecine environmental skirmishes are likely. Territoriality-ecological wars to some extent have already arrived. Recall that Yemen is ripe for environmental disaster and particularly the disappearance of its water table in its capital, Sanaa. Coincidentally, there is a great deal of warlike behavior bubbling to the surface in Yemen in 2016. There are raging battles between various groups, Al-Qaeda, the Houti rebels, and only the president and his entire cabinet resigned. The president fled to Saudi Arabia only to return with new armaments and troops.[71] [72]

Media war reporting does not currently spotlight the environmental underpinnings to these conflicts. One exception, though, is Thomas Friedman. In a *New York Times* op-ed, he eloquently described how conflicts in the Middle East have very significant climate change determinants:

> The past few years have seen a number of significant social, economic, environmental and climatic changes . . . up to 60 percent of Syria's land experienced one of the worst droughts and most severe set of crop failures in its history . . . "nearly 75 percent . . . suffered total crop failure." The United Nations reported that more than 800,000 Syrians had their livelihoods wiped out by these droughts, and many were forced to move to the cities to find work. .
>
> If climate projections stay on their current path, the drought situation in North Africa and the Middle East is going to get progressively worse, and you will end up witnessing cycle after cycle of instability that may be the impetus for future authoritarian responses. . . . A key point is that it's now increasingly clear that the climate models that had been predicting the countries surrounding the Mediterranean would start to dry out were correct. . . . *The Beirut Daily Star* in February, pointed out that twelve of the world's fifteen most water-scarce countries—Algeria, Libya, Tunisia, Jordan, Qatar, Saudi Arabia, Yemen, Oman, the United Arab Emirates, Kuwait, Bahrain, Israel and Palestine—are in the Middle East, and after three decades of explosive population growth these countries are "set to dramatically worsen their predicament.[73]

In Syria today, 250,000 people have died due to the civil war,[74] and four million sought refuge in Jordan, Turkey, and now Europe.[75] [76] Underneath these conflicts lurks the haunting shadow of climate change.

While we expect environmental and territorial skirmishes to increase, we have not offered any reprieve or rescue from the psychic immune system, so far, so let us now turn our attention to that.

The Hero Archetype and the Artificial Psychic Immune System

Sometimes, especially in a crisis for survival, the innate psychic immune system activates the hero archetype. If you recall the altruistic hero-archetype is considered part of the ancestral inheritance of every human being. It is the human analogue to the biological altruism seen from honeybees to flycatchers.

To Jung, it rises out of the depths of the collective unconscious, and this "imprint" becomes manifest in certain individuals who then perform quite extraordinary feats which rescue or save individuals, groups, nations, or even humanity from danger.

In the case of nuclear confrontations and mistakes, the role of Vasili Arkhipov and Stanislav Petrov certainly are instructive: two unsung heroes who prevented all out nuclear war and probably a nuclear winter.

Albert Einstein and Robert Oppenheimer played a role in the United States getting a nuclear capability before Hitler did. How fortuitous these intrepid heroes were not employed by the SS!

If one follows these implications with respect to climate change, we should see a sprinkling of Nobel Prize winners appearing who help, at least partially, to invent us out of this dilemma with radically newer technologies that haven't even been divined.

One incipient hero is K. R. Sridhar, president of Bloom Energy. His firm invented a fuel cell that promises cheap, clean, and abundant energy.[77] Such innovations should be expected to radically change the planet's environmental profile as surely as the atomic bomb changed the profile of World War II.

One prediction from the theory of the psychic immune system, then, is that humankind might be seeing a few Henry Fords, Thomas Edisons, Igor Sikorskys, and Eli Whitneys coming into view to provide humanity with important transformative technologies.

When speaking of technological advances, we are talking about the artificial psychic immune system and its congregation of conscious, rational, and deliberative strategies to defuse threat. The efforts of the artificial psychic immune system should increase exponentially with global warming.

There has already been some success. The development of the LED electric light which uses one-fifth the energy of the original light bulb has done "more to meet growth in America's energy needs than the combined contributions of oil, coal, natural gas and nuclear power."[78]

There is also a likelihood of a breakthrough in fusion research as well so that the planet might retreat from burning fossil fuels entirely. A significant advance in fusion would put an end to the fossil fuel age which got humanity into this predicament in the first place.

An experimental reactor called the ITER project is currently under development in France.

> The ITER project aims to make the long-awaited transition from experimental studies of plasma physics to full-scale electricity-producing fusion power plants. The ITER fusion reactor itself has been designed to produce 500 megawatts of output power from 50 megawatts of input power, or ten times the amount of energy put in. The machine is expected to demonstrate the principle of producing more energy from the fusion process than is used to initiate it, something that has not yet been achieved with previous fusion reactors.[79]

There are other fusion developments too. Lockheed-Martin made a surprise announcement in 2015:

> Lockheed Martin Corp said on Wednesday it had made a technological breakthrough in developing a power source based on nuclear fusion, and the first reactors, small enough to fit on the back of a truck, could be ready for use in a decade. . . . Tom McGuire, who heads the project, said he and a small team had been working on fusion energy at Lockheed's secretive Skunk Works for about four years, but were now going public to find potential partners in industry and government for their work. Initial work demonstrated the feasibility of building a 100-megawatt reactor measuring seven feet by 10 feet, which could fit on the back of a large truck, and is about 10 times smaller than current reactors.[80]

Two other private firms, General Atomics and Tri Alpha Energy are reporting advances in fusion,[81] along with heavy hydrogen breakthroughs at the University of Gothenburg.[82]

With the mobilization of the artificial psychic immune system, major advances can be expected in geothermal,[83] solar power, perovskite, wave transmitting solar satellites,[84] geoengineering, stellerator fusion systems,[85] solar radiation management,[86] algae and wood waste, battery storage technology, microsupercapacitors,[87] flow battery and lithium air battery technology,[88] [89] tidal lagoons,[90] hydrogen fuel cells, molten salt storage,[91] hydrogen electrocatalysis,[92] [93] methane cracking,[94] bacterial engineering, minirotor turbines,[95] nonphotonic crystals,[96] cultured and in vitro meat agriculture,[97] vertical farming,[98] artificial photosynthesis,[99] pervaporation desalination,[100] and myriad other clean energy alternatives.[101] All of these will progressively impact global warming.[102]

These are predictions for the future, however. Today the United States spends only 1/400th as much on global warming research as it spends on defense, but this situation will appreciably change.[103]

The intervention of the psychic immune system will take yet another form beyond activation of hero archetypes and miraculous inventions from the wellspring of the artificial psychic immune system.

Cooperation, Reciprocity, and Mass Psychology

Another "instinctive" aspect of the psychic immune system is cooperation. From the thumping of the prairie dog, to the screech of the chimpanzee lookout, the animal kingdom is brimming with social networks whose function is to protect the group and the species, through cooperative, affiliative behavior.

To parse out implications of how this will impact global warming, we would expect a huge ground swell of collective consciousness far beyond anything we have seen to date. A mobilization of consciousness means galvanized, unified, and integrated mass movements focused on protecting the human race from peril.

This could take the form, initially, of rebellion and militancy. The massive Japanese protests against the Fukushima nuclear accident may be symptomatic—and simultaneously a harbinger of things yet to unfold. To recall Victor Hugo: "Nothing is stronger than an idea whose time has come." Militancy and rebellion spanning the globe, and far more contagious than the Arab Spring, could easily swell into a planetary insurgency.

If the Arab Spring erupted across Tunisia, Libya, Egypt, Qatar, Jordan, The Emirates, and Syria in only months, occasioned, primarily, by the increase in the price of bread,[104] mass demonstrations focused on the global warming crisis could metastasize just as quickly.

Demands by all peoples across the globe form themselves into myriad mass movements, and these protests result in drastic changes in collective, political behavior. Hard-fisted, steely economic demands are spawned demanding, for example, that every country boycott major polluters, or cease trade with countries which continue to use coal-fired power plants.

Angry rebellions materialize from all quarters of the planet. Mass movements are like magma swirling under the crust of consciousness until they erupt into an inferno. Any eruption of mass psychology today is only in its infancy, but we have already seen incipient demonstrations against climate change in New York and London in 2014, however timid they may have been. In 2015, Norwegian pension funds divested themselves of all of their coal holdings.[105] Already over four hundred institutions have similarly removed fossil fuel holdings from their portfolios.[106] These are early symptoms of such mass movements that can be expected.

America's Experience with Mass Psychology

Recall that the United States was not attacked on its own soil by Hitler. As the war was taking hold in Europe, Charles Lindbergh urged America to stay out. There was a huge isolationist mood in the United States in 1941 which was organized into a political movement called "America First." Joseph Kennedy, ambassador to England, cautioned against America entering the war as well.

But that is not how history unraveled. Something else kicked in. America responded with incredible, unmistakable, and unpredicted mettle marshaling its entire economy toward the defeat of the menace which was threatening Europe and the Pacific.

The "innate releasing" stimulus was the attack on Pearl Harbor. From that moment forward, Americans changed. Draft boards did not have to find recruits. They were overwhelmed with volunteers.

Americans might have chosen a different path, following Lindbergh's advice, and meandered across their verdant hills in comfortable isolationism until the Nazis finally got around to attacking Miami. But other forces gathered under the mantle of American consciousness—which

Pearl Harbor aroused, activated, and marshaled—so that America rather instantly changed. Even Charles Lindbergh changed and tried to enlist.[107]

This was a collective event infecting the vast majority of the citizenry. Perhaps this is why Jung called war a psychic "epidemic." There was palpable contagion.

When survival is threatened, the physical immune system is activated and mobilized, but so is the psychic immune system. The cortisol-adrenaline rush courses through the entire population. There is every reason to believe such a process will occur during the unfolding global warming crisis. But it is not here yet.

Global warming's Pearl Harbor has not arrived, and the innate releasing event has not come to pass. When it does, the psychic immune system will be aroused in a way few have considered.

What we can see today, however, is that consciousness is growing. The voice of the "null" cited the high level of denial, particularly among the elite, the top 1-percenters in the United States, and in the corporate media, but a recent September, 2014, poll shows that more than half of Americans now say global warming is caused by human behavior. Admittedly that is meager, but it is still "the highest level ever recorded by a national poll."[108]

In 2015, a Stanford University poll showed 48 percent were "likely to vote for a candidate who supports fighting climate change."[109] A second 2015 study shows that close to two-thirds of Americans, 63 percent, would support limiting carbon emissions from power plants.[110] Clearly America is a long way off from any Pearl Harbor shock-and-awe stimulus which releases public opinion from its shackles of doubt and resistance, but there is at least some incipient momentum. Indeed, the recent 2015 Paris Climate Accord, at least according to Thomas Friedman of the *New York Times*, is a "big, big, deal."[111]

Ronald Reagan's Fantasy

When Ronald Reagan met with the USSR's Mikhail Gorbachev in 1985 to negotiate peace, he made an unusual remark that impressed his Russian counterpart:

> How easy his task and mine might be in these meetings that we held if suddenly there was a threat to this world from some other species from another planet outside in the universe. We'd forget all the little local differences that we have between our countries. . . . an "alien threat [to the Earth] from outside this world" coming from "another planet," which would eventually help all people recognize the common bond which "unites all the members of humanity."[112]

Reagan was anticipating the kind of collective reciprocity and cooperative resolve which would occur if there was a threat to our species. Global warming is exactly that, and, moreover, there is every reason to expect that, at some point, a psychic threshold will be crossed where precisely this cooperative, nonviolent, altruistic reciprocity will rise out of the psychic immune system.

Earlier, we discussed evidence that empathy and compassion had an innate component seen in infants as early as seventy-two hours after birth. Lest we forget, empathic, compassionate, and cooperative behaviors are just as hard-wired as territoriality and aggression, and no less essential for group survival.

Reagan's fantasy of a galvanizing moment—or covenant—which calls out the "common bond between all members of humanity," is not just a wished-for outcome. There is strong empirical reason to believe such a watershed of cooperative and mutually beneficent behavior will be "released" when the crisis facing humanity crosses this threshold. Even Pope Francis alluded to it in 2015.[113]

To picture this process more directly, we can imagine unusual and sudden changes in our lives. A new political resolve happens rapidly. It is not confined to the United States but becomes global in scope. Geopolitical militancy grips humanity. The conventional world is turned upside down. People are willing to sacrifice and give of themselves to meet the threat to themselves, their children, and their future in the same way that Russians and Americans and countless others were prepared for sacrifice at the dawn of World War II.

Here are some examples of what such an eruption might look like in specific terms and policies impacting not only Americans, but all citizens of the world.

- Rationing of Red Meat: 14 percent of the world's greenhouse gases come from cows and the methane they produce.[114] No one in the U.S. Congress has ever proposed rationing red meat, the cessation of export of red meat, or the culling of America's cattle herd, much less the global cattle herd, but revolutionary and militant actions come center stage to initiate extreme emergency measures. Suddenly, red meat is in short supply worldwide, and so are cows. Just as Americans in World War II had no difficulty accepting rationing, so too will they accept such draconian measures willingly and even enthusiastically.
- Rationing of Electricity: 33 percent of greenhouse gas emissions come from electricity generation.[115] Today, no one in Washington, DC, or other world capitals is making any proposal to ration electricity, but in World War II there was an expression "There's a war on you know," and sugar, butter, gasoline, meat, and other commodities were rationed.[116] The same mental attitude can be ex-

pected, and electricity rationing will not only be proposed, but even welcomed. "There's a war on you know."

- Carbon Taxes and Trade Prohibitions: Stiff implementation of global carbon taxes, inclusive of the United States, Europe, and China are put into effect by world parliaments.[117] [118] These burdensome carrying charges bring coal burning down to levels not seen in decades. There is currently no public consensus on carbon taxes today, but after the psychic immune system is aroused, measures like carbon taxes will become quickly engraved in law. Legislation will cross the desks of dozens of governments and international trade organizations prohibiting dealings with gross polluters like China or the United States—unless and until they convert coal-fired plants to cleaner fuels.[119] This may be met with resistance or even war, but China has a $3 trillion hard currency surplus which stands ready to rescue its export markets through immediate coal plant conversions and pollution abatement.[120]

  By the way, some progress has already appeared on this front.[121] By converting coal plants to natural gas, the United States in 2015 reduced the CO2 from its power plants to a twenty-seven-year low.[122]

  > For the first time ever, natural gas trumped coal as the top source of electric power generation in the U.S. In April, roughly 31 percent of electric power generation came from natural gas, whereas coal accounted for 30 percent, according to a recent SNL Energy report. It's a dramatic difference from April 2010, when coal accounted for 44 percent of the mix and natural gas just 22 percent.[123]

  In 2016, U.S. coal production actually reached its lowest level in thirty years.[124] And in another pleasant surprise, Britain announced it will shutter all of its coal-fired plants by 2015.[125]
- Wind Farming: Massive development of wind farms supported cooperatively by dozens of countries begins on a scale never before seen—similar to efforts made by the United Kingdom presently.
- Solar Farms: Environmentalist, Lester Brown, suggested that if an area of one hundred square miles of the Nevada desert witnessed the construction of the largest solar farm ever built, a project which would cost well over a trillion dollars, the amount of electricity generated could be enough to power the entire United States on a sunny day. Elon Musk has similarly forwarded an idea for a massive solar farm in Texas he calls "the blue square."[126] A similar hypothetical plan was proposed for Europe called Desertec,[127] arguing that solar farms in the Sahara could supply the entire European Union, even the world, with ample electricity.[128]

Other rational speculations by Mark Jacobson, an engineer at Stanford and the Deep Decarbonization Pathways Project estimate that 156,000 wind turbines could be built by 2050 and that the world itself could operate on 100 percent renewable power by that time. The cost of erecting a wind turbine is similar to the cost of the oil and gas industry drilling new wells.[129]

Suddenly, such "fantasies," which today have virtually no popular support, leave drawing boards to reappear as genuine engineering projects toward which the world community is moving—and, by the way, almost as rapidly as General Motors converted its factories from building cars to bombers in World War II.

- Nuclear Options: The construction of nuclear power plants and the temporary deployment of mini-nuclear power plants known as small modular reactors[130] to generate electricity gain considerable momentum. Despite the fact that nuclear power has inherent dangers, the use of this technology in the emergency atmosphere of global warming becomes necessary. In 2015 wind and solar power only accounted for 2 percent of the world's energy. New voices appear advocating modern, safer, and advanced nuclear plants to replace fossil fuels.[131] Intriguing designs, like sodium based, molten salt, or liquid metal reactors enter the discussion.[132] [133] Even the esteemed Intergovernmental Panel on Climate Change issued a call for four hundred more reactors "as part of an overall effort to bring more carbon-free energy sources online faster."[134] And noted environmentalists like James Hanson and Stewart Brand have even endorsed these proposals.[135]
- Conservation: Mandated cutbacks in emissions of black carbon, soot, methane, and hydroflurocarbons[136] globally are introduced, enforced, and supported by aroused mass psychology.

Such changes, unheard of currently—and many seemingly politically incorrect in the present era—would produce a rapid, solid, and far-reaching turnaround in human affairs.

New technologies, plus the currently missing political resolve, will attenuate this catastrophe-in-waiting, and the firing up of the psychic immune system will carry forward with this mission aggressively. Once aroused, it will move forward as rapidly as the Manhattan Project did in World War II.[137] [138]

Whatever course, or multiple courses, the psychic immune system adopts, it is worth remembering from prior chapters that the length of time of *Homo sapiens'* most barbarous and dark episodes (world war, genocides, tyrannies) was about thirty-seven years. That is how long it took, on average, to bring human-induced savageries and ruthlessness to an end as the psychic immune system, both in its conscious and unconscious dimensions, rallied its resources to attack these psychic epidemics over the course of the last two thousand years.

If we date the actual "catastrophic" onset of the coming global warming crisis to be 2020—the most reasonable date when summer arctic ice will be completely gone—then thirty-seven years from that moment, the psychic immune system might have already completed its work, and the problem of global warming *solved.* That's right, *solved!*

In other words, if the most massive impacts of global warming begin in 2020, the psychic immune system, if it exists at all, should take roughly thirty-seven years—until 2057—to work its magic, activate its archetypes, enlist its mercurial antibodies, and ignite mass psychology, revolutions, climate insurgencies, boycotts—and inventions—to snuff out this existential threat.

If we wished to propose a more conservative estimate, and added one standard deviation to this calculation, the crisis should be defused by the end of this century.

There is a long litany of crises humanity has faced and survived, miraculously, and, if the psychic immune system played a role then, we should not expect it to let us down this time either. The global warming threat is a perfect *in situ* experimental test of the theory.

We do not know exactly how it works, except that it has both innate and adaptive constituents. It will manifest in its conscious (artificial) dimension in the form of technological breakthroughs and the implementation of global policies and prohibitions. But we should also see it appear in its autonomic and more unconscious incarnations as a cooperative magnet of mass psychology, grassroots contagion, and unexpected collective consensus and solidarity.

The null hypothesis vision critiqued the psychic immune system theory, because there was no bell-shaped curve. There was no peak, or any predicted diminution in the curve of greenhouse gas emissions down to baseline. It only remarked that CO2 levels were increasing and increasing and it legitimately asked where the crest and inflection point of this supposed bell-shaped curve is? But that point of view misses the point.

The epidemic is still in its infancy. The disease is gathering momentum. It is ascending. It will ultimately crest, like a severe fever, and fall into remission as predicted. Let us not forget that the woof and warp of the psychic immune system is that it is a positive, healing, and rescuing force, and, so the prognosis is thoroughly optimistic.

But it is still an invisible system. We cannot see the guts of how it operates. Few psychologists are working in this area. Epigenetic research is so new little can be said which is not speculative. It is as mysterious and hidden to contemporary academic psychology as dark matter is to physics today.

But physics can observe the effects of dark matter. Galaxies don't fly apart when they should—unless there is more gravitation, more matter, and thus, more dark matter holding them together. Even though they have never seen it, they have good reason to suppose dark matter exists.

Psychology too may not be able to see its own dark matter either, and we may not be able to observe how the psychic immune system actually operates, but we can see its effects.

We observed them with the disappearance of the gulags, the cessation of the An Lushan rebellion, the end of the racist slaughter in King Leopold's Congo, the termination of the Ottoman slaughter of Armenians and Greeks at the hands of the three pashas, the winding down of the atrocities of Maoism, the end of the barbarities of Timur and Genghis Khan, the closing of Pol Pot's killing fields, and the record of twenty-near nuclear miscalculations which could have unleashed a nuclear winter, but didn't.

And we saw its effects in bringing to a close the darkest moment in human history, the scourge of Nazism and the premeditated murder of over six million human beings, an atrocity never before committed by our species.

Although we have never seen the psychic immune system, its effects will be observable and felt in due course in the venue of global warming if for no other reason than this is the greatest threat humanity has faced, and the greatest plague it ever incubated.

The species has had fevers before. According to the Bulletin of Atomic Scientists, it has been in critical condition at least four times in the last seventy years. Each time, the fever declined. Each time the patient survived. Each time the human race sighed with relief, and the crisis passed.

There is no reason to believe the psychic immune system will not wage a furious battle across the entire landscape of human consciousness—and unconsciousness—to achieve the same outcome and preserve and protect the denizens of this planet.

In the presentation of this view of the psychic immune system, there is one anecdotal piece of evidence that we might consider too as an addendum to this presentation: In 2013, during the Boston Marathon, terrorists set off a bomb which killed three people and injured and maimed 145 others. Comedian Patton Oswalt wrote a poignant reaction to the tragedy. Curiously, it also is a very personal statement about the theory of the psychic immune system. Here is Patton Oswalt's compelling commentary about the Boston bombings:

> Boston. Fucking horrible! I remember when 9/11 went down, my reaction was, "Well, I've had it with humanity." But I was wrong. I don't know what's going to be revealed to be behind all of this mayhem. One human insect or a poisonous mass of broken sociopaths.
>
> But here's what I DO know. If it's one person or a HUNDRED people, that number is not even a fraction of a fraction of a fraction of a percent of the population on this planet. You watch the videos of the carnage and there are people running TOWARDS the destruction to

> help out. This is a giant planet and we're lucky to live on it, but there are prices and penalties incurred for the daily miracle of existence. One of them is, every once in awhile, the wiring of a tiny sliver of the species gets snarled and they're pointed toward darkness. But the vast majority stands against that darkness and, like white blood cells attacking a virus, they dilute and weaken and eventually wash away the evildoers and, more importantly the damage they wreak. This is beyond religion or creed or nation. We would not be here if humanity were inherently evil. We'd have eaten ourselves alive long ago. So when you spot violence, or bigotry, or intolerance or fear or just garden-variety misogyny, hatred or ignorance, just look it in the eye and think, "The good outnumber you, and we always will."[139]

We might offer Mr. Oswalt our thanks for his humanity and perspective which artfully expresses the very essence of the theory of the psychic immune system. There is a fundamental and ubiquitous positive force operating in the ether of the human condition, and Patton Oswalt exquisitely described it.

CONCLUSION

Ban Ki-moon, secretary general of the United Nations has warned, "Science has spoken. There is no ambiguity in their message. Leaders must act. Time is not on our side."[140] Global warming presents an interesting opportunity. It may take a while before all the data is in, but it is arguably the greatest crisis the human race ever created for itself, and we can only hope something inside us exists which will come to our rescue.

This is not hyperbole. A study published in 2010 estimated that the number of deaths related to global warming exceeds five million people per year.[141] In China 350,000 to 500,000 die prematurely as a result of the toxicity in the air and water.[142] A study by the Institute of Physics puts the number of deaths from air pollution alone at two million annually.[143]

What will life be like in 2030? Oxfam predicts that by that date one hundred million deaths are to be expected if drastic measures are not taken—that is only fourteen years from now.[144] Another study commissioned by twenty countries called the Climate Vulnerable Forum, estimated one hundred million deaths by 2030 as well.[145] On top of that the World Bank recently argued that over one hundred million poor will be newly admitted to the ranks of "extreme poverty" by 2030 due to climate change.[146]

If these estimates are even reasonably close, this would be the *largest* human-induced catastrophe in the 160,000-year history of our species. Until now, World War II held that record with sixty million deaths. The coming cataclysm is nearing *twice* the magnitude of World War II.

It is hard to imagine that after poring over history books and the ancient hordes that ravaged civilization from Genghis Khan, to Atilla, to

Pol Pot, to African genocides, the gravest catastrophe awaits us, now, in this lifetime, in this era. That is a very sobering thought.

The *Bulletin of Atomic Scientists* in January 2015, moved the Doomsday Clock up saying, "the threat of climate change and nuclear war posed a very serious threat to modern society. Their symbolic clock is now set at three minutes to midnight, but while they say it is not too late to avert disaster 'the window for action is closing rapidly.'" [147]

If someone announced that the Great Depression is coming, for sure, or another World War was definitely in the pipeline—without a doubt—in the next fourteen years, what would we do? Would we try to buy insurance? Would we move? Would we protect our children in some way? Would we buy gold, or stash more money in our mattresses?

Whatever the reaction, the catastrophe awaiting is predicted to be close to *twice as severe* as anything humanity has endured up to this time, twice as horrific, twice as painful. To author Ross Gelbspan, "Absent the rapid mobilization of climate advocates at every level—and the pooling of all their energy, creativity, and resources into a coordinated, no-holds-barred campaign—we will soon be crossing the threshold into climate hell." [148]

We listened carefully to the voice of the null hypothesis that called the psychic immune system a mirage and an invisible hobgoblin. Its conclusions were disquieting to the extreme. The only way the global warming crisis would be mitigated was through plague, world war, or global depression. It presented no bromide, no rescue, and the news from that perspective was as bad as could be imagined.

The second voice, however, lifted our spirits considerably and actually proposed a date when all the resources, conscious and unconscious of the human psychic immune system rally all that is necessary to defuse and defeat this crisis.

In this theory, in fact, it is precisely the psychic immune system which played a role in suppressing all of the man-made follies in human history, and it should be fully expected to play out its defensive, positive, healing role to vanquish this menace as well.

So, from inside the global warming laboratory, where the biggest crisis spawned by *Homo sapiens* is propagating, will we see nothing? Will there be no abatement, no resolution? Will it just be greedy, anarchic ants clawing for ever-dwindling crumbs the earth can supply as the planet warms humanity to extinction? Or will we see something else?

Scientists at CERN broke into wild applause when they saw the first experimental evidence that the seventy-year search for the invisible Higgs boson had been proven. It had been seen and measured. Finally, the greatest hidden variable in the history of physics was observed.

Within this century, hopefully, we too will break into applause when we see the first experimental confirmation of psychology's most extraordinary hidden variable—the invisible psychic immune system—and cheer that it successfully mobilized humankind to defeat the gravest threat our species ever faced.

The golden age is before us, not behind us.[149]
—William Shakespeare

NOTES

1. Alex Kirby, "Elephants Eat their Way to Equilibrium," BBC News, March 8, 2001, http://news.bbc.co.uk/2/hi/science/nature/1208970.stm.
2. Brian Merchant, "Record Breaking CO2 Emissions Levels Put World on Track for Worst-case Warming Scenarios," Treehugger, June 3, 2011, http://www.treehugger.com/corporate-responsibility/record-breaking-co2-emissions-levels-put-world-on-track-for-worst-case-warming-scenarios.html.
3. Justin Gillis and John Broder, "With Carbon Dioxide Emissions at Record High, Worries on How to Slow Warming," *New York Times*, December 2, 2012.
4. Justin Gillis and David Jolly "Slowdown in Carbon Emissions Worldwide, but Coal Burning Continues to Grow," *New York Times*, November 18, 2013.
5. Brendan Koerner, "The Other Greenhouse Gases," The Green Lantern, November 27, 2007, http://www.slate.com/articles/health_and_science/the_green_lantern/2007/11/the_other_greenhouse_gases.html.
6. Katherine Bagley, "Where the Presidential Candidates Fall on Climate Change," InsideClimateNews, August 7, 2015. A second study (2015) corroborates that methane leaks are 3 times higher than prior estimates.http://insideclimatenews.org/news/20150128/methane-leaks-gas-pipelines-far-exceed-official-estimates-harvard-study-finds]\].
7. John Schwartz, "Study Finds Low Cost in Reducing Methane Emissions," *New York Times* April 22, 2015.
8. Coral Davenport, "Study Finds Methane Leaks Negate Benefits of Natural Gas as a Fuel for Vehicles," *New York Times*, February 13, 2014.
9. Michael Wines, "Emissions of Methane in U.S. Exceed Estimates," *New York Times*, November 25, 2013.
10. Matt McGrath, "Greenhouse Gas Levels Rising at Fastest Rate Since 1984."
11. Andrew Kramer, "Russia Preparing Patrols of Arctic Shipping Lanes," *New York Times*, September 14, 2013.
12. Andrew E. Kramer. "Polar Thaw Opens Shortcut for Russian Natural Gas," *New York Times*, July 24, 2013.
13. M. F.Moonzajer, *Love, Hatred, and Madness*, 1000 quotes, Goodreads, accessed 2015, https://www.goodreads.com/work/quotes/34971951-love-hatred-and-madness.
14. Mark Lander and John Broder, "Obama Outlines Ambitious Plan to Cut Greenhouse Gasses," *New York Times*, June, 25, 2013.
15. The UN International Panel on Climate Change recommends far more drastic action: Alister Doyle, "Industrialized Nations Should Cut Emissions by Between 25 and 40 percent Below 1990 levels by 2020"; Alister Doyle, "UN Draft Sounds Alarm,"

Reuters, April 1, 2014, http://news.yahoo.com/u-n-draft-sounds-alarm-world-looks-set-133629870.html.

16. Coral Davenport, "New Limit for Smog-causing Emissions isn't as Strict as Many had Expected," *New York Times* October 1, 2015.

17. Alex Morales, "US CO2 Output Projected to be Above 1990 Level in 2030," *Bloomberg Business*, June 4, 2014, http://www.bloomberg.com/news/2014-06-04/u-s-co2-output-projected-to-be-above-1990-level-in-2030.html?cmpid=yhoo.

18. Justin Gillis, "Climate Talks Avoid Scientists' Idea of 'Carbon Budget,'" *New York Times*, November 28, 2015.

19. Bjorn Lomborg, "The Paris Climate Deal Won't Even Dent Global Warming," *New York Post*, February 22, 2016.

20. Edward Wong, "China Exports Pollution to U.S., Study Finds," *New York Times*, January 20, 2014.

21. "Meet the Family," Walmart blog, accessed 2015, http://walmart1percent.org/family/.

22. Nicholas Kristoff, "It's Now the Canadian Dream," *New York Times*, May 14, 2014, http://www.nytimes.com/2014/05/15/opinion/kristof-its-now-the-canadian-dream.html?.

23. Charles Babinton and Jennifer Agiesta, "13 percent of Americans Approve of Congress," *Huffington Post*, December 11, 2013, http://www.huffingtonpost.com/2013/12/11/congress-approval-ratings_n_4424718.html.

24. Charles Mahtesian, "2012 Reelection Rate: 90 percent," Politico, December 13, 2012, http://www.politico.com/blogs/charlie-mahtesian/2012/12/reelection-rate-percent-151898.html.

25. "Democratic Party ID Drops in 2010, Tying 22-Year Low," Gallup, January 5, 2011.

26. Egberto Willies, "Extreme GOP Gerrymandering Responsible for Tea Party Extremist" *Daily Kos*, October 10, 2013, http://www.dailykos.com/story/2013/10/11/1246244/-Extreme-GOP-Gerrymandering-Responsible-For-Tea-Party-Extremist-VIDEO#.

27. Martha Moore, "Governors: Big Wins for Republicans," *USA Today*, November 5, 2014.

28. "The Affluent Ante up for the Presidency," New York Times Editorial Board, *New York Times*, August 14, 2015.

29. Josh Harkinson, "America's 100 Richest People Control More Wealth than the Entire Black Population," *Mother Jones*, December 2, 2015.

30. Chuck Collins, "Twenty Billionaires Have More Wealth than Half U.S. Households," *Huffington Post*, December 2, 2015.

31. Marc Wiersum, "China's Manufacturing Wages Rise to $7000 per Year," Market Realist, April 22, 2014.

32. Coral Davenport, "McConnell Urges States to Help Thwart Obama's War on Coal," *New York Times* March 19, 2015.

33. Coral Davenport, "Senate Votes to Block Obama's Climate Change Rules," *New York Times*, November 17, 2015.

34. Glenn Kessler, "How did Mitch McConnell's Net Worth Doar?" *Washington Post*, May 22, 2014.

35. Paul Krugman, "Republicans' Climate Change Denial," *New York Times*, December 4, 2015.

36. *New York Times* editorial: "The Court Blocks Efforts to Slow Climate Change," February 11, 2016.

37. Dylan Byers, "Glenn Beck Makes More Money than Gaga," Politico, June 26, 2013, http://www.politico.com/blogs/media/2013/06/glenn-beck-makes-more-money-than-gaga-167145.html.

38. "Bill O'Reilly Net Worth," Celebs net worth, accessed 2015, http://getnetworth.net/bill-oreilly-net-worth/.

39. Kristina Bravo, "Guess Who's Been Secretly Funding a Famous Climate Change Denying Scientist?" Takepart, February 21, 2015, http://news.yahoo.com/guess-secretly-funding-famous-climate-change-denying-scientist-232619796.html.

40. Bravo, "Guess Who's Been Secretly Funding a Famous Climate Change Denying Scientist?"

41. Naomi Oreskes, "Exxon's Climate Concealment," *New York Times*, October 9, 2015.

42. Robert Stavins, "Climate Realities," *New York Times*, September 20, 2014.

43. Edward Wong "In Step to Lower Carbon Emissions, China will Place a Limit on Coal Use in 2020," *New York Times*, November 24, 2014.

44. Chris Buckley, "China Burns Much More Coal than Reported," *New York Times*, November 3, 2015.

45. Andrew Revkin, "A Closer Look at the Technical and Behavioral Barriers to Action on Global Warming," *New York Times*, August 19, 2013.

46. Justin Gillis, "Ending its Summer Melt, Arctic Sea Ice Sets a New Low that Leads to Warnings," *New York Times*, September 19, 2012.

47. Katia Moskvitch, "Mysterious Siberian Crater Attributed to Methane," *Nature*, July 31, 2014, http://www.nature.com/news/mysterious-siberian-crater-attributed-to-methane-1.15649.

48. Quote is from William Burns an energy analyst cited in Peter Galuskca, "With China and India Ravenous for Energy, Coal's Future Seems Assured," *New York Times*, November 12, 2012.

49. Note that a recent study in Delhi shows that half of the 4.4 million schoolchildren in the city have "irreversible lung damage from poisonous air." The city's air is now more than twice as polluted as Beijing. Gardiner Harris, "Holding your Breath in India," *New York Times*, May 29, 2015.

50. Michael Forsythe, "China's Coal Dependency Threatens Efforts to Curb Warming," *New York Times*, May 12, 2014.

51. Gardiner Harris, "Coal Rush in India Could Tip Balance on Climate Change," *New York Times*, November 17, 2014.

52. Ellen Barry and Coral Davenport, "India Announces Plan to Lower Rate of Greenhouse Gas Emissions," *New York Times* October 2, 2015.

53. Michael Snyder, "If Economic Cycle Theorists are Correct, 2015 to 2020 will be Devastating for the U.S." ZeroHedge, May 13, 2014, http://www.zerohedge.com/news/2014-05-13/if-economic-cycle-theorists-are-correct-2015-2020-will-be-devastating-us.

54. Michael Synder, "14 Experts Predict Economic Catastrophe for 2014 and Beyond," Douglas Ross Journal, accessed 2015, http://directorblue.blogspot.mx/2013/12/14-experts-predict-economic-catastrophe.html.

55. Anna Bernasek, "What the Nation got for $800 billion," *New York Times* August 3, 2013.

56. Ron Paul, "Audit the Federal Reserve," RonPaul.com, 2008, http://www.ronpaul.com/misc/congress/legislation/111th-congress-200910/audit-the-federal-reserve-hr-1207/.

57. "What is Quantitative Easing," *The Economist*, March 9, 2015.

58. Ron Paul, "Don't be Fooled by the Federal Reserve's Anti-audit Propaganda," Ron Paul Institute, March 8, 2015, http://www.ronpaulinstitute.org/archives/featured-articles/2015/march/08/don-t-be-fooled-by-the-federal-reserve-s-anti-audit-propaganda/.

59. Barry Eichengreen and Kris Mitchener, "The Great Depression as a Credit Boom Gone Wrong," August 2003, http://elsa.berkeley.edu/~eichengr/research/bisconferencerevision5jul30-03.pdf.

60. "Global CO2 Emissions from 1995 to 2013," The statistics portal, accessed 2016, http://www.statista.com/statistics/276629/global-co2-emissions/.

61. Kevin Schultz, "Carbon Dioxide Emissions Rise with Rebounding Economy," *Scientific American*, June 6, 2014.

62. "Carbapenem-resistant Enterobacteriaceae in Healthcare Settings," CDC, February 23, 2015, http://www.cdc.gov/HAI/organisms/cre/.

63. Sarah Knapton, "E. coli has Developed Resistance to Last-line of Antibiotics, Warn Scientists," *The Telegraph*, November 19, 2015.

64. WHO (October 28, 2005), "H5N1 avian influenza: timeline" Dec 13, 2011, http://www.who.int/influenza/human_animal_interface/avian_influenza/H5N1_avian_influenza_update.pdf.

65. Laura Sanders, "Bird Flu Leaves Tracks in Brain," *Science News*, March 10, 2012.

66. Tina Hesman Saey, "MERS Outbreak Picks up Pace," *Science News*, May 31, 2014.

67. "Arctic Sea Ice Reaches Maximum Extent on Record," Prediction of the National Snow and Ice Data Center (NSIDC), February 25, 2015, http://nsidc.org/arcticseaicenews/2015/03/2015-maximum-lowest-on-record/.

68. Paul Ehrlich, "The Biological Effects of Nuclear War," Quest for Peace, accessed 2015, http://www.independent.co.uk/environment/climate-change/climate-change-could-force-1-billion-from-their-homes-by-2050-817223.html.

69. Claudia Dreifus, "A Chronicler of Warnings Denied," *New York Times*, October 27, 2014.

70. Carl Sagan, "The Nuclear Winter," Cooperativeindividualism, 1983, http://www.bibliotecapleyades.net/ciencia/ciencia_uranium16.htm.

71. Nick Paton Walsh and Laura Smith-Spark, CNN, "Yemen's President, Cabinet Resign," January 23, 2015, http://www.cnn.com/2015/01/22/world/yemen-violence/.

72. "Yemen's President Flees to Saudi Arabia," *The Week*, March 26, 2015.

73. Joe Romm, "Must-Read: Tom Friedman on Climate Change and the 'Other Arab Spring,'" ClimateProgress, April 8, 2012, http://thinkprogress.org/climate/2012/04/08/460221/tom-friedman-on-climate-change-and-the-other-arab-spring/.

74. Chris York and George Bowden, "Syria Civil War Death Toll Paints a Horrifyingly Complex Picture," *Huffington Post UK*, October 31, 2015.

75. "Syria: Refugees Brace for More Bloodshed," *The News* 24 (March 12, 2012).

76. Jethro Mullen, "Syrian Refugee Population Above 4 million," CNN, July 10, 2015, http://www.cnn.com/2015/07/09/middleeast/syria-refugee-crisis-united-nations/index.html,

77. "Tech Pioneers Who Will Change Your Life", *Time*, December 17, 2009.

78. Ralph Cavanagh, "Good News on Energy," *New York Times*, November 23, 2014.

79. Daniel Clery, "After ITER Other Obstacles for Fusion Power," Science Insider, January 17, 2013.

80. Andrea Shalal, "Lockeed Says Makes Breakthrough on Fusion Energy Project," Reuters, October 15, 2014.

81. Daniel Clery, "Mystery Company Blazes a Trail in Fusion Technology," *Science*, October 15, 2015.

82. "Near Term Commercial Fusion Power Possible," September 25, 2015, http://nextbigfuture.com/2015/09/near-term-commercial-fusion-power.html.

83. "Highly Porous Non-precious Bimetallic Electrocatalysts for Efficient Hydrogen Evolution," *Nature Communications* 6, Article number: 6567 DOI: 10.1038/ncomms7567.

84. "Japanese Space Scientists Make Wireless Energy Breakthrough," Phys.Org, March 12, 2015, http://phys.org/news/2015-03-japan-space-scientists-wireless-energy.html.

85. Jessica Orwig, "Germany is About to Start up a Monster Machine that Could Revolutionize the Way We Use Energy," *Business Insider*, October 30, 2015.

86. Henry Fountain, "Panel Urges Research on Geonengineering as a Tool Against climate change," *New York Times*, Feb 10, 2015,

87. Zhong-Shuai Wu, Khaled Parvez, et al., "Graphene Based in Plane Microsupercapacitors with High Power and Energy Densities," Nature Communications, August 2013, doi:10.1038/ncomms3487.

88. "A Battery Made of Iron Could Improve the Economy of Solar and Wind Power," *MIT Technology Review*, accessed 2015, http://www.technologyreview.com/tagged/flow-battery/.

89. William Pentland, "Lithium-air Battery Breakthrough may Mean the End for Gasoline," *Forbes* October 31, 2015.

90. Rebecca Harrington, "Europe has Adopted Clean Energy with Such Gusto that it's Created a Strange New Problem," *Business Insider* March 31, 2016.

91. Ivan Penn, "Santa Monica Firm Says it has Found a Way to Salt Away Electricity, Literally," *Los Angeles Times*, March 20, 2016.

92. "Hypersolar Surpasses Critical Threshold to Split Water Molecules for Renewable Hydrogen Fuel Production," CNN Monday, September 15, 2015.

93. "Cobalt Atoms on Graphene, A Powerful Combo," The Next Big Future, October 28, 2015, http://nextbigfuture.com/2015/10/cobalt-atoms-on-graphene-powerful-combo.html.

94. Michael McDonald, "Breakthrough in Hydrogen Cracking Could Create Clean Fuel," *Oil Price*, December 21, 2015.

95. Todd Alhart, "This Scientist's got the Power Plant in his Hands," GE Reports, May 15, 2016, http://www.gereports.com/this-scientists-got-the-power-plant-in-his-hands/.

96. Thomas Burton, "New Solar Cell Devices Surpasses Theoretical Efficiency Limit," Energy and Clean Energy Technology Matters, June 2016.

97. D.J. Siegelbaum, "In Search of a Test-Tube Hamburger", *Time*, April 23, 2008.

98. Dickson Despommier, The Vertical Farm, 2011 (New York: St. Martin's Press).

99. Joint Center for Artificial Photoysynthesis, JCAP, accessed 2015, http://solarfuelshub.org/.

100. Zongli Xie, Mang Hoang, et al, Sol-gel Derived Poly(vinyl alcohol)/Maleic Acid/Silica Hybrid Membrane for Desalination by Pervaporation, Journal of Membrane Science, 2011, 383.

101. Ucilla Wang, "Super Efficient Perovskites are Dazzling Solar Cell Researchers," GIGAOM, November 28, 2014. See also "What is Geoengineering?" Oxford Geoengineering Programme, 2015. See also Electra Therm, "ElectraTherm Technology Generates Power from Wood Waste," Biomass, September 17, 2014.

102. Scientists estimate that the U.S. alone would save $1 billion annually if CO2 could be kept below 500 ppm. "Carbon Cuts Could save U.S. Farmers Billions of Dollars." *Science News*, September 19, 2015.

103. Kroth, *Duped!* ibid.

104. David Rosenberg, "Food and the Arab Spring," Rubin Center, October 27, 2011, http://www.gloria-center.org/2011/10/food-and-the-arab-spring/.

105. James Stewart, "King Coal, Long Besieged, is Deposed by the Market," *New York Times*, August 6, 2015.

106. Damian Carrington and Emma Howard, "Institutions Worth $2.6 trillion Have Pulled out of Fossil Fuels," *The Guardian*, September 22, 2015.

107. J. Kroth, *The Lindbergh Kidnapping: Mobs, Mass Psychology and Myth* (Cupertino, CA: Genotypc, 2010).

108. Marjorie Connelly, "Global Warming Concerns Grow," *New York Times*, September 22, 2014.

109. Coral Davenport and Marjorie Connelly, "Most Americans Support Government Action on Climate Change, Poll Finds," *New York Times*, Januar 30, 2015.

110. Giovanni Russonello, "Two-thirds of Americans want U.S. to Join Pact." *New York Times* November 30, 2015.

111. Thomas Friedman, "Paris Climate Accord is a Big, Big Deal," *New York Times*, December 16, 2015.

112. Lucy Scantamburlo, August 9, 2015, http://www.ufodigest.com/news/1206/gorbachev.html see also A Hovni, "The shocking truth: Ronald Reagan's obsession with an alien invasion," Feb. 1995,http://www.theforbiddenknowledge.com/hardtruth/ronald_reagan_ufo.htm.

113. From Pope Francis: "The Earth, our home, is beginning to look more and more like an immense pile of filth. . .Yet all is not lost. Human beings, while capable of the worst, are also capable of rising above themselves, choosing again what is good, and making a new start." . . . The climate is a common good, belonging to all and meant for all. . . . We need to strengthen the conviction that we are one single human family. . . . We must regain the conviction that we need one another, that we have a shared responsibility for others and the world, and that being good and decent are worth it." Daniel Burke, "5 Powerful Quotes from the Pope's Encyclical," June 18, 2015, http://www.cnn.com/2015/06/18/world/pope-encyclical-quotes/.

114. Jacob Silverman, "Do Cows Pollute as Much as Cars?" Howstuffworks, accessed 2015, http://science.howstuffworks.com/zoology/methane-cow.htm.

115. "Sources of Greenhouse Gas Emissions," EPA, July 21, 2015, http://www.epa.gov/climatechange/ghgemissions/sources.html.

116. "World War II Rationing on the U.S. Homefront," accessed 2015, http://www.ameshistory.org/exhibits/events/rationing.htm.

117. Deiter Helm, "To Slow Warming, Tax Carbon," *New York Times*, November 11, 2012.

118. Eduardo Porter, "Counting the Cost of Fixing the Future," *New York Times*, September 10, 2013.

119. See also Andrew Revkin, "Energy Agency Sees Global Coal Boom Unabated, Europe's Binge Temporary," *New York Times*, December 18, 2012.

120. Martin Weitzman, professor of economics at Harvard and co-author of Climate Shock believes a carbon tax of $50 per ton might have a significant and immediate impact. Eduardo Porter, "Climate Deal Badly Needs a Big Stick," *New York Times*, June 2, 2015.

121. Note also that President Obama revised his prior plans and proposed in 2015 that CO2 emissions be cut to 32 percent below 2005 levels. It is not likely to pass, but it does show an increasing level of seriousness in some quarters of the U.S. government. See Richard Revesz and Jack Lienke, "Obama takes a Crucial Step on Climate Change," *New York Times*, August 3, 2015.

122. "U.S. Carbon Pollution from Power Plants Hits 27-year Low," *New York Times*, August 5, 2015.

123. Morgan Brennan, "Natural Gas Tops Coal as Top Source of Electricity in US," CNBC, July 14, 2015, http://www.cnbc.com/2015/07/14/natural-gas-tops-coal-as-top-source-of-electric-power-generation-in-us.html.

124. Associated Press, "Coal Production Falls to Lowest Volume in 3 Decades," *New York Times*, January 8, 2016.

125. "UK's Coal Plants to be Phased out within 10 Years," BBC News, November 18, 2015.

126. Andrew Smith, "Fact Checking Elon Musk's Blue Square." U.S. Energy Institute Blog, May 21, 2015, http://blogs.ucl.ac.uk/energy/2015/05/21/fact-checking-elon-musks-blue-square-how-much-solar-to-power-the-us/.

127. Charis Michelsen, "Solar Energy from the Sahara Desert Could Power the World, But Will It?" Clean Technica, December 14, 2010, http://cleantechnica.com/2011/12/14/solar-energy-from-the-sahara-desert-could-power-the-world-but-will-it/.

128. A recent MIT study reports a trillion watts of electricity can be generated from solar power fields using technology available today. Lucas Mearian, "MIT Says Solar Power Fields with Trillion Watts of Capacity are on the Way," Computerworld, May 6, 2015, http://www.computerworld.com/article/2919134/sustainable-it/mit-says-solar-power-fields-with-trillions-of-watts-of-capacity-are-on-the-way.html.

129. Justin Gillis, "A Path for Climate Change, Beyond Paris," *New York Times*, November 30, 2015.

130. Eduado Porter's essay on the huge supply of coal, and the fact that only 6 percent of U.S. energy comes from renewable sources, makes the argument that nuclear energy is the most propitious investment for any kind of rapid decrease in U.S. consumption of coal to occur. Even with a carbon tax of $30 per metric ton of CO2, still

neither wind nor solar could outcompete coal. See "Coming Full Circle in Energy, to Nuclear," *New York Times*, August 20, 2013. Environmentalist Jim Hansen makes a similar argument and asserts that only1 to 2 percent of renewables are satisfying energy demands, and that nuclear energy is the most likely solution for the next half century. See Andrew Revkin, "Jim Hansen Presses the Climate Case for Nuclear Energy," *New York Times*, July 23, 2013.

131. Peter Thiel, "The New Atomic Age we Need," *New York Times*, November 27, 2015.

132. Matthew Wald. "Betting on the Need, Scientists Work on Lighter, Cleaner Nuclear Energy," *New York Times*, December 15, 2014.

133. "Liquid Metal Cooled Reactors," Lucas Mearian, "MIT says solar power fields with trillion watts of capacity are on the way," Computerworld, May 6, 2015, http://www-pub.iaea.org/MTCD/publications/PDF/te_1569_web.pdf.

134. Stephen Edelstein, "Nuclear Waste Could Offer Carbon-free Energy, Scientists Suggest," Yahoo News, February 26, 2015, http://news.yahoo.com/nuclear-waste-could-offer-carbon-free-energy-scientists-133004675.html.

135. Richard Muller, "Nuclear Power—Not Electric Cars—will Change our Future," Observer Business & Teach, April 5, 2016.

136. Durwood Zaelka, "Going Beyond Carbon Dioxide," *New York Times*, December 6, 2012.

137. Matthew Wald, "From Harvard, A Cheaper Storage Battery," *New York Times*, January 8, 2014.

138. "Genetic Bacterial Engineering Could Herald New Era of Biofuels," *Reuters*, accessed 2015, http://news.yahoo.com/video/genetic-bacterial-engineering-could-herald-153031847.html.

139. Patton Oswalt, "The Good Outnumber You and We Always Will," *Huffington Post*, June 15, 2013, http://www.huffingtonpost.com/patton-oswalt/patton-oswalt_b_3088337.html.

140. Justin Gillis, "UN Panel Issues its Starkest Warning yet on Global Warming," *New York Times*, November 2, 2014.

141. Patricia Levy, "Climage Change Kills 5 million People Every Year," News.Mic, December 27, 2012, http://mic.com/articles/21419/climate-change-kills-5-million-people-every-year.

142. Malcolm Moore, "China's 'Airpocalypse' Kills 350,000 to 500,000 Each Year," *The Telegraph*, January 7, 2014.

143. "Air Pollution Responsible for More than 2 million Deaths Worldwide Each Year," *Science News*, July 12, 2013, http://www.sciencedaily.com/releases/2013/07/130712084455.htm.

144. "Climate Change Deaths Could Total 100 million by 2030 if World Fails to Act," *Reuters*, November 25, 2012, http://www.huffingtonpost.com/2012/09/26/climate-change-deaths_n_1915365.html.

145. "Climate Change Deaths Could Total 100 million by 2030 if World Fails to Act."

146. "Climate Change Could Result in 100 million Poor, World Bank Report Says," *Science*, November 9, 2015.

147. Rachel Reilly, Victorial Woollaston, et al., "Doomsday Clock Reads 11:57. Atomic Scientists Move Minute Hand Two Minutes Forward," *Daily Mail*, February 4, 2015, http://www.dailymail.co.uk/sciencetech/article-2921899/Doomsday-Clock-reads-11-57-Atomic-scientists-minute-hand-two-minutes-forward-say-closest-point-disaster-decades.html#ixzz3PayoDvCQ Original Source: Bulletin of Atomic Scientists, February 4, 2015, https://www.google.com/?gws_rd=ssl#q=BAS+Bullentin+of+Atomic+Scientists.

148. Reilly, Woollaston, et al., "Doomsday Clock Reads 11:57."

149. Henry IV, Part I, line 2551, *The Complete Works of William Shakespeare*, accessed 2015, http://www.opensourceshakespeare.org/search/search-results.php.

Bibliography

Aberbach, David. *The European Jews, Patriotism and the Liberal State, 1789–1939* (New York: Routledge, 2012).

Able Archer Escalation. Althistory, http://www.militaryeducation.org/10-most-epic-tank-battles-in-military-history/.

Abraham, Karl. *On Character and Libido Development* (New York: W. W. Norton, 1966) 66.

Abu-Musa, A., L. Kobeissi, A. Hannoun, et al. "Effect of War on Fertility: A Review of the Literature," (2008) PMID: 18644222 [PubMed - indexed for MEDLINE].

Adams, Stephen. "Happiness Gene Discovered," *The Telegraph* December 20, 2013.

Ahmed, Emin. *Turkey in the World War* (New Haven, CT: Yale University Press, 1930).

Alberts, Bruce, Alexander Johnson et al. "Lymphocytes and the Cellular Basis of Adaptive Immunity," *Molecular Biology of the Cell,* 4th ed. (New York: Garland Science, 2002) http://www.ncbi.nlm.nih.gov/books/NBK26921/.

Alex, Dan. "Second World War History." Accessed 2015. http://www.secondworldwarhistory.com/world-war-2-statistics.asp.

Amos, Jonathan. "Deep Ice Tells Long Climate Story," BBC News, September 4, 2006. http://news.bbc.co.uk/2/hi/science/nature/5314592.stm

Anand, Vatsal. "Can Dengue Transfer from Person to Person, " *OnlyMyHealth,* Oct. 2012, http://www.onlymyhealth.com/is-dengue-fever-contagious-1301653693

Arango, Tom. "In Struggle for National Identity, Iraqis Rally Around Many Flags." *New York Times,* December 22, 2014.

Arya Wilson. "Iraq: West's Failed Democracy Project," *International Policy Digest,* June 16, 2014.

Asfura-Heim, Patricio, and Ralph Espach. "The Rise of Mexico's Self-defense Forces," *Foreign Affairs,* July/August 2013.

Associated Press. "Coal Production Falls to Lowest Volume in 3 Decades," *New York Times,* January 8, 2016.

Atkins, Matthew. "The US Army's Ambitious Fight against PTSD," *Science,* March 13, 2013, http://www.popsci.com/technology/article/2013-02/us-armys-ambitious-fight-against-ptsd.

Atomic Archive, National Science Digital Library, http://www.atomicarchive.com/Company/Company.shtml.

Austin Alchon, Suzanne. A Pest in the Land: New World Epidemics in a Global Perspective. (Albuquerque: University of New Mexico Press, 2003) 21.

Babinton, Charles, and Jennifer Agiesta. "13 percent of Americans Approve of Congress," *Huffington Post,* December 11, 2013, http://www.huffingtonpost.com/2013/12/11/congress-approval-ratings_n_4424718.html.

Bagley, Katherine. "Where the Presidential Candidates Fall on Climate Change," InsideClimateNews, August 7, 2015. http://insideclimatenews.org/news/20150128/methane-leaks-gas-pipelines-far-exceed-official-estimates-harvard-study-finds]\].

Bakalar, Nicholas. "Stress May Affect Fertility, *Well* (2014). http://well.blogs.nytimes.com/2014/03/24/stress-may-affect-fertility/?_r=2.

Baker, Robin. *Sperm Wars* (London: Fourth Estate, 1996). http://www.robin-baker.com/books/sperm-wars/.

Ball, Jerry. "Employee Fire and Life Safety," National Fire Protection Association, 2001. http://www.nfpa.org/~/media/Files/Safety%20information/For%20consumers/Occupancies/Evacuation.pdf.

Bargh, John, and Ezequiel Morsella. "The Unconscious Mind," *Perspectives in Psychological Science* 3 (2008): 73–79.
Barnard, Anne. "Death Toll from War in Syria now 470,000 Group Finds," *New York Times*, February 11, 2016.
Barringer, Felicity. "Climate Change will Disrupt Half of North America's Bird Species, Study Says," *New York Times*, September 8, 2014.
Barro, Robert, and Jong-Wha Lee. "Educational Attainment in the World, 1950-2010, VOX, May 18, 2010. http://www.voxeu.org/article/educational-attainment-world-1950-2010.
Barry, Ellen, and Coral Davenport. "India Announces Plan to Lower Rate of Greenhouse Gas Emissions," *New York Times*, October 2, 2015.
Barsh, David. "Is There a War Instinct?" *Aeon*, October. 15 2012. http://aeon.co/magazine/society/human-beings-do-not-have-an-instinct-for-war/.
Battuta's Travels. *Part Three, Persia and Iraq*.
Bekoff, Mark. "Give Peace a Chance: We Do Not Have to Go to War," *Psychology Today*, March 14, 2013. http://www.psychologytoday.com/em/120246
Benedictow, Ole J. *The Black Death, 1346–1353: The Complete History*. (Woodbridge, UK, Boydell Press, 2004).
Bergland, Christopher. "Evolutionary Biology of Altruism," *Psychology Today*, December 25, 2012.
Bernasek, Anna. "What the Nation Got for $800 Billion." *New York Times*, August 3, 2013.
Bernstein, Dennis, J. "Iraq and the Oil Wars," Consortiumnews, August 17, 2014. https://consortiumnews.com/2014/08/17/iraq-and-the-oil-wars/.
Bingham, Amy. "Stock Market History: the 10 Worst Days," *ABC News*, August 9, 2011.
"Biologists Discover Why 10 Percent Of Europeans Are Safe From HIV Infection." *Science Daily*. April 3, 2005.
Black, Ian. "Iranian Air Force Bombs ISIS Targets in Iraq, says Pentagon," *The Guardian*, December 3, 2014.
Blake, John. "The New Threat: Racism Without Racists," CNN, November 27, 2014. http://www.cnn.com/2014/11/26/us/ferguson-racism-or-racial-bias/.
Blight, James, and Janet Lang. *The Fog of War* (New York: Rowman & Littlefield, 2005) 58.
Bloomberg, B. "Psychosocial Adaptatiaon and Cellular Immunity in Breast Cancer Patients," *Journal of Psychosomatic Research* (2009): 67.
Bonanno, G. "Loss, Trauma and Human Resilience: Have we Underestimated the Human Capacity to Thrive after Extremely Aversive Events," *American Psychologist* 59 (2004).
Bonnano, G. A. "Resilience to Loss in Bereaved Spouses, Bereaved Parents, and Bereaved Gay Men." *Journal of Personality and Social Psychology* 88 (2005).
Booth, Robert. "Discovery of Higgs Boson Rated Year's Top Scientific Achievement by Science," AAAS, December 2012. http://www.guardian.co.uk/science/2012/dec/20/top-scientific-discoveries-higgs-boson.
Borenstein, Seth. "Absurdly Hot October as Earth sets 8th Heat Record this Year." AP, November 19, 2015.
———. "Science Academies Explain Global Warming Reality," *Associates Press*, February 26, 2014.
Borning, Alan. "Computer System Reliability and Nuclear War," 2001. http://www-ee.stanford.edu/~hellman/Breakthrough/book/chapters/borning.html.
Bornstein, Seth. "World Becoming Less Violent," *Huffington Post*, December 22, 2011. http://www.huffingtonpost.com/2011/10/22/world-less-violent-stats_n_1026723.html.
Bouchard, Thomas. "Genetic Influence on Human Psychological Traits," Current Directions in Psychological Science, (2004), Casey Kazan, "The happiness gene—is it

inherited," (2008) http://www.dailygalaxy.com/my_weblog/2008/11/the-happiness-i.html.

Boyle, J. A., ed. *The Cambridge History of Iran: Volume 5, The Saljuq and Mongol Periods.* (Cambridge, UK, Cambridge University Press, 1968).

Brennan, Morgan. "Natural Gas Tops Coal as Top Source of Electricity in US," CNBC, July 14, 2015. http://www.cnbc.com/2015/07/14/natural-gas-tops-coal-as-top-source-of-electric-power-generation-in-us.html.

Brian Greene, Brian. "How the Higgs Boson Was Found," *Smithsonian Magazine,* August 2013, p. 27.

Brooks, Arthur. "A Formula for Happiness," *New York Times,* December 14, 2013.

Brooks, David. "Why Elders Smile, "*New York Times,* December 4, 2014.

Brown, Lester. *World on the Edge,* (Colorado: Earth Policy Institute, January 2011), location 30.

Browning, E. S. "Exorcising Ghosts of October Past," *Wall Street Journal,* October 15, 2007.

Bruner, Robert, and Sean Carr. *The Panic of 1907: Lessons Learned from the Market's Perfect Storm (*Hoboken, NJ: John Wiley & Sons, 2007).

Buckley, Chris. "China Burns Much More Coal Than Reported," *New York Times,* November 3, 2015.

Burton, Thomas. "New Solar Cell Devices Surpasses Theoretical Efficiency Limit," Energy and Clean Energy Technology Matters, June 2016.

Byers, Dylan. "Glenn Beck Makes More Money than Gaga," Politico, June 26, 2013. http://www.politico.com/blogs/media/2013/06/glenn-beck-makes-more-money-than-gaga-167145.html.

Cabneca, Anna. "Why Do I Feel Disconnected? The Cortisol-Oxytocin Connection." Accessed 2015. http://www.saragottfriedmd.com/why-do-i-feel-disconnected-the-cortisol-oxytocin-connection/.

Cacioppo, J. D. "Autonomic, Neuroendocrine, and Immune Responses to Psychological Stress." *Psychological Beitrage* (2000): 42.

Callaway, Ewen. "Fearful Memories Haunt Mouse Descendants," *Nature,* December 2013. http://www.nature.com/news/fearful-memories-haunt-mouse-descendants-1.14272.

Callaway, Ewen. "Genghis Khan's Genetic Legacy has Competition," *Nature,* January 23, 2015.

Campbell, Thomas. "World Cup Final Breaks Records Worldwide for TV Broadcasters, July 14, 2014. http://www.iptv-news.com/2014/07/world-cup-final-breaks-re cords-worldwide-for-tv-broadcasters/.

Carl Estabrook, Carl. "Israel and the US War on Iraq," Counterpunch, February 26, 2003. http://www.counterpunch.org/2003/02/26/israel-and-the-us-war-on-iraq/.

Carrington, Damian, and Emma Howard. "Institutions Worth $2.6 trillion have Pulled Out of Fossil Fuels," *The Guardian,* September 22, 2015.

Cavanagh, Ralph. "Good News on Energy." *New York Times,* November 23, 2014.

CDC. Cited in Liz Szabo, "CDC: Vaccines Save Hundreds of Thousands of Lives," *USA Today,* April 24, 2014.

Chan, Cherie. "Soil Contamination Found Near Huge Mine in Western China," *New York Times,* June 12, 2015.

Chaplin, Charlie. The Great Dictator, https://www.youtube.com/watch?v=W2ft Z1g4FtE.

Charney, Evan, and Roger Chapman, eds. *Culture Wars: An Encyclopedia of Issues, Voices, and Viewpoints* (Armonk, NY: M. E. Sharpe, 2009)."History and Debate on Flag Burning," Debate.org, accessed 2015,

Charpentier, Marie, Delphine Deubel, and Patricia Peignot. "Relatedness and Social Behaviors in Cercopithecus solatus." *International Journal of Primatology* 29 (2008): 487–95.

Chavan, Nandini, and Qutub Jehan Kidwai. *Personal Law Reforms and Gender Empowerment: A Debate on Uniform Civil Code.* (India: Hope India Publications, 2006).

Choi, Charles. "A Small Nuclear War Could Trigger Catastrophic Cooling," 2014. http://news.yahoo.com/small-nuclear-war-could-trigger-catastrophic-cooling-181056235.html.

Chomsky, Noam. Interviewed by Tavis Smiley, NPR, 2003. http://www.chomsky.info/interviews/20031119.htm.

Christian, Bennett. "Rape in a Lawless Land." *The Guardian*, March 27, 2010.

Civil, Miguel. "The Law Collection of Ur-Namma." *Cuneiform Royal Inscriptions and Related Texts in the Sch ø yen Collection*, edited by A. R. George, 2011, 221–86,

Clay, Janet. "The Inheritance of Acquired Immunity." Accessed 2015. http://jeb.biologists.org/content/12/1/49.full.pdf.

Clery, Daniel. "After ITER Other Obstacles for Fusion Power," *Science Insider*, January 17, 2013.

Clery, Daniel. "Mystery Company Blazes a Trail in Fusion Technology," *Science*, October 15, 2015.

Clodfelter, Michael. *Warfare and Armed Conflicts—A Statistical Reference to Casualty and Other Figures, 1500–2000.* 2nd ed, (New York: McFarland & Co., 1998).

Clover, R., T., Abell, L. Crawford, et al. "Family Functioning and Stress as Predictors of Influenza B Infection." *The Journal of Family Practice* (1989): 28.

Coghlan, Benjamin, Pascal Ngoy, et al. "Morality in the Democratic Republic of Congo, an Ongoing Crisis." Accessed 2015. http://www.rescue.org/sites/default/files/migrated/resources/2007/2006-7_congomortalitysurvey.pdf.

Cohen, Stan. *America's Home Front During World War II*, 1991. http://www.ameshistory.org/exhibits/events/rationing.htm.

Collins, Chuck. "Twenty Billionaires Have More Wealth than Half U.S. Households," *Huffington Post*, December 2, 2015.

Connelly, Mark. "Global Warming Concerns Grow," *New York Times*, September 22, 2014.

Cooper, Helene. "U.S. Strategy in Iraq Increasingly Relies on Iran," *New York Times*, March 5, 2015.

Cossins, Dan. "How HIV Destroys Immune Cells," *The Scientist*, 2013. http://www.the-scientist.com/?articles.view/articleNo/38739/title/How-HIV-Destroys-Immune-Cells/.

Coyne, Jerry. "Why Evolution is True." Blog at Wordpress, 2011. http://whyevolutionistrue.wordpress.com/2011/09/26/epigenetics-again-will-it-cause-a-revolution-in-evolution/.

Crabtree, Steve. "U.S. Confidence in Police about Average for Wealthy Countries," Gallup, July 29, 2015. http://www.gallup.com/poll/180227/confidence-police-average-wealthy-countries.aspx.

Craig, Jeffrey. "The New Science of Epigenetics and the Possibilities for Resilience," ABC, 2015. http://www.abc.net.au/tv/life/stories/s2994579.htm.

Crawford, Jack. "The Missing 100 Million," 2015.

Cumming-Bruce, Nick. "UN Reports Nearly 19,000 Iraqi Civilian Deaths in 22 months," *New York Times*, January 19, 2016.

Daly, M., and M. Wilson. "Child Abuse and Other Risks of Not Living with Both Parents." *Ethology and Sociobiology* (1985): 6, 197.

Danielle, Britni. "75 Percent of White People Do Not Have any Nonwhite Friends," Takepart, July 2015. http://www.takepart.com/article/2014/08/28/75-percent-white-people-have-no-nonwhite-friends.

Daphna Birenbaum, Carmeli. "Prevalence of Jews as Subjects in Genetic Research: Figures, Explanation, and Potential Implications," *American Journal of Medical Genetics* (2004): 130.

Davenport, Coral. "Senate Votes to Block Obama's Climate Change Rules," *New York Times*, November 17, 2015.

Davenport, Coral. "Study Finds Methane Leaks Negate Benefits of Natural Gas as a Fuel for Vehicles." *New York Times*, February 13, 2014.

Davenport, Coral, and Marjorie Connelly. "Most Americans Support Government Action on Climate Change, Poll Finds." *New York Times,* January 30, 2015.

Davenport, Coral. "McConnell Urges States to Help Thwart Obama's War on Coal." *New York Times,* March 19, 2019.

Davenport, Coral. "New Limit for Smog-Causing Emissions Isn't as Strict as Many Had Expected." *New York Times,* October 1, 2015.

Davenport, Coral. "Senate Rejects Human Role in Climate Change," *New York Times,* January 22, 2015.

deMause, Lloyd. *Foundations of Psychohistory,* 1982. Accessed 2015. http://www.geocities.ws/kidhistory/found/p271x290.htm.

"Demographic Consequences of the Great Leap Forward in China's Provinces," *Population and Development Review* 13, no. 4 (1987): 639–70.

Dennen, J., and V. Falger, eds. *Sociobiology and Conflict: Evolutionary Perspectives on Competition, Cooperation, Violence and Warfare* (London: Chapman and Hall, 1990).

Despommier, Dickson. *The Vertical Farm* (New York: St. Martin's Press, 2011).

DeWitte, Sharon. "Health in Post-Black Death London 1350–1538," *American Journal of Physical Anthropology* (April 17, 2014).

Dobbs, Michael. "Cuban Missile Crisis," *New York Times,* 2015. http://topics.nytimes.com/top/reference/timestopics/subjects/c/cuban_missile_crisis/index.html.

Dotings, Randy. "Genetic HIV Resistance Deciphered," 2005. http://www.wired.com/medtech/health/news/2005/01/66198?currentPage=all.

Douglass, James *JFK and the Unspeakable,* (New York: Orbis Books, 2010) 109.

Dreifus, Claudia. "A Chronicler of Warnings Denied," *New York Times,* October 27, 2014.

Dummett, Mark. "King Leopold's Legacy of DR Congo violence," 2004. http://news.bbc.co.uk/2/hi/africa/3516965.stm.

Eaaswarkhanth, M., B. Dubey, et al. "Micorsatellite Diversity Delineates Genetic Relationships of Shia and Sunni populations," *Hum Biol* 81, no. 4 (August 2009): 427–45. doi: 10.3378/027.081.0403.

Edelstein, Stephen. "Nuclear Waste Could Offer Carbon-free Energy, Scientists Suggest," Yahoo News, February 26, 2015. http://news.yahoo.com/nuclear-waste-could-offer-carbon-free-energy-scientists-133004675.html.

Edwards, Erica. "Resilience in Aging," Arizona Center on Aging, 2012. http://aging.arizona.edu/sites/default/files/resilience_in_aging_0.pdf.

Edwards, Philip. "Plumage Variation, Territoriality and Breeding Displays of the Golden Plover pluvialis Apricaria in Southwest Scotland," *International Journal of Avian Science* (April, 2008). http://onlinelibrary.wiley.com/doi/10.1111/j.1474-919X.1982.tb03747.x/abstract.

Ehrlich, Robert. *Waging Nuclear Peace* (New York: Suny Press, 1985) 272.

Eichengreen, Barry, and Kris Mitchener. "The Great Depression as a Credit Boom Gone Wrong," August 2003. http://elsa.berkeley.edu/~eichengr/research/bisconf erencerevision5jul30-03.pdf.

Epp, Charles, and Steven Maynard-Moody. "Driving While Black," *Washington Monthly,* February 2014. http://www.washingtonmonthly.com/magazine/january_february_2014/ten_miles_square/driving_while_black048283.php?page=all.

Euronews. 2011. http://www.euronews.com/2011/06/17/back-in-the-day-united-states-and-soviet-union-create-a-hotline/.

Fadel, Leila, and Hussein Kadhim. "Some Sunni Muslims Won't Salute New Flag," McClatchy DC, January 25, 2008. http://www.mcclatchydc.com/2008/01/25/25471/some-sunni-muslims-wont-salute.html.

Fajnzylber, Pablo, Daniel Lederman, and Norman Loayza. "Inequality and Violent Crime," *Journal of Law and Economics,* 45 (April 2002). http://siteresources.worldbank.org/DEC/Resources/Crime%26Inequality.pdf.

Fan, Maureen, and Ariana Cha. "China's Capital Cases Still Secret, Arbitrary" The Washington Post, 2008.

Faulkner, J., M. Schaller, et al. "Evolved Disease–Avoidance Mechanisms and Contemporary Xenophobic Attitudes," *Group Processes and Intergroup Relations* 7 (2004): 333–53.

Ferner, Matt. "Snowpack in Sierra Nevada at 500 year low." *Huffington Post*, September 14, 2015. Original source: Soumaya Belmecheri, Flurin Babst, et al., "Multicentury Evaluation of Sierra Nevada Snowpack," *Nature Climate Change* doi:10.1038/nclimate2809.

First Encyclopaedia of Islam: 1913–1946 (New York: Brill, 1993). http://books.google.com/books?id=ro--tXw_hxMC&dq=timur+buried+4000+christians+alive&source=gbs_navlinks_s.

Fischer, Benjamin B. "A Cold War Conundrum: The 1983 Soviet War Scare." Central Intelligence Agency, March 17, 2007. https://www.cia.gov/library/center-for-the-study-of-intelligence/csi-publications/books-and-monographs/a-cold-war-conundrum/source.htm#HEADING1-12.

Fletcher, Ian. *Free Trade that Doesn't Work*. Washington, DC, U.S. Business and Industry Council, 2010, location 199.

Fletcher, Roly and Martin Milton. "Being Aggressive: An Existential Phenomenological Critique on the Psychological Literature on Human Aggression. Accessed 2015. http://www.academia.edu/1108345/Being_Aggressive_An_existential-phenomenological_critique_of_the_psychological_literature_on_Human_Aggression.

Forbes, Viv. "Clearing the Smog of Beijing with 'Coal by Wire," Canada Free Press, August 4, 2008. http://www.canadafreepress.com/index.php/article/4274.

Forden, Geoffrey. "False Alarms in the Nuclear Age," Nova, 2001. http://www.pbs.org/wgbh/nova/military/nuclear-false-alarms.html.

Forsythe, Michael. "China's Coal Dependency Threatens Efforts to Curb Warming," *New York Times*, May 12, 2014.

Fouchier, R. A., T. Kuiken, M. Schutten, et al. "Aetiology: Koch's Postulates Fulfilled for SARS virus." *Nature* (2003): 423.

Fountain, Henry. "Panel Urges Research on Geonengineering as a Tool Against Climate Change," *New York Times*, February 10, 2015.

Francis, John M. *Iberia and the Americas Culture, Politics, and History: A Multidisciplinary Encyclopedia*. (Santa Barbara, CA: ABC-CLIO, 2005).

Friedman, Richard. "The Feel-Good Gene," *New York Times*, March 6, 2015.

Friedman, Thomas. "Paris Climate Accord is a Big, Big Deal." *New York Times*, December 16, 2015.

———. "The Market and Mother Nature," *New York Times*, January 8, 2013.

———. "The Scary Hidden Stressor," *New York Times*, March 2, 2013.

———. "The World's Hot Spot," *New York Times*, August 19, 2015.

———. "The Other Arab Spring," *New York Times*, April 2012.

Fromm, M., B., Stocks, and R. Servranckx, et al. "Smoke in the Stratosphere: What Wildfires have Taught Us about Nuclear Winter" *Eos, Transactions, American Geophysical Union* (Washington, DC: American Geophysical Union, 2006).

Fruehwald, Edwin. "A Biological Basis of Rights," *Southern California Interdisciplinary Law Journal* 195, 2010.

Galbraith, Kate. "Wildfires and Climate Change," *New York Times*, September 4, 2013.

Gardner, Amanda. "Many Obese Americans Struggle with Stigma," Health Day, August 2012. http://consumer.healthday.com/vitamins-and-nutritional-information-27/obesity-health-news-505/many-obese-americans-struggle-with-stigma-discrimination-poll-finds-667697.html.

Gardner, Amanda. "Genes May Play a Key Role in Stress," Health.com, September 19, 2012.

Gelbspan, Ross. "The Big Name Game," *Grist* magazine, July 31, 2002.

General Overview of the Effects of Nuclear Testing CTBTO. Retrieved 2015. http://www.ctbto.org/nuclear-testing/the-effects-of-nuclear-testing/general-overview-of-theeffects-of-nuclear-testing/.

Genzlinger, Neil. "Same Cuba Crisis, Different Angles 50 Years Later." World News, 2012. http://article.wn.com/view/2012/10/22/Same_Cuba_Crisis_Different_Angles_50_Years_Later/.

Ghandi, Mahatma. *An Autobiography: The Story of My Experiments with Truth* (Boston: Beacon Press, 1990). http://www.un.org/events/nonviolence/2008/.

Gholipour, Bahar. "Here's a Look at the 3 Front Runners," *Live Science*, January 12, 2015. http://news.yahoo.com/ebola-vaccines-heres-look-3-front-runners-070326797.html.

Gholipour, Behar. "Vaccination has Saved 732,000 Children's Lives since 1994," Livescience, April 24, 2014. http://www.livescience.com/45111-national-vaccination-effects.html.

Gibbon, Edward. *Decline & Fall of the Roman Empire*. vol. 3&6 (London: Stahan, and Cadell, 1776).

Gierloff, Maryann. "Positive Emotions and Immune Response to Influenza in Medically Stable Older Adults." *Dissertation Abstracts International* (2013): 73.

Gillis, Justin. "Ending its Summer Melt, Arctic Sea Ice Sets a New Low that Leads to Warnings." *New York Times*, September 19, 2012.

———. "Study Indicates a Greater Threat of Extreme Weather," *New York Times*, April 27, 2012.

———. "A Path for Climate Change, Beyond Paris," *New York Times*, November 30, 2015.

———. "Climate Talks Avoid Scientists' Idea of 'Carbon Budget," *New York Times*, November 28, 2015.

———. "Ending its Summer Melt, Arctic Sea Ice Sets a New Low that Leads to Warnings." *New York Times*, September 19, 2012.

———. "Not Even Close: 2012 Was the Hottest Ever in U.S." *New York Times*, January 8, 2013.

———. "Scientists Report Faster Warming in Antarctica." *New York Times*, December 23, 2012.

———. "UN Climate Panel Endorses Ceiling on Global Emissions." *New York Times*, September 27, 2013.

———. "UN Panel Issues its Starkest Warning Yet on Global Warming." *New York Times*, November 2, 2014.

———. "Zika Could be Omen of Global Warming Threat," *New York Times*, February 18, 2016.

———. "In Sign of Warming, 1600 Years of Ice in Andes Melted in 25 years." *New York Times*, 2013.

———. "Heat-trapping Gas Passes Milestone, Raising Fears." *New York Times*, 2013.

Gillis, Justin, and David Jolly. "Slowdown in Carbon Emissions Worldwide, but Coal Burning Continues to Grow." *New York Times*, November 18, 2013.

Gillis, Justin, and John Broder. "With Carbon Dioxide Emissions at Record High, Worries on How to Slow Warming." *New York Times*, December 2, 2012.

Gilmore, Margaret. "Global Warming Disease Warning," BBC News, June 18, 1999. http://news.bbc.co.uk/1/hi/sci/tech/372219.stm.

Ginsberg, Mitch. "Dayan Pushed PM Meir to Use Nuclear Weapons in '73 war," *The Times of Israel*, October 3, 2013.

Gladstone, Rick. "Former Lord's Resistance Army Commander Appears at War Crimes Court," *New York Times*, January 26, 2015.

Gladstone, Rick. "26 Percent of World's Adults are Anti-Semitic Survey Finds," *New York Times*, May 13, 2014.

Goldberg, Dave. "Ask a Physicist: Why Believe in Dark Matter" *io9*, May 2010. http://io9.com/5528758/ask-a-physicist-why-believe-in-dark-matter.

Goldin, Semion. Antisemitism and Pogroms in the Military (Russian Empire), in: 1914-1918-online. International Encyclopedia of the First World War, edited by Ute Daniel, Peter Gatrell, Oliver Janz, Heather Jones, Jennifer Keene, Alan Kramer, and Bill

Nasson, issued by Freie Universität Berlin, Berlin 2014-10-08. DOI: http://dx.doi.org/10.15463/ie1418.10283.

Gooding, P, A. Hurst, J. Johnson, and N. Tarrier. "Psychological Resilience in Young and Older Adults." *Int Journal of Geriatric Psychiatry*, 3, 2012.

Gorebel, J., and R. Hinde. *Aggression and War: Their Biological and Social Bases.* (London: Cambridge University Press, 2012).

Gorman, James. "Animals Die in Large Numbers, and Researchers Scratch Their Heads," *New York Times*, January 18. 2016.

Gorman, James. "Scientists Predict Widespread Extinction by Global Warming," *New York Times*, January 8, 2004.

Gorman, James. "Ants That Can Flow Like a Fluid or Move like a Solid." *New York Times*, December 16, 2013.

Grady, Denise. "Happiness Doesn't Bring Good Health, Study Finds." *New York Times*, December 9, 2015.

Grady, Denise. "T-cell Therapy Puts Leukemia Patients in Extended Remission," *New York Times*, October 15, 2014.

Greenwald, A. G., and M. R. Banaji. "Implicit Social Cognition: Attitudes, Self-esteem, and Stereotypes," *Psychological Review* 102 (1995): 4-27.

Griffis, Margaret. "Casualties in Iraq," Antiwar.com, May 2015. http://antiwar.com/casualties/.

Grossman, David. *On Killing: the Psychological Cost of Learning to Kill in War and Society*, 2009. http://www.amazon.com/On-Killing-Psychological-Learning-Society/dp/0316040932.

Grossman, David. "Aggression and Violence," Killology research group, 2000. http://www.killology.com/article_agress&viol.htm.

Haker, H., and W. Rossler. "Empathy in Schizophrenia: Impaired Resonance." *Eur Arch Psychiatry Clin Neurosci*, September 6, 2009.

Halverson, M. "Native American Beliefs and Medical Treatments during the Smallpox Epidemics: an Evolution." Archiving Early America, 1995. http://www.earlyamerica.com/review/2007_summer_fall/native-americans-smallpox.html.

Hammen, R. "Age and Gender as Determinants of Stress Exposure and Reactions in Youngsters." *Child Development*, 3, 1999.

Handwerk, Brian. "Global Warming Could Cause Mass Extinctions," *National Geographic News*, April 2006.

Hanioglu, Sukru. *Ataturk: an Intellectual Biography*, (Princeton, NJ: Princeton University Press, 2011) 129.

Hanninen, O., M. Farago, and E. Monos. "Ignaz Philipp Semmelweis, the Prophet of Bacteriology," *Infection Control* 4, no. 5 (September/October 1983): 367–70.

Harkinson, Josh. "America's 100 Richest People Control More Wealth than the Entire Black Population," *Mother Jones*, December 2, 2015.

Harrington, Rebecca. "Europe has Adopted Clean Energy with such Gusto that it's Created a Strange New Problem," *Business Insider*, March 31, 2016.

Harris, Gardiner. "Coal Rush in India Could Tip Balance on Climate Change," *New York Times*, November 17, 2014.

———. "Holding Your Breath in India." *New York Times*, May 29, 2015.

———. "India Warns Kashmiris to Prepare for Nuclear War." *New York Times*, January 22, 2013.

———. "Steps Set for Livestock Antibiotic Ban," *New York Times*, March 24, 2012.

Hart, Peter. "In Denial on Climate Change," FAIR, May 1, 2007. http://www.fair.org/index.php?page=3418.

Hartmann, H., W. Bruere, et al. "General Adaptation Syndrome(Seyle) in Cattle," 1976. http://www.ncbi.nlm.nih.gov/pubmed/793558.

Hays, Jeffrey. "Tartars and Mongols," 2012. http://factsanddetails.com/asian/cat65/sub423/item2692.html.

Heather, Jamie. "T-cell receptors Part One," 2013. http://jamimmunology.blogspot.com/2013/02/TCR-part-1-the-immtroduction.html.

Heilprin, John. "Wildlife Populations Plummet for 3,000 Species," Associated Press, September 30, 2014.
Helm, Deiter. "To Slow Warming, Tax Carbon," *New York Times*, November 11, 2012.
Henry IV, Part I, line 2551. *The Complete Works of William Shakespeare*. Accessed 2015. http://www.opensourceshakespeare.org/search/search-results.php.
Hersh, Seymour. *The Third Temple:The Story Behind the Vanunu Revelation*, (New York: Amana Books, 1989) 147.
Hesman Saey, Tina. "Glu Immunity Prompted, Years Later." *Science News* September 21, 2013.
Hinde, Robert. *Psychological Bases of War*. http://www.unc.edu/depts/diplomat/AD_Issues/amdipl_7/hinde3.html.
"The History of Russia." http://www.parallelsixty.com/history-russia.shtml.
Hodgson, K, and P. McGuffin. "The Genetic Basis of Depression," *Current Topics in Behavioral Neuroscience*, 2013. http://www.researchgate.net/publication/230733447_The_Genetic_Basis_of_Depression.
Hoffman, David. Washington Post Foreign Service, 1999. http://www.washingtonpost.com/wp-srv/inatl/longterm/coldwar/shatter021099b.htm.
Hogan, Jenny. "Unseen Universe: Welcome to the Dark Side." *Nature* 448, no. 7151 (2007): 240–45.
Hook, Leslie. "China Smog Cuts 5.5 Years from Average Life Expectancy," CNBC, July 8, 2003. http://www.cnbc.com/id/100871380.
Hopkin, Michael. "Did Black Death Boost HIV Immunity in Europe," *Nature* (March 11, 2005): doi:10.1038/news050307-15.
Horwitz, Richard. "American's Problems with Global Warming,"*American Studies* 45, no. 1 (spring 2004): 5–37.
Hovni, A. "The Shocking Truth: Ronald Reagan's Obsession with an Alien Invasion," February 1995. http://www.theforbiddenknowledge.com/hardtruth/ronald_reagan_ufo.htm/
Howell, Elizabeth. "Earth Lost Half its Trees to Humans," Live Science, September 3, 2015.
Hsueh-Ling, Janice, Samuel Ken-En Gan, et al. "Understanding the T cell Immune Response in SARS Coronavirus Infection," *Emerging Microbes & Infections* 1 (2012): doi:10.1038/emi.2012.26.
Hubbuch, Chris."False Alarm: How a Bear Nearly Started a Nuclear War," LaCrosseTribune.com. http://lacrossetribune.com/news/false-alarm-how-a-bear-nearly-started-a-nuclear-war/article_bc6f4da6-a89c-5d7d-bf0a-e41150753b62.ht.
Hunt, Greg, Gro Amdan, et al. "Behavioral Genomics of Honeybee Foraging," April 2007. http://www.ncbi.nlm.nih.gov/pmc/articles/PMC1829419/.
Hurley, Dan. "Grandma's Experiences Leave a Mark on your Genes," Discover, June 25, 2015. http://discovermagazine.com/2013/may/13-grandmas-experiences-leave-epigenetic-mark-on-your-genes.
Hutchinson, Alex. "Epigenetics and Fitness," *Runner's World*, September 22, 2014. http://www.runnersworld.com/health/epigenetics-and-fitness.
Isachenov, Vladimir. Cultura Cubana, 2002. https://groups.yahoo.com/neo/groups/culturacubana/conversations/topics/7583.
Jamail, Dahr. "Western Oil Firms Remain as U.S. Exits Iraq," Al Jazerra, January 2012. http://www.aljazeera.com/indepth/features/2011/12/2011122813134071641.html.
Janeway, C., P. Travers, M. Walport, et al. *Inherited Immunodeficiency Diseases* (New York: Garland Science, 2001).
Johnson, Dominic and Monica Duffy Toft. "Grounds for War: the Evolution of Territorial Conflict," *Journal of International Security* 38 (2014) 7–38.
Joint Center for Artificial Photoysynthesis, JCAP. Accessed 2015. http://solarfuelshub.org/.
Jolly, David. "United Nations Group Warns on Emissions." *New York Times*, November 5, 2013.
Jonathan, Fenby. "Mao's Great Famine by Frank Dikötter," *Guardian*, September 2010.

Jones, Nathan. "One Misstep Could Trigger a Great War," 2009. http://gradworks.umi.com/1465450.pdf.
Jung, Carl J. *Psychological Reflections* (Princeton, NJ, Princeton University Press, 1973).
———. *The Collected Works.* (New York: Routledge, 2015) 4434.
Kagan, Harman. *The Psychological Immune System.* (Bloomington, IN: Author House, 2006) 20.
Kaktuna, Michiko. "Cataclysm has Arrived: Man's Inhumanity to Nature." *New York Times*, February 3, 2014.
Kardasz, Frank. "Common Ground, World Religions," Ethics training for Law Enforcement. Accessed 2015. http://kardasz.org/Ethics_CommonReligiousBeliefs.html.
Katie McGhee, and Alison Bell. "Paternal Care in a Fish: Epigenetics and Fitness Enhancing Effects on Offspring," Proceedings B, The Royal Society, September 17, 2014. DOI: 10.1098/rspb.2014.1146.
Kazan, Casey. "The Happiness Gene—Is It Inherited?" 2008. http://www.dailygalaxy.com/my_weblog/2008/11/the-happiness-i.html.
Kazan, Ogla. "The Antibiotics Problem in Man," *Atlantic*, 2015. http://www.theatlantic.com/health/archive/2015/03/the-next-big-antibiotic-resistance-threat/388430/.
Keeling, Matthew. "The Mathematics of Disease." Accessed in 2015. https://plus.maths.org/content/mathematics-diseases?sa=X&ved=0CCYQ9QEwCGoVChMIt4LRoqH3xgIVT5aICh23Ngo_. Graphic courtesy of Matthew Keeling, Zoology Department, Cambridge University.
Keltner, Dacher. "The Compassionate Instinct," Greater Good, March 1, 2004. http://greatergood.berkeley.edu/article/item/the_compassionate_instinct#sthash.Uy8hyZ4H.dpuf.
Kendler, K., and C. Prescott. *Genes, Environment, and Psychology* (New York: Guilford Press, 2007) 71.
Kennedy, S. *The Prager Handbook on Stress and Coping* (Santa Barbara, CA: Greenwood Publishing, 2007).
Kent, Mary Mederois. "Most Americans Marry Within their Race," PRB, August 2010. http://www.prb.org/Publications/Articles/2010/usintermarriage.aspx.
Kent, Sarah. "Iraq's Oil Output Surges to Highest Level in over 30 years," *Wall Street Journal,* March 14, 2014. http://www.wsj.com/articles/SB10001424052702304914904579438860227481506.
Kessler, Glenn. "How Did Mitch McConnell's Net Worth Soar?" *Washington Post,* May 22, 2014.
Khan, Chagatai. "On the Nuclear Edge by Seymour Hersh," 2009. http://chagataikhan.blogspot.ca/2009/05/on-nuclear-edge-by-seymour-m-hersh.html.
KHOU staff. "Texas Mom Jumps in Front of Car to Save Child," KHOU.com, February 1, 2013. http://www.khou.com/story/news/local/texas/2014/07/22/11954144/.
Kick, Russ, ed. *Everything you Know is Wrong* (New York: The Disinformtion Company, 2007) location 4667.
Kiernan, Ben. "The Original Cambodian"*New Internationalist*, 1993, 242.
Kils, U. "The ecoSCOPE and dynIMAGE: Microscale Tools for In Situ Studies of Predator-prey Interactions." *Arch Hydrobiol Beih* 36 (1992): 83–96.
Kim, Meeri. "Study Finds that Fear can Travel Quickly through Generations," *Washington Post*, December 7, 2013. http://www.washingtonpost.com/national/health-science/study-finds-that-fear-can-travel-quickly-through-generations-of-mice-dna/2013/12/07/94dc97f2-5e8e-11e3-bc56-c6ca94801fac_story.html.
King, Simon. "Reflex Reactions, our Body's Rapid Defence Mechanism," Positive Health, 2010. http://www.positivehealth.com/article/chiropractic/reflex-reactions-our-body-s-rapid-defence-mechanism.
Kinzer, Stephen. "A Kinder, Gentler Tamerlane Inspires Uzbekistan," *New York Times*, November 10, 1997.M

Kirby, Alex. "Elephants Eat Their Way to Equilibrium," BBC News, March 8, 2001. http://news.bbc.co.uk/2/hi/science/nature/1208970.stm.
Kluger, Jeffrey. "The Turning Point," *Time,* April 3, 2006.
Kluger, Jeffrey. "Americans Flunk Science Again," *Time,* April 22, 2014.
Knapton, Sarah. "E. Coli has Developed Resistance to Last-line of Antibiotics Warn Scientists," *Telegraph,* November 19, 2015.
Koch, Wendy. "U.S. Carbon Emission Rise Despite Obama Climate Plan," *USA Today,* September 26, 2014. http://www.usatoday.com/story/money/business/2014/09/26/us-carbon-emissions-rise-despite-obama-climate-plan/16276811/.
Koerner, Brendan. "The Other Greenhouse Gases," The Green Lantern, November 27, 2007. http://www.slate.com/id/2178595/.
Koerth-Baker, Maggie. "Want to Understand Mortality? Look to the Chimps," *New York Times,* June 25, 2013.
Kohn, George. *Encyclopedia of Plague and Pestilence,* (New York: Infobase Publishing, 2007).
Kolata, Gina. *The Flu: the Story of the Great Influenza Pandemic* (New York: Touchstone, 1999).
Kolbert, Elizabeth. Quotes, *New Yorker,* April 25, 2005.
Korean War FAQ. http://www.zzwave.com/cmfweb/history/faq7.shtml.
Kramer, Andrew. "Russia Preparing Patrols of Arctic Shipping Lanes."
Kramer, Andrew, E. "Polar Thaw Opens Shortcut for Russian Natural Gas," *New York Times,* July 24, 2013.
Kristof, Nicholas. "Our Biased Brains," *New York Times,* May 7, 2015.
Kristoff, Nicholas. "It's now the Canadian Dream," *New York Times,* May 14, 2014. http://www.nytimes.com/2014/05/15/opinion/kristof-its-now-the-canadian-dream.html?.
Kroth, Jerry. "Saloth Sar," *Omens and Oracles: Collective Psychology in the Nuclear Age* (New Haven, CT: Praeger, 1991).
———. *Duped: Delusion, Denial, and the End of the American Dream* (Cupertino, CA: Genotype, 2013) 11.
———. *Psychology Underground* (Akron, OH: Academic Press, 2001).
———. *The Lindbergh Kidnapping: Mobs, Mass Psychology and Myth* (Cupertino, CA: Genotype, 2010).
Krugman, Paul. "Republicans' Climate Change Denial," *New York Times,* December 4, 2015.
Lamb, Harold. *Genghis Khan Emperor of All Men.* http://www.goodreads.com/book/show/224038.Genghis_Khan.
Lander, Mark, and John Broder. "Obama Outlines Ambitious Plan to Cut Greenhouse Gasses," *New York Times,* June, 25, 2013.
Lane, R., and L. Nadel. *Cognitive Neuroscience of Emotion* (New York: Oxford University Press, 1999).
Lang, Phillip. *Science: Antiquity and its Legacy* (London, I. B. Tauris, 2015) 25.
Larner, George, and Michael Dobbs. "New Tapes Reveal Depth of Nixon's Anti-Semitism," *Washington Post,* October 6, 1999.
Larsin, Kud, G. Vazov, K. Krumov and J. Schneider. *Advances in International Psychology* (Sofia: Kassel University Press. 2013) 142.
Larson, Eric. "China's Growing Coal Use is World's Greatest Problem" Climate Central, January 27, 2014. http://www.climatecentral.org/blogs/chinas-growing-coal-use-is-worlds-growing-problem-16999.
Lawing, Charles. "Loving v. Virginia and the Hegemony of 'Race.'" PDF, 2000. http://www.charlielawing.com/modhist_lovingv.virginia.pdf.
Leahy, Robert. "Are We Born to be Afraid," *Psychology Today,* May, 2009. https://www.psychologytoday.com/blog/anxiety-files/200805/are-we-born-be-afraid.
Lebedev, Anastasiya. MosNews, "The Man Who Saved the World Finally Recognized," 2004. http://web.archive.org/web/20110721000030/http://www.worldcitizens.org/petrov2.html.

Leber, Rebecca. "Just Two Percent of Canadians Deny Climate Change," ClimateProgress, August 16, 2012. http://thinkprogress.org/climate/2012/08/16/697911/canada-climate-change/.
LeDeux, Joseph. "'Run, Hide, Fight' is not How Our Brains Work," *New York Times*, December 18, 2015.
LeDeux, Joseph. *The Emotional Brain* (New York: Simon & Schuster, 1996).
Lehrman, Gilder. Institute of American History. Accessed 2015. http://www.gilderlehrman.org/history-by-era/slavery-and-anti-slavery/resources/facts-about-slave-trade-and-slavery.
Leveridge, Brett. "David Rakoff," Salon.com, 2001. http://www.brettnews.com/clips/rakoff.html.
Levin, Dan. "Study Links Polluted Air in China to 1.6 Million Deaths a Year," *New York Times*, August 13, 2015.
Levy, Patricia. "Climate Change Kills 5 Million People Every Year," News.Mic, December 27, 2012. http://mic.com/articles/21419/climate-change-kills-5-million-peo ple-every-year.
Lewis, Tanya. "Twins Separated at Birth Reveal Staggering Influence of Genetics," Yahoo News, August 11, 2014. http://news.yahoo.com/twins-separated-birth-reveal-staggering-influence-genetics-182019977.html
Li-Ching, Hsu, Lin Sheue-Rong, et al. "Ethnic Differences in Immune Responses to Hepatitis B vaccine," *American Journal of Epidemiology*, 143, 1996.
Li, Mia. "Chinese City's Pollution Goes Off the Charts." *New York Times*, October 20, 2013.
Lind, Michael. "The Wars that Really are About the Oil," *The Spectator*, August 30, 2014.
Lomborg, Bjorn. "The Paris Climate Deal Won't Even Dent Global Warming," *New York Post*, February 22, 2016.
Long, Larissa. "Older Adults Less Sensitive to the Effects of Stress," Whole Health, 2011. http://www.wholehealthinsider.com/newsletter/older-adults-less-sensitive-effects-stress/.
Low, Bobbi. *Why Sex Matters: A Darwinian Look at Human Behavior* (Princeton, NJ: Princeton University Press, 2000).
MacDonald, Kevin. "A Social Identity Theory of anti-Semitism." Accessed 2015. http://www.kevinmacdonald.net/chap1.pdf.
MacFarquhar, Roderick, and Michael Schoenhals. Glossary of Names and Identities in Mao's Last Revolution (Cambridge, MA: Harvard University Press, 2006).
Macrae, Fiona. "Why You Can't Ignore a Baby's Cry," November 1, 2012. Lifestyle/family/baby-toddler http://www.iol.co.za/lifestyle/family/baby-toddler/why-you-ca nt-ignore-a-babys-cry-1415929.
Mahtesian, Charles. "2012 Reelection Rate: 90 percent," Politico, December 13, 2012. http://www.politico.com/blogs/charlie-mahtesian/2012/12/reelection-rate-percent-151898.html.
Manfredini, Fabio, Oksana Rba-Grognuz, et al. "Sociogenomics of Cooperation and Conflict During Colony Founding in the Fire Ant Solenopsis invicta," Plos, August 8 2013. DOI: 10.1371/journal.pgen.1003633.
Marion, Lloyd. "Soviets Close to Using A-Bomb in 1962 Crisis, Forum is Told," Boston Globe 2002, A20.
Marshall, Andrew. "The National Security State and the Assassination of JFK." http://www.globalresearch.ca/the-national-security-state-and-the-assassination-of-jfk/22071.
Marshall, S. L. A. *Men Against Fire: the Problem of Battle Command*. 2000. http://www.amazon.com/Men-Against-Fire-Problem-Command/dp/0806132809.
Martin, Ben. "Fight or Flight," Psyche Central, 2013. http://psychcentral.com/lib/fight-or-flight/00030.
Matthews, Chris. "Wealth Inequality in America: It's Worse Than You Think," *Fortune*, October 31, 2014. http://fortune.com/2014/10/31/inequality-wealth-income-us/.

Max, Arthur. AP, "2010 on Track to be of the 3 Hottest Years on Record," *San Francisco Chronicle*, December 31, 2010.

May, Timothy. *The Mongol Conquests in World History* (London: Reaktion Books, 2012).

McDonald, Michael "Breakthrough in Hydrogen Cracking Could Create Clean Fuel," *Oil Price*, December 21, 2015.

McDonald, Nicole, and Danial Messinger. "The Development of Empathy." Accessed 2015. http://www.psy.miami.edu/faculty/dmessinger/c_c/rsrcs/rdgs/emot/McDonald-Messinger_Empathy%20Development.pdf.

Mcdougal, Sam. "Humans are Nicer than We Think," Motherboard, March 8, 2012. http://motherboard.vice.com/blog/humans-are-nicer-than-we-think.

McGrath, Matt. "Greenhouse Gas Levels Rising at Fastest Rate Since 1984," BBC, September 9, 2014. http://www.bbc.com/news/science-environment-29115845.

McKown, Delow. Cited at http://www.goodreads.com/quotes/17434-the-invisible-and-the-non-existent-look-very-much-alike.

McLendon, Russell. "7 Examples of Animal Democracy," Mother Nature Network, November 4, 2012. http://www.mnn.com/earth-matters/animals/photos/7-examples-of-animal-democracy/cockroaches.

McNamee, David. "Global Life Expectancy has Increased by 6 Years since 1990," *Medical News Today*, December 2014.

McNeil, Donald. "U.S. Becomes More Vulnerable to Tropical Diseases like Zika," *New York Times*, January 4, 2016.

Mearsheimer, John, and Stephen Walt, *The Israeli Lobby and U.S. Foreign Policy*, (New York: Farrar, Straus and Giroux, 2007).

Medred, Craig. "Expert Predicts Ice-free Arctic by 2020 as UN Releases Climate Report," *Alaska Dispatch News*, November 2, 2014.

Melnick, Meredith. "CDC: 20% of Gay Men are HIV-positive, but Nearly Half Don't Know It," *Time*, September 26, 2010. http://healthland.time.com/2010/09/26/study-20-of-homosexual-men-are-hiv-positive-but-only-half-know-it/.

Melon, Maurizio, and Guiseppe Testa. "Scrutinizing the Epigenetics Revolution," BioSocieties, 2014. http://www.palgrave-journals.com/biosoc/journal/v9/n4/full/biosoc201422a.html.

Merchant, Brian. "Record Breaking CO2 Emission Levels Put World on Track for Worst-Case Warming Scenarioes," Treehugger, Junr 3, 2011. http://www.treehugger.com/corporate-responsibility/record-breaking-co2-emissions-levels-put-world-on-track-for-worst-case-warming-scenarios.html.

Messenger, Stephen. "Climate Refugees Could Number 1 Billion by 2050," Treehugger, December 8, 2009. http://www.treehugger.com/corporate-responsibility/climate-refugees-could-number-1-billion-by-2050.html.

Michelsen, Charis. "Solar Energy from the Sahara Desert Could Power the World, but Will it?" Clean Technica, December 14, 2010. http://cleantechnica.com/2011/12/14/solar-energy-from-the-sahara-desert-could-power-the-world-but-will-it/.

Middleton, Kim. "Fight or Flight or Just Chill," Birds and More Birds, 2012. http://kimmiddleton.com/blog/45597/fight-or-flight-or-just-chill.

Midlarsky, Manus I. *The Killing Trap: Genocide in the Twentieth Century*. (Cambridge: Cambridge University Press, 2005),342–43.

Miller, Angela. *Violence and Abuse in Society*, (Santa Barbara, CA: ABC-Clio, 2010) 445.

Milton, S. H. "'Gypsies' as Social Outsiders in Nazi Germany." In *Social Outsiders in Nazi Germany*, Robert Gellately and Nathan Stoltzfus (Princeton, NJ: Princeton University Press, 2001) 216, 231.

Min, Ariel. "World's Tropical Forests Vanishing More Rapidly than Previously Thought," PBS Newshour, March 2, 2015. http://www.pbs.org/newshour/rundown/worlds-tropical-forests-vanishing-rapidly-previously-thought/.

Mohamed, Besheer. "Who are the Kurds?" The Christian Century, Sepember 4, 2014. http://www.christiancentury.org/article/2014-09/who-are-iraqi-kurds.

Moir, Anne. "Brainsexmatters," 2015. http://www.brainsexmatters.com.

Montana, Sam. "The History of Stock Market Panics," Knoji, 2010. https://stocks.knoji.com/the-history-of-stock-market-panics/.

Mooney, Chris. "Global Warming is Now Slowing Circulation of the Oceans with Dire Consequences," *Washington Post,* March 23, 2015.

Mooney, Chris. "Scientists are Floored by What's Happening in the Arctic Right Now," *Washington Post,* February 18, 2016.

Moonzajer, M. F., "Love, Hatred, and Madness, 1000 Quotes,"Goodreads. Accessed 2015. https://www.goodreads.com/work/quotes/34971951-love-hatred-and-madness.

Moore, Harry. "Exceptional Sperm Cooperation in the Wood Mouse." *Nature* 418 (2002): 174–77.

Moore, Malcolm. "China's 'Airpocalypse' Kills 350,000 to 500,000 Each Year," *Telegraph,* January 7, 2014.

Moore, Martha. "Governors: Big Wins for Republicans," *USA Today,* November 5, 2014.

Morales, Alex. "US CO2 Output Projected to be Above 1990 Level in 2030," *Bloomberg Business,* June 4, 2014. http://www.bloomberg.com/news/2014-06-04/u-s-co2-output-projected-to-be-above-1990-level-in-2030.html?cmpid=yhoo.

Morgan, David. *The Mongols and Global History* (New York: Blackwell Publishing, 2007).

Morgenstern, Madeline. "How Many People Own Guns and is Gun Ownership Declining?" *The Blaze,* March 19, 2013. http://www.theblaze.com/stories/2013/03/19/how-many-people-own-guns-in-america-and-is-gun-ownership-actually-declining.

Morris, Nigel. "Climate Change Could Force 1 Billion from Their Homes by 2050," *Independent,* August 6, 2015. http://www.independent.co.uk/environment/climate-change/climate-change-could-force-1-billion-from-their-homes-by-2050-817223.html.

Moskowitz, Clara. "Dark Matter Still Hiding: Latest Experimental Sweep Comes up Empty," *Scientific American,* October 30, 2013.

Moskvitch, Katia. "Mysterious Siberian Crater Attributed to Methane," *Nature,* July 31, 2014. http://www.nature.com/news/mysterious-siberian-crater-attributed-to-methane-1.15649.

Motluk, Alison. "Close Family Smells Worse Than A Stranger," *Daily News,* August 22, 2002. http://www.newscientist.com/article/dn2705-close-family-smells-worse-than-a-stranger.html#.VKMWBSgzfTI.

Mower, Lawrence. "Most Burglaries Go Unsolved," *Las Vegas Review Journal,* February 10, 2008. http://www.reviewjournal.com/news/most-burglaries-go-unsolved.

Mullainathan, Sendhil. "Racial Bias, Even when we have Good Intentions." *New York Times,* January 3, 2015.

Mullen, Jethro. "Syrian Refugee Population Above 4 Million," CNN, July 10, 2015. http://www.cnn.com/2015/07/09/middleeast/syria-refugee-crisis-united-nations/index.html.

Muller, Richard. "Nuclear Power—Not Electric Cars— Will Change our Future, Observer Business & Teach, April 5, 2016.

Murphy, Caryle. "Lingering Gulf War Mystery: How many Iraqis really died?" *Washington Post,* June 30, 1991.

Nagraj, Aarti. "Top 10 Countries with the World's Biggest Oil Reserves," *Gulf Business,* April 14, 2013.

Navarro, Peter, and Greg Autrey. *Death by China* (New York: Pearson FT Press, 2011).

Neave, N. and S. Wolfson. "Testosterone, Territoriality, and the 'Home Advantage," *Physiological Behavior* 2 (2003): 169–75 .

Neimark, Neil. "Fight or Flight vs. Relaxation Response." Accessed 2015. http://www.relaxationresponse.org/fightorflight.htm.

Nelson, Randy, ed. *Biology of Aggression.* (Oxford: Oxford University Press, 2006).

Nelson, Randy, and Silvana Chiavegatto. "Molecular Basis of Aggression," *Trends in Neurosciences* 24, no. 12 (2001): 713–19.

New World Encyclopedia, 2015. http://www.newworldencyclopedia.org/entry/An_Lushan.

Newport, Frank. "Americans' Global Warming Concerns Continue to Drop," Gallup, March 11, 2010. http://www.gallup.com/poll/126560/americans-global-warming-concerns-continue-drop.aspx.

Nicholls, H. "Pandemic Influenza: The Inside Story." *Biology* 4, 2006.

Nicolle, David. *The Mongol Warlords: Genghis Khan, Kublai Khan, Hulegu, Tamerlane* (New York: Firebird, 1990) 2. http://www.biblio.com/book/mongol-warlords-genghis-khan-kublai-khan/d/707025332.

Nirenberg, David. *Communities of Violence,* (Princeton, NJ: Princeton University Press, 2015).

Norberg, Joakim. "Fearful Attention" Stockholm University, 2012. http://www.diva-portal.org/smash/get/diva2:576589/FULLTEXT01.pdf.

Norris, D., J. W. Ngambi, et al. "Genetic Selection for Docility," *Journal of Animal and Plant Sciences,* 24 (2014): 13–18.

Norris, Robert S., and Hans M. Kristensen. "Global Nuclear Stockpiles, 1945–2006," *Bulletin of the Atomic Scientists* 62, no. 4 (July/August 2006): 64–66.

North, Anna. "Why Misleading Americans about Climate Change is Dangerous," *New York Times,* August 11, 2015.

Norton-Taylor, Michael, and Ewen MacAskillk. "A Litany of Failure, but No One to Blame" *Guardian,* July 14, 2004.

Numlock, Tab. "Flags are the Equivalent of Bird Plummage," Flags Forum, January 2010. http://www.flagsforum.com/viewtopic.php?f=20&t=1005.

Nussbaum Cohen, Debra. "Poll: American Jews with Disabilities Excluded from Community," *Haaretz,* July 31, 2015. http://www.haaretz.com/jewish-world/jewish-world-news/.premium-1.547310.

O'Connor, Anahad. "The Claim: Yawning is Contagious Between Dogs and Their Owners," *New York Times,* August 21, 2013.

Oreskes, Naomi. "Exxon's Climate Concealment," *New York Times,* October 9, 2015.

———. "The Scientific Consensus on Climate Change," *Science* 3 (December 2004).

Orwig, Jessica. "Germany is About to Start Up a Monster Machine that Could Revolutionize the Way we Use Energy," *Business Insider,* October 30, 2015.

Osborne, Hannah. "Happy 80th Birthday Jane Goodall: Inspirational Quotes from the Lady of the Apes," *Business Times,* April 3, 2014.

Oswalt, Patton. "The Good Outnumber You and We Always Will," *Huffington Post,* June 15, 2013. http://www.huffingtonpost.com/patton-oswalt/patton-oswalt_b_3088337.html.

Over, Mead. "Five Steps to Reduce the Economic Impact of Ebola, Center for Global Development, 2014. http://www.cgdev.org/blog/five-steps-reduce-economic-impact-ebola.

Paez, Juan Andres. "Racial Discrimination in Latin America: the 'Pigmentocracy' Approach," *Dejustica,* December 2014. http://dejusticiablog.com/2014/12/09/racial-discrimination-in-latin-america-the-pigmentocracy-approach/.

Palma, Felix. *A Map of the Sky: a Novel* (New York: Simon & Schuster, 2011).

Pappas, Stephanie. "Black Death Likely Altered European Genes," Live Science, 2014.

Pappas, Stephanie. "Black Death Survivors and their Descendants went on to Live Longer," *Scientific American,* May 2014. http://www.scientificamerican.com/article/black-death-survivors-and-their-descendants-went-on-to-live-longer/.

Paton Walsh, Nick, and Laura Smith-Spark, CNN, "Yemen's President, Cabinet Resign," January 23, 2015. http://www.cnn.com/2015/01/22/world/yemen-violence/.

Paul, Ron. "Don't be Fooled by the Federal Reserve's Anti-Audit Propaganda," Ron Paul Institute, March 8, 2015. http://www.ronpaulinstitute.org/archives/featured-articles/2015/march/08/don-t-be-fooled-by-the-federal-reserve-s-anti-audit-propaganda/.

———. "Audit the Federal Reserve," RonPaul.com, 2008. http://www.ronpaul.com/misc/congress/legislation/111th-congress-200910/audit-the-federal-reserve-hr-1207/.

Paye-Layley, Jonathan. "Ebola Outbreak: Quarantine Camps in West Africa at Breaking Point," *Independent,* August 1, 2015.
Payne, Ed. "Pentagon: US to Begin to Train and Equip Moderate Syria Rebels, CNN, January 16, 2015.
Pearson, Racheal. "Disease Threat from Immigrant Children Wildly Overstated," Observer, July 10, 2014.
Peirls, R."Wolfgang Ernst Pauli, 1900–1958." *Biographical Memoirs of Fellows of the Royal Society,* 1960 .
Penn, Ivan. "Santa Monica Firm Says it has Found a Way to Salt Away Electricity, Literally," *Los Angeles Times,* March 20, 2016.
Pensac Schwartz, Teresa. *Holocaust Forgotten,* 2012. http://www.holocaustforgotten.com/non-jewishvictims.htm.
Pentland, William. "Lithium-air Battery Breakthrough May Mean The End for Gasoline," *Forbes,* October 31, 2015.
Peterson, Dale, and Richard Wrangham. *Demonic Males: Apes, and the Origin of Human Violence* (New York: Mariner Books, 1997) 115.
Pfingstein, Max. "Mongolians and their Contributions to Western Civilization," Study.com. Accessed 2015. http://education-portal.com/academy/lesson/mongolians-and-their-contributions-to-western-civilization.html#lesson.
Philips, Alan. "20 Mishaps That Might Have Started Accidental Nuclear War," 1998. http://nuclearfiles.org/menu/key-issues/nuclear-weapons/issues/accidents/20-mishaps-maybe-caused-nuclear-war.htm.
Philos1. "Beyond PTSD: the Moral Casualties of War," Daily Kos, June 15, 2007.
Pinger, Nathan. "Home Field Advantage: the Facts and the Figures," *Business,* March 4, 2014.
Pinker, Steven. Cited on "Its a Kids World, "PBS, Scientific American Frontiers," episode 505. http://www.pbs.org/saf/transcripts/transcript505.htm.
Plumer, Brad. "After Years of Decline, U.S. Carbon Emissions Rose 2 Percent in 2013," *Washington Post,* January 13, 2014.
Plumer, Brad. "Carbon-Dioxide Levels in the Atmosphere Rose at a Record Pace in 2013," World Meteorological Association. Accessed in 2015. http://www.vox.com/2014/9/9/6126245/carbon-dioxide-levels-in-the-atmosphere-rose-at-a-record-pace-in-2013.
Poppick, Laura. "Warming From Arctic Sea Ice Melting More Dramatic Than Thoughts," LiveScience, February 17, 2014. http://news.yahoo.com/warming-arctic-sea-ice-melting-more-dramatic-thought-202504784.html.
Porter, Eduardo. "Counting the Cost of Fixing the Future," *New York Times,* September 10, 2013.
———. "Climate Deal Badly Needs a Big Stick," *New York Times,* June 2, 1015.
Prawdin, Michael. *The Mongol Empire* (Brunswick, NJ: Transaction Publishers, 2009) 224.
Pring, Luke. "Empire History," 2015). http://empirehistory.weebly.com/timurid-empire.html.
Pulliam, H. Ronald. "On the Advantages of Flocking," *Journal of Theoretical Biology* 38 (February 1973).
Purdy, Michael. "Immune System Memory Cells have Trick for Self Preservation," 2012. http://news.wustl.edu/news/pages/23214.aspx.
Pusey, Anne. "Mechanisms of Inbreeding Avoidance in Nonhuman Primates," *Pedophilia,* 1990. http://link.springer.com/chapter/10.1007%2F978-1-4613-9682-6_8#close.
Pusey, S. "Mechanisms of Inbreeding Avoidance in Nonhuman Primates," Pedophilia, 1990. http://link.springer.com/chapter/10.1007%2F978-1-4613-9682-6_8#close.
Radkov, D. V. *Schooling in the Ecology of Fish* (New York: Halstead Press, 1973).
Raioff, Janet. "Studies See 4 Degrees of Warming," *Science News,* December 18, 2010.
Raloff, Janet. "Empty Nets," *Science News,* June 4, 2005, 167.
Ray, C. Clairborne. "The Roots of BRCA1 Mutations for Ashkenazi Jews," *New York Times,* October 12, 2015.

Rennell, Tony. "September 26th, 1983: The Day the World almost Died," Daily Mail, 2007. http://www.dailymail.co.uk/news/article-505009/September-26th-1983-The-day-world-died.html. Based on the documentary "1983 The Brink of Apocalypse," BBC.

Revkin, Andrew. "A Closer Look at the Technical and Behavioral Barriers to Action on Global Warming," *New York Times* August 19, 2013.

Rice, Doyle. "Report: 97 Percent of Scientists Say Man-made Climate Change is Real," *USA Today*, June 22, 2010.

Roberts, Sam. "NATO War Games Unwittingly put Soviets and US on 'Hair Trigger' in 83 Analysis Suggests." *New York Times*, November 9, 2015.

Roboc, Alan, Luke Oman, and Georgiy Stenchikov. "Nuclear Winter Revisited," *Journal of Geophysical Research*, 2007. http://onlinelibrary.wiley.com/doi/10.1029/2006JD008235/abstract.

Rogers, Kara. "Inclusive Fitness," *Encyclopedia Britanica*, Accessed 2015. http://www.britannica.com/EBchecked/topic/1710067/inclusive-fitness.

Rogers, Simon and Lisa Evans. World Carbon Dioxide Emissions Data by Country: China Speeds Ahead of the Rest," *Guardian*, January 31, 2011. http://www.guardian.co.uk/news/datablog/2011/jan/31/world-carbon-dioxide-emissions-country-data-co2.

Rogozinski, Jan. *A Brief History of the Caribbean* (New York: Putnam, 2001).

Rokke, Doug. "Gulf War Casualties," Trapock Peace Center, Rense.com, September 30, 2002. http://www.rense.com/general29/gulf.htm.

Romeo, Stefano, Julia Kozlitina, Chao Xing, et al. "Genetic Variation in PNPLA3 Confers Susceptibility to Nonalcoholic Fatty Liver Disease," *Nature Genetics*, 2008, 40, 1461–1465.

Romm, Joe."Must-Read: Tom Friedman on Climate Change and the 'Other Arab Spring," ClimateProgress, April 8, 2012. http://thinkprogress.org/climate/2012/04/08/460221/tom-friedman-on-climate-change-and-the-other-arab-spring/.

Romm, Joseph."Experts Debunk Polls Claiming Fewer Americans Believe in Climate Change," *Grist*, November 16, 2011. http://www.grist.org/climate-change/2011-11-16-experts-debunk-polls-claiming-fewer-americans-believe-in-climate.

Ropelk, David. "An End to War vs. the Animal Instinct to Survive," *Huffington Post*, 2010. http://www.huffingtonpost.com/david-ropeik/an-end-to-war-vs-the-anim_b_595282.html.

Roscoe, P. "Intelligence, Coalitional Killing, and the Antecedents of War," *American Anthropologist* 109, no. 3, (2007): 485–95.

Rosenbaum, Ron. *How the End Begins*. (New York. Simon & Schuster, 2011).

Rosenberg, David. "Food and the Arab Spring," Rubin Center, October 27, 2011. http://www.gloria-center.org/2011/10/food-and-the-arab-spring/.

Rosenberg, Mike. "Time to Partition Iraq?" Doing Business on the Earth Blog, June 23, 2014. http://blog.iese.edu/doing-business/2014/06/23/time-to-partition-iraq/#sthash.cyfAHIfM.Ql2kpmAP.dpuf.

Rosenthal, Elizabeth. "Burning Fuel Particles do More Damage to Climate than Thought, Study Says," *New York Times*, January 15, 2013.

Rossabi, Morris. "The Mongols in World History," http://www.google.com/search?client=safari&rls=en&q=collapse+of+mongols&ie=UTF-8&oe=UTF-8.

Rossiter, S., G. Jones, R. Ransome, and E. Barratt. "Relatedness Structure and Kin-Biased Foraging in the Greater Horseshoe Bat." *Behavioral Ecology and Sociobiology* 51, 2002.

Rowan, Karen. "Why Baby's Hungry Cry Tugs at Women (But Not Men)," Live Science, 2013. http://www.livescience.com/36964-baby-cries-women-men-brains.html.

Russonello, Giovanni. "Two-thirds of Americans Want U.S. to Join Pact." *New York Times*, November 30, 2015.

Sack, Kevin, Sheri Fink, et. al. "How Ebola Roared Back," *New York Times*, December 29, 2014.

Sagan, Carl. "The Nuclear Winter," Cooperativeindividualism, 1983. http://www.bibliotecapleyades.net/ciencia/ciencia_uranium16.htm.
Sagan, Scott D. *The Limits of Safety: Organizations, Accidents, and Nuclear Weapons* (Princeton, NJ: Princeton University Press, 1993) 79.
Samuel, Henry. "Soviet Plan for Nuclear Attack Unearthed," *Telegraph*, 2007. http://www.telegraph.co.uk/news/uknews/1563692/Soviet-plan-for-WW3-nuclear-attack-unearthed.html.
Sanders, Laura. "Bird Flu Leaves Tracks in Brain," *Science News* March 10, 2012.
Scantamburlo, Lucy. August 9, 2015. http://www.ufodigest.com/news/1206/gorbachev.html.
Scheiber, Noam/ "Fake Cover Letters Expose Bias Against Disabled," *New York Times*, November 2, 2015.
Schlosser, Eric. *Command and Control* (New York, Penguin Press, 2013) 292.
Schmid, B., E. Buntgen, et. al. "Climate-driven Introduction of the Black Death and Successive Plague Reintroductions into Europe," 2010. PNAS, doi: 10.1073/pnas.1412887112, http://www.pnas.org/content/112/10/3020.abstract.
Schollser, Eric. "Nuclear Weapons: an Accident Waiting to Happen," *Guardian*, 2013.
Schrock Simring, Karen. "Age Brings Happiness," *Scientific American*, April 11, 2013. http://www.scientificamerican.com/article/age-brings-happiness/.
Schultz, Kevin. "Carbon Dioxide Emissions Rise with Rebounding Economy," *Scientific American*, June 6, 2014.
Schuster, Mike. "Nixon Considered Nuclear Option against N. Korea," NPR, 2010. http://www.npr.org/templates/story/story.php?storyId=128337461.
Schwalm, Christopher. "Hundred-Year Forecast: Drought." *New York Times*, August 11, 2012.
Schwartz, John. "Study Finds Low Cost in Reducing Methane Emissions." *New York Times*, April 22, 2015.
Scribbler, Robert. "CO2, Earth's Global Thermostat Dials up to Record 401.6 ppm" Robertscribbler.com http://robertscribbler.com/2014/03/14/co2-earths-global-thermostat-dials-up-to-record-401-6-ppm-daily-value-in-march/.
Shah, Anup. "World Military Spending," *Global Issues*, June 30, 2013. http://www.globalissues.org/article/75/world-military-spending.
Shalal, Andrea. "Lockeed Says Makes Breakthrough on Fusion Energy Project," Reuters, October 15, 2014.
Shaller, Marc. "The Behavioral Immune System," April 9, 2014. http://anthropology.ua.edu/blogs/primatereligion/2014/04/09/the-behavioral-immune-system/.
Shaller, Mark. "The Behavioral Immune System: How Unconscious Fears of Infection Shape Many Aspects of our Psychology." *Scientific American*, November 20, 2014. 1–3.
Sherwood, Harriet. "Global Refugee Figure Passes 50m for First Time Since Second World War," *Guardian*, June 2014.
Sherwood, Ross. "US Plan to Attack Iran with Nuclear Weapons Devised under Bush," Global Research 2012, http://www.globalresearch.ca/obama-prepares-protracted-afghanistan-occupation/5308984.
Shultz, Colin. "Globally Deaths from War and Murder are in Decline, *Smithsonian.com*, March 21 2014. http://www.smithsonianmag.com/smart-news/globally-deaths-war-and-murder-are-decline-180950237/#wutvjswK1pGr4bvS.99.
Siegel, Matt, and Colin Packham. "Australia Swelters After Record Hot 2013," Reuters, January 3, 2014. http://ca.news.yahoo.com/australia-swelters-record-hot-2013-farmers-slaughter-cattle-044230636.html.
Silverman, Jacob. "Do Cows Pollute as Much as Cars?" Howstuffworks. Accessed 2015. http://science.howstuffworks.com/zoology/methane-cow.htm.
Sinor, Denis. "Inner Asia: History, Civilization, Languages; A Syllabus" (Bloomington: Indiana University, 1969).

Smith, Andrew. "Fact checking Elon Musk's Blue Square," U.S. Energy Institute Blog, May 21, 2015. http://blogs.ucl.ac.uk/energy/2015/05/21/fact-checking-elon-musks-blue-square-how-much-solar-to-power-the-us/.

Smith, Jeremy, and Alex Dixon. "Birds do it. Bats do it," The Greater Good, 2009.

Smith, Kendall, "Louis Pasteur, the Father of Immunology?" PMC, U.S. National Library of Medicine, 2012. http://www.ncbi.nlm.nih.gov/pmc/articles/PMC3342039/.

Snyder, Michael. "If Economic Cycle Theorists are Correct, 2015 to 2020 will be Devastating for the U.S." ZeroHedge, May 13,2014. http://www.zerohedge.com/news/2014-05-13/if-economic-cycle-theorists-are-correct-2015-2020-will-be-devastating-us.

Snyder, Timothy. "Hitler vs. Stalin: Who Killed More?" *New York Review of Books,* July 2011. http://www.nybooks.com/articles/archives/2011/mar/10/hitler-vs-stalin-who-killed-more/?pagination=false.

Solis, Marcus. "Woman Who Saved Man in Hudson River Speaks Out," WABC-TV, September 9, 2014. http://7online.com/news/woman-who-saved-child-in-hudson-river-speaks-out/298690/.

Solomon, Christopher. "When Birds Squawk, Other Species Seem to Listen," *New York Times,* May 18, 2015.

Solomon, S., Gian-Kasper Plattner, et. al. "Irreversible Climate Change due to Carbon Dioxide Emissions," Proc Natl Acad Sci USA, February 10, 2009. 106(6): 1704–1709.

Sovacool, Benjamin K. "A Preliminary Assessment of Major Energy Accidents, 1907–2007," *Energy Policy* 36 (2008).

Soviet Nuclear Test Summary. 2001. Nuclearweaponarchive.org.

Stannard, David. *American Holocaust* (New York: Oxford University Press, 1992), http://www.amazon.com/American-Holocaust-Conquest-New-World/dp/0195085574.

Stavins, Robert. "Climate Realities," *New York Times,* September 20, 2014.

Stephens, Tim. "Study Shows how Epigenetic Memory is Passed across Generations," UC Santa Cruz Newscenter, September 18, 2014. http://news.ucsc.edu/2014/09/epigenetics.html.

Stewart, James. "King Coal, Long Besieged, is Deposed by the Market," *New York Times,* August 6, 2015.

Strom, Stepani. "Report on U.S. Meat Sounds Alarm on Resistant Bacteria," *New York Times,* 2013.

Synder, Michael. "14 Experts Predict Economic Catastrophe for 2014 and Beyond," Douglas Ross Journal. Accessed 2015. http://directorblue.blogspot.mx/2013/12/14-experts-predict-economic-catastrophe.html.

Szczepanski, Kallie. "What Was the An Lushan Rebellion?" 2015. http://asianhistory.about.com/od/ancientchina/f/What-Was-The-An-Lushan-Rebellion.htm See also: http://ozebook.com/wordpress/archives/26016 .

Tacoma, E., and L. Huey. "Psychic Distress and the Immune Response." *Life Sciences,* 1985, 36.

Taubengerger, J., and D. Morens. "1918 Influenza: the Mother of All Pandemics," Centers for Disease Control and Prevention, 2006.

Tavernise, Sabrina. "Antibiotics in Livestock: FDA Finds Use is Rising." *New York Times,* October 2, 2014.

Tavernise, Sabrina. "Suicide Rates hit a 30-year High in the United States," *New York Times,* April 21, 2016.

Thiel, Peter. "The New Atomic Age We Need," *New York Times,* November 27, 2015.

Thomas, Ken. "Why Do Honeybees Die After They Sting," EarthSky, June 2011. http://earthsky.org/earth/why-do-bees-die-after-they-sting-you.

Thompson, Graham, Peter Hurd, et al. "Genes Underlying Altruism," *Biology Letters,* October 2013. http://rsbl.royalsocietypublishing.org/content/9/6/20130395.

Thornhill, Randy, Steven Gangestad, et al. "Major Histocompatibility Complex Genes, Symmetry, and Body Scent Attractiveness in Men and Women," *Behavioral Ecology* 14 (2003): 668–78.

Thornhill, Ted. "Raped, Tortured, Forced to Watch Beheadings, then Beaten when they Tried to Kill Themselves: Yazidi Girls Reveal the Hell they Endured during ISIS Captivity," Daily Mail, October 1, 2014. http://www.dailymail.co.uk/news/article-2776268/Raped-tortured-forced-watch-beheadings-beaten-tried-kill-Yazidi-girls-reveal-hell-endured-witnessed-ISIS-captivity.html.

Thurtle, Estelle. "10 Ridiculous Theories about Ebola Crisis," Listverse, October 2014. http://listverse.com/2014/10/10/10-disturbing-conspiracy-theories-about-the-ebola-crisis/.

Tiger, Lionel. *Men in Groups*, (New York: Transaction, 1971) 232.

Timor, Rajkai. "The Timurid Empire and the Ming Ching China," doctoral dissertation. Accessed 2015. http://doktori.btk.elte.hu/hist/rajkai/diss.pdf.

Tina Hesman Saey. "MERS Outbreak Picks Up Pace," *Science News*, May 31, 2014.

Todar, Kenneth. *Online Textbook of Bacteriology*. Accessed 2015. http://textbookofbacteriology.net/adaptive.html.

Tony, Long. "Jan. 17, 1966: H-Bombs Rain Down on a Spanish Fishing Village," *WIRED* January 17, 2008.

Toth, Tim. "A Nuclear World," *Chicago Tribune*, October 26, 2012 .http://articles.chicagotribune.com/2012-10-26/opinion/ct-perspec-1026-nuke-20121026_1_test-ban-nuclear-warheads-doomsday-clock.

Toth, Toth. "The Cuban Missile Crisis and Nuclear Testing, CBTBO, 2012. http://www.ctbto.org/press-centre/highlights/2012/the-cuban-missile-crisis-and-nuclear-testing.

Trotsky, Leon. *The History of the Russian Revolution*, 1932. Cited at https://www.marxists.org/archive/trotsky/1930/hrr/ch48.htm.

Trotta, Daniel. "Iraq War Costs U.S. More than $2 Trillion: Study." Reuters, March 14, 2013. http://www.reuters.com/article/2013/03/14/us-iraq-war-anniversary-idUSBRE92D0PG20130314.

Turvey, Stuart and David Briode. "Innate Immunity," 2011. http://www.ncbi.nlm.nih.gov/pmc/articles/PMC2832725/.

Uffalussy, Jennifer. "ISIS Beheadings, Plane Crashes: Why We Should Avoid Images that Can't be Unseen," *Yahoo Health*, February 4, 2015. https://www.yahoo.com/health/isis-beheadings-plane-crashes-why-we-should-110078169512.html.

Underhill, Richard. "Guard Bees Protect the Hive," The Peace Bee Farmer Blog, August 21, 2009. http://peacebeefarm.blogspot.com/2009/08/guard-bees-protect-hive.html.

Upshur, Jiu-Hwa Lo. "An Lushan's Rebellion." In *Encyclopedia of World History: The Expanding World, 600 CE to 1450*, vol. 2., edited by Marsha E. Ackermann, Michael Schroeder, Janice J. Terry, Jiu-Hwa Lo Upshur, and Mark F. Whitters (New York: Facts On File, Inc., 2008).

Vaidyanathan, Gayathri. "2014 to be Hottest Year Ever Measured," *Scientific American*, December 4, 2014.

van Rensberg, Theunis Janen. "Large Hadron Collider Detects Higgs Boson Particle," BWTH blog, July 4, 2012. http://www.bandwidthblog.com/2012/07/04/large-hadron-collider-detects-higgs-boson-particle/.

Vanga, G., and V. G. Westover. "Origin of the 1918 Spanish Influenza Virus: a Comparative Genomic Analysis," *Molecular Phylogenetics and Evolution* 47, no. 3 (2008): 1100–10.

Vergano, Dan. "Half-million Iraqis Died in War, Study Says," *National Geographic*, October 16, 2013.

Vergano, Dan. "Mystery of 1918 Flu that Killed 50 Million Solved," *National Geographic*, 2014. http://news.nationalgeographic.com/news/2014/04/140428-1918-flu-avian-swine-science-health-science/.

Vicount, James Bryce, and Arnold Toynbee. *The Treatment of Armenians in the Ottoman Empire, 1915–1916: Documents Presented to Viscount Grey of Falloden, Uncensored Edition*, edited by Ara Sarafian (Princeton, NJ: Gomidas Institute, 2000).

Vidal, John. "Global Warming Causes 300,000 Deaths a Year says Kofi Annan Think-tank," *Guardian,* May 29, 2009. http://www.guardian.co.uk/environment/2009/may/29/1.
Vine, David. "The United States Probably Has more Foreign Military Bases than any Other People, Nation or Empire in History," *The Nation,* September 14, 2015.
Vitelli, Romeo. "Can Happiness be Genetic," *Media Spotlight,* February 25, 2013.
Vlet, Elizabeth. "Illegal Immigrants Bring Risk of Ebola and Global Array of Viral Illnesses" CP Opinion, August 2014. http://www.christianpost.com/news/illegal-immigrants-bring-risk-of-ebola-and-global-array-of-viral-illnesses-124329/.
Voros, C. "Commercial Bottom Trawling and Deep Sea Corals," June 2006. http://jrscience.wcp.muohio.edu/fieldcourses06/PapersMarineEcologyArticles/CommercialBottomTrawlingaA.html.
Wald, Matthew. "Betting on the Need, Scientists Work on Lighter, Cleaner Nuclear Energy," *New York Times,* December 15, 2014.
Wald, Matthew. "From Harvard, a Cheaper Storage Battery," *New York Times,* January 8, 2014.
Walden, Bruce. "The Ecology of Kin Recognition," *Annual Review of Ecology and Systematics,* 1988, 1543–71.
Waldman, Katy. "Is Anybody Watching My Do-gooding?" *Slate,* October 20, 2014. http://www.slate.com/articles/health_and_science/medical_examiner/2014/10/psychology_of_heroism_and_altruism_what_makes_people_do_good_deeds.html.
Walsh, Bryan. "Plan B- How to Stop Global Warming," *Time,* January 4, 2008.
Waters, Ethan. "DNA is Not Destiny: the New Science of Epigenetics" Discover, November 2006. http://discovermagazine.com/2006/nov/cover.
Watt-Cloutier, Sheila. *Sierra Club Currents* 6, no. 54 (March 2007).
Wayman, Eric. "Polar Ice Sheets Shrinking Overall." *Science News,* March 9, 2013.
Weber, Mark. "Iraq, a War for Israel," Institute for Historical Review. Accessed 2015.
Weber, Tom. "Faulty Intelligence," *UMaine Today Magazine,* October 2007. http://www.magarchive.umaine.edu/issues/v7i5/intelligence.html.
Wellerstien, Alex. "About Those Nukes in Cuba," The Nuclear Secrecy blog, 2012. http://blog.nuclearsecrecy.com/2012/10/25/about-those-nukes-in-cuba/.
WGBH Educational. "Double Immunity," 2001. http://www.pbs.org/wgbh/evolution/library/10/4/l_104_05.html.
Whitfield, Philip. "Plumage Variability and Territoriality," *Animal Behavior* 34 (October 1986): 1471–82.
Wiersum, Marc. "China's Manufacturing Wages Rise to $7000 Per Year," Market Realist, April 22, 2014.
William, Tompson. *J. Khrushchev: A Political Life* (New York: St. Martin's Press, 1995).
Williams, Ray. "Why We Love Bad News," *Psychology Today,* December 2010. http://www.psychologytoday.com/blog/wired-success/201012/why-we-love-bad-news.
Willies, Egberto. "Extreme G0P Gerrymandering Responsible for Tea Party Extremist" Daily Kos, October10, 2013. http://www.dailykos.com/story/2013/10/11/1246244/-Extreme-GOP-Gerrymandering-Responsible-For-Tea-Party-Extremist-VIDEO#.
Wilson, James. "What is Adrenal Fatigue?" Accessed 2015. https://www.adrenalfatigue.org/who-is-dr-wilson.
Wines, Michael. "Emissions of Methane in U.S. Exceed Estimates," *New York Times,* November 25, 2013.
Wolford, Ben. "Global Carbon Emissions Keep Rising; Expected to Reach New Record in 2013," *International Science Times,* November 18, 2013. http://www.isciencetimes.com/articles/6342/20131118/global-carbon-emissions-keep-rising-expected-reach.htm.
Wong, Edward. "Air Pollution Linked to 1.2 million Premature Deaths in China." *New York Times,* April 1, 2013.
Wong, Edward. "Hundreds of Chinese Cities Don't Meet Air Standards, Report Finds." *New York Times,* April 21, 2015.

Wong, Edward. "China Exports Pollution to U.S. Study Finds." *New York Times*, January 20, 2014.

Wong, Edward. "In Step to Lower Carbon Emissions, China will Place a Limit on Coal Use in 2020," *New York Times*, November 24, 2014.

Wood, Archie. 2004. http://everything2.com/title/accidental+nuclear+war.

Wood, Shawn Paul. "Bad News: Negative Headlines Get Much More Attention," PRNewser, February 2014. http://www.mediabistro.com/prnewser/bad-news-negative-headlines-get-much-more-attention_b85912.

World War graphic. Developed from data at Persuade Me Politics. Accessed 2015. https://persuademepolitics.wordpress.com/2015/07/30/now-most-peaceful-time-in-world-history/.

Wright, Robert. "Why Some Physicists Bet Against the Higgs Boson" *Atlantic*, July 17, 2012.

Wynne Parry. "Oceans Turning Acidic Faster Than Past 300 Million years," Live Science, March 2, 2012. http://news.yahoo.com/oceans-turning-acidic-faster-past-300-million-years-164401538.html.

X. Yu et al. "Neutralizing Antibodies Derived from the B cells of 1918 Influenza Pandemic Survivors," Nature 455 (2008): 532–36.

Xie, Zongli, Hoang, Mang, et al. Sol-gel Derived Poly(vinyl alcohol)/Maleic Acid/Silica Hybrid Membrane for Desalination by Pervaporation, Journal of Membrane Science, 2011, 383.

Yale Genocide Studies Program. 1994–2008. http://www.yale.edu/cgp/.

Yang Jisheng. "China's Great Shame," *New York Times*, November 13, 2012.

Yepiskoposian, Levon, Ashto Margarian, et al. "Genetic Affinity Between the Armenian Yezidis and the Iraqi Kurds," *Iran and the Caucases* 14 (2010): 37–42.

York, Bridget. "The Nuclear Age of Peace?" 2013. https://prezi.com/fmrrixfxj5na/the-nuclear-age-of-peace/.

York, Chris, and George Bowden. "Syria Civil War Death Toll Paints a Horrifyingly Complex Picture," *Huffington Post UK*, October 31, 2015.

Zaelka, Durwood. "Going Beyond Carbon Dioxide," *New York Times*, December 6, 2012.

Zaid Al-Ali. "How Maliki Ruined Iraq," *Foreign Policy*, June 19, 2014.

Zhaobao, J., T Wenhua, et al. "Are the Elderly More Vulnerable to the Psychological Impact of Natural Disasters' BMC Public Health, 2010. http://www.biomedcentral.com/1471-2458/10/172.

Zhong-Shuai Wu, Khaled Parvez, et al. "Graphene Based in Plane Microsupercapacitors with High Power and Energy Densities," Nature Communications, August 2013. doi:10.1038/ncomms3487.

Zimmer, Carl. "More Than Half of Entire Species of Saigas Gone in Mysterious Die-off," *New York Times*, November 2, 2015.

———. "In 1918 Flu Pandemic, Timing was a Killer," *New York Times*, April 30, 2014.

———. "Is Patriotism a Subconscious Way for Humans to Avoid Disease," *Discover*, March 2009. http//discovermagazine.com/2009/mar/17-is-patriotism-a-subconscious-way-for-humans-to-avoid-disease.

———. "Ocean Life Faces Mass Extinction," *New York Times*, January 15, 2015.

———. "Parents May Pass Down More than Just Genes, Study Suggests," *New York Times*, December 3, 2015.

———. "Unraveling Why Some Mammals Kill off Infants." *New York Times*, November 13, 2014.

Zisels, Josef, and Halyna Kharaz. "Will Holodomor Receive the Same Status as the Holocaust?" "Maidan" Alliance, 2012. http://eng.maidanua.org/.

Zsolt, Laszlo, Balaz Rosivall, et al. "Determinants of Male Territorial Behavior in a Hungarian Flycatcher Population," *Behavioral Ecology Sociobiology* 60 (2006): 663–71.

Zyga, Lisa. "Dark Matter May be an Illusion Caused by a Quantum Vacuum," Phys.org, August 11, 2011. http://phys.org/news/2011-08-dark-illusion-quantum-vacuum.html.

Index

5HT, 100
5-HTTLPR, 90

Able Archer, 57, 58, 65
acetophenone, 134
adaptive immune system, 32, 80, 133
adrenaline, 86, 119, 169
aggression, 94, 99, 100, 103, 177
agouti mice, 135
AIDS, 7, 37, 174
Alexins, 32, 33
alpha fish, 98
altruism, 111, 116, 121, 176, 195
Andropov, Yuri, 57
An Lushun, 12
Antarctic ice sheet, 211, 218
antigen, 19, 71, 79, 80, 140
anti-Semitism,, 132, 143, 144
archetype of the hero, 121, 237
Arctic Methane Apocalypse, 229, 233
Arctic Ocean, 211, 230
Ardrey, Robert, 95, 104, 178
Arkhipov, Vasili, 56, 63, 70, 71, 72, 122
artificial immune system, 81, 176
artificial psychic immune system, 163, 164, 173, 176, 178
Ataturk, 16, 25
Auschwitz, 22, 24, 40
autonomic, 34, 36, 147, 163, 196

B-52, 52, 59, 72, 91
Bargh, Joseph, 106
Biogram, 97, 105
black carbon, 217, 244
Black Death, 5, 7, 35, 234
Boesch, Christophe, 112
Bonanno, G. A., 132, 133
Brezhnev, Leonid, 54, 57
Brown, Lester, 210, 218, 243
bubonic plague, 5, 8, 9
Buchner, Hans, 32
Bulletin of Atomic Scientists, 70, 246, 248

Cambodian genocide, 18
Campbell, Joseph, 121
carbon taxes, 243
Castro, Fidel, 69
CCR5 gene, 8, 35
Cheney, Dick, 66, 188
Chenshan, Lin, 54, 63
China : and nuclear weapons,3.63: and pollution, 216, 217, 232, 243; and Red Guards, 23; and SARS, 81
Chomsky, Noam, 47, 72
CIA, 52, 53
Cinderella effect, 142
coal, 216, 217, 232, 238, 240, 243
collective : flight responses, 89, 90; hysteria, 172, 173; insanity, 38, 68; psyche, 121; psychology, 126; self-preservative instinct, 227; unconscious, 9, 83, 121
competition, 85, 94, 105, 119
COMT gene, 119
Congolese genocide, 15, 21
cooperation, 111, 116, 166, 195, 239
Cordon Sanitaire, 34
cortisol, 86, 88, 119, 241
Coyne, Jerry, 139
Cuban Missile Crisis, 50, 51, 55, 66, 68
cystic fibrosis, 93

Darwin, 114, 116, 139
DEFCON, 49, 50, 52, 57
deforestation, 213
deMause, Lloyd, 142
Dengue fever, 175, 214
dominance, 111; and aggression, 100, 112, 122, 126; and males, 102, 106; and reproduction, 103; and

territoriality, 95, 97, 166, 196
Doomsday Clock, 70, 248
Dulles, Allen, 66

Ebola, 153, 155, 164, 175
Einstein, Albert, 2, 49, 238
Eisenhower, Dwight D., 43, 66
empathy, 118; and altruism, 114, 195; and biology, 87, 116; and compassion, 154, 242; and neurology, 117
epigenetics, 134, 135; and learning, 153; and toxins, 136; and trauma, 137
epiphenomenon, 85, 97, 140, 152, 173
Eros, 83

Feynman, Richard, 207
fight-flight, 85, 86, 87, 89, 172, 173
Fukushima, 240

Gang of Four, 24, 40
Genghis Khan, 13, 14, 20, 25, 41, 184, 247
genocide, 15, 16, 18, 19, 21, 38
geo-engineering, 239
Ghandi, 25, 42, 43
Gillis, Justin, 230
Global Carbon Project, 229
Global Humanitarian Forum, 220
golden rule, 165
Goodall, Jane, 132, 164

Hamilton, W. D., 141, 154, 155
Hansen, James, 217
heritability, 90, 91, 153
hero archetype, 121, 176
Himmler, Heinrich, 44, 112
HIV, 8
home team advantage, 103, 104
homeostasis, 41, 42, 89, 189, 199, 229, 236

ICBM, 50, 51, 53, 58, 64
immunity, 5, 8, 19; artificial, 81; adaptive, 131, 132; innate, 35, 36, 80; psychological, 138; and self-preservation, 34, 120
incest avoidance, 93, 169
innate releasing' stimulus, 97
intraspecies killing, 122, 165, 166, 199
Israel, 48, 56, 57, 190
ITER, 238

Jung, Carl, 10, 21, 83, 121, 133

Kagan, Harman, 120, 129n44, 129n46
Keeling, Matthew, 35
Kennedy, John F., 51, 65, 66, 67
Khmer Rouge, 18, 21, 24
Khrushchev, 22, 55, 68, 69, 183
kin recognition, 143, 144, 148
kin selection, 142, 144
King Leopold, 15, 21, 26
Kosygin, Alexei, 54
Kubla Khan, 20

lithium air battery technology, 239
lymph nodes, 33, 79, 80

MacArthur, Douglas, 66
Macmillan, Harold, 50
malaria, 31, 80, 214
Maoism, 18, 23, 26, 40, 246
Marshall, S.L.A., 123
Maslennikov, Ivan, 56
mass psychology, 89, 239, 240, 244, 245
Mauna Loa Observatory, 219
McNamara, Robert, 55, 63, 67, 68
media, 125, 152, 155, 156, 174
Meir, Golda, 56
Middle East, 23, 190, 213, 237
Mongol empire, 11, 12, 13, 20, 25, 41

Nagasaki, 47
NATO, 50, 57
Nesler, Ellie, 169, 171
neuroception, 87
neuroscience, 134, 135, 152
Nixon, Richard, 66, 144
nonviolence, 22, 42, 111, 165, 166, 176, 196, 199, 236
NORAD, 49, 50, 51, 52, 53
nuclear winter, 48, 49, 56, 59, 63, 236

oxytocin, 118, 119
optimism, 82, 91, 93, 126
Oswalt, Patton, 246

Ottoman Empire, 16, 25, 38, 187, 192, 217
Oxfam, 241

Pakistan, 47, 48, 49, 58, 59, 210
pandemic, 6, 9, 37, 40, 41, 88, 199
parasites, 33, 147
pathogen-avoidant strategies, 148, 149
pathogens, 33, 80, 81, 146, 151, 153
Pauli, Wolfgang, 2
Pearl Harbor, 98, 240
perovskite, 239
Petrov, Stanislav, 53, 64, 70, 71, 238
phylogenetic, 19, 63, 94, 114, 176
phylogeny of gangs, 101
physical immune system, 72, 79–83, 155
Pinker, Steven, 24, 127, 168
Pigmentocracies , 149
Pol Pot, 18, 21, 24, 26, 39, 43, 246
Potter, William, 57
prairie dog, 113, 141, 176, 239
prejudice, 146, 147, 154, 155, 174
psychic epidemics, 6, 23, 43–44, 194, 197, 228, 244
psychic memories, 9
psychoneuroimmunology, 82
Pusey, Anne, 94

Rakoff, David, 111
rational actor hypothesis, 64, 66, 70
rationing, 242
Reagan, Ronald, 57, 241, 242
remission, 35, 37, 38, 40, 41, 190, 193, 196, 197
resilience, 132, 132–133
resistance, 19, 23, 40, 124, 133, 229
"Ring around the Rosy", 22
Roberts, Paul, 82
Rosenbaum, Ron, 57
Roscoe, Paul, 124
Russell, Bertrand, 67, 69, 70

SARS, 36, 81, 234
Savitsky, 56, 70, 73
schooling fish, 96, 115
self/nonself, 139, 143, 154, 155
self-preservative instinct, 20, 33, 44, 71, 114
self-preservative system, 8, 19, 33, 38, 44, 47
Shaller, Mark, 151, 174
sickle cell anemia, 80, 93
Skinner, Michael, 136
slave trade, 14, 38
smallpox, 8, 31, 163
Snyder, Timothy, 17
solar farms, 239, 243
Soviets, 54, 55, 57, 63, 64, 65, 68
Spanish flu, 8, 9, 19, 40, 131, 193, 194
Stalin, 18, 22, 23, 183, 196
Stalinism, 17, 23, 40
Stannard, David, 5
Stephens, Walter, 99, 171
stress hormones, 88, 119, 152
surrender rituals, 102
swine flu, 8, 175, 234

T cell, 8, 33, 37
territoriality, 85–111, 116, 191, 197, 199
testosterone, 104, 105
The Great Famine, 18, 24
Thucydides, 31, 32, 43
thymus, 33, 79
Tiger, Lionel, 101
Timur, 12, 14, 18, 20, 41, 196
tolerance, 173, 174, 176, 246
totem, 103, 106
Truman, Harry S., 66
Turkey, 14, 25, 38, 50, 55, 64, 209, 237
Twain, Mark, 21

unconscious: attitudes, 150; and autonomic processes, 19, 50; bias, 149; and fight-flight, 89; and immunity, 36; mind, 106
Us versus Them, 142, 145, 150, 165, 174, 193

Vaughn, Victor, 6
Vetter, David, 42
violence, 21, 99, 126, 139, 166, 195, 196

wind farming, 243
Wilson, E. O., 116
worker bees, 120, 151
World War I, 16

World War II : and GM,11.139: and nuclear weapons, 47; and Stalin, 17; and territoriality, 228; and violent deaths, 196

xenophobia, 144, 145, 147, 174, 175

About the Author

Jerry Kroth is associate professor emeritus in the graduate counseling psychology program at the Santa Clara University in California and a member of the International Psychohistorical Association. He has written twelve books on counseling, psychology, child sexual abuse, learning disorders, metapsychology, transpersonal psychology, and research methodology. He has also written and presented over seventy-five papers on anxiety, child development, mass psychology, synchronicity, experimental studies of the dream process, the psychology of propaganda, and collective psychology. To view more of his work, visit his website, collectivepsych.com, or check out his numerous online lectures that are available on YouTube and iTunes U.

www.ingramcontent.com/pod-product-compliance
Ingram Content Group UK Ltd.
Pitfield, Milton Keynes, MK11 3LW, UK
UKHW041633031026
15587UKWH00001B/251

9 781498 528917